# Holistic Solutions for Anxiety & Depression in Therapy

# HOLISTIC SOLUTIONS FOR ANXIETY & DEPRESSION IN THERAPY

*Combining Natural Remedies with Conventional Care*

PETER B. BONGIORNO

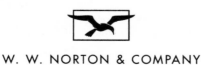

W. W. NORTON & COMPANY
New York • London

For information about permission to reproduce selections from this book, write to
Permissions, W. W. Norton & Company, Inc., 500 Fifth Avenue, New York, NY 10110

For information about special discounts for bulk purchases, please contact
W. W. Norton Special Sales at specialsales@wwnorton.com or 800-233-4830

Manufacturing by Courier Westford
Production manager: Leeann Graham

**Library of Congress Cataloging-in-Publication Data**

Bongiorno, Peter B.
  Holistic solutions for anxiety & depression in therapy : combining natural remedies
with conventional care / Peter B. Bongiorno. — First edition.
      pages cm
  "A Norton Professional Book."
  Includes bibliographical references and index.
  ISBN 978-0-393-70934-6 (hardcover)
  1. Anxiety—Alternative treatment.   2. Depression, Mental—Alternative
treatment.   3. Holistic medicine.   4. Traditional medicine.   I. Title.   II. Title:
Holistic solutions for anxiety and depression in therapy.
  RC531.B66 2015
  616.85'22—dc23        2014029926

ISBN: 978-0-393-70934-6

W. W. Norton & Company, Inc., 500 Fifth Avenue, New York, N.Y. 10110
www.wwnorton.com
W. W. Norton & Company Ltd., Castle House, 75/76 Wells Street, London W1T 3QT

1 2 3 4 5 6 7 8 9 0

*This book is dedicated firstly to the patients who teach me something valuable everyday. Their courage is my inspiration. I want to also dedicate this book to the mental health practitioners that I have the honor to work with in order to create a true team care approach. Together, we have learned that working in an integrative fashion truly creates the best results. Finally, this book is co-dedicated to the tireless laboratory and clinical researchers running trials and pouring over statistics to learn how lifestyle and natural medicines work. Without that hard and often unrewarded work, the information for this book would not be available.*

# Contents

# CONTENTS

# Acknowledgments

To my best friend, wife, and fellow naturopathic doctor Pina LoGiudice, who is the grounding center from which I can traverse out. To the Bongiornos and LoGiudices who love me and my family without reserve. To Andrea Costella at Norton, whose vision conceived this project, and whose gentle guidance allowed it to take form. Also, to Norton's Kathyrn Moyer for allowing me to feel safe and secure with transition; and Trish Watson, who spent an amazing amount of time bringing things to a usable form. Finally, to Joy Sanjek, LCSW, a beloved clinician whose invaluable time, insight and feedback is greatly appreciated.

# Introduction

## Why Holistic Care for Anxiety and Depression?

Insanity: doing the same thing over and over again and expecting different results.

*About a year before writing this book, I worked with a 42-year-old father of two; let's call him Jason. Jason came in for his sixth monthly follow-up visit. He had been dealing with depression for most of his adult life. An avid athlete in his youth, by the time he was twenty-four he began to experience low mood and low-grade depression. This was around the time he started having severe difficulties in his family life, specifically discussing difficulties with his drug-addicted brother and aging alcoholic parents. He suddenly began to have a very hard time playing soccer, a game he loved. For almost two decades he avoided athletic events and fought the "dark cloud," as he put it, that kept him from enjoying sports, going out dancing, or even just being social with friends. While functional at his job as an engineer, he was labeled "dysthymic" by his psychiatrists and bounced from medication to medication, with equivocal results. At the time we began to work together, he was also working with a psychotherapist, as well as a psychopharmacologist, and believed he would always be somewhat depressed, for that was his "nature."*

*Jason's most recent therapist decided to refer him to me for a more holistic view and to see if there were any physical reasons that might be contributing Jason's mood challenges. After taking his full history and completing a round of blood tests, we learned that Jason's vitamin D and ferritin (iron storage) levels were abysmally low. We also found out through the blood tests that he had a low-grade reaction to gluten (a protein from wheat) that was likely contributing to the slightly high inflammation in his body. I referred him to a hematologist and gastrointestinal doctor to check on the low iron. Once it was clear that no gastrointestinal or hematologic problems were the cause of low iron, I encouraged him to eat more iron-containing foods and gave him low doses of an easy-to-absorb iron supplement with herbs that help absorption. I also recommended vitamin D3 and had him avoid all gluten and wheat products. We also adjusted his sleep schedule and added more vegetables and anti-inflammatory foods (e.g., fish and olive oil) to his diet. After working with these recommendations for about 4 months, his mood gradually lifted. He even went back to working out, and now he is excitedly considering getting back on a local men's soccer team this coming summer. I suspect he will be able to wean off his current medications within the next few months.*

*Jason had difficulty absorbing iron. His vitamin D was low because he avoided the sun after his medical doctor told him sunlight would cause skin cancer, even though he had no known increased risk for skin cancer. Because he did not have digestive issues, laboratory tests for gluten sensitivity were never performed. After we added a gentle but absorbable iron, his red blood cells' ability to carry oxygen improved, which helped both Jason's mood and energy. Giving him vitamin D likely balanced inflammation in his body and supported his mood. Having Jason eliminate gluten foods and adding anti-inflammatory foods also lowered inflammation in the body. Inflammation in the body translates to more brain inflammation—a contributor to poor mood in susceptible individuals.*

*At our last visit, Jason asked me a very reasonable question: "After almost 20 years of going from doctor to doctor, why didn't anyone think to check and do these things?" My answer was simple: "Because conventional care rarely looks at the body as a whole." Often, when we look at the body holistically, we can elicit much more information to help support the body's healing ability.*

Jason's story is an example of a type of patient I typically work with: someone with a long-term mood disorder who has tried many forms of medication and has had limited success. I am lucky, for in my New York practice I work alongside like-minded therapists, social workers, psychologists, and psychiatrists who look to me to assess, from a more holistic perspective, the physical reasons for a person's mood issues. In a team care spirit, I rely on them for their expertise to monitor patients' safety, work on improving their psychological well-being, and consider pharmaceutical options when absolutely necessary. Together, we create a full complementary and alternative medicine (CAM) perspective that allows patients full opportunity to heal and provides a small community in which patients feel safe to share concerns, change patterns, and heal.

Most therapists I have the honor to work with in this team care approach tell me that most of their clientele are either interested in or are already using some type of natural remedy or holistic modality. However, I have also heard that, whether it be the latest diet craze, acupuncture, fish oil, vitamin D, St. John's wort, or some new "miracle mood cure," often the therapist does not feel familiar enough with these remedies to give an opinion, and some have confided in me their concern for drug-nutrient-herb interactions. Even more overarching is the safety concern that their clients may inappropriately use these remedies in lieu of more potent and necessary conventional care. This book will help orient you regarding these concerns and give you a holistic framework to help see where safe and effective use of CAM can fit with your clients' concerns.

As a clinician, you probably have noticed that anxiety and depression rank as the top reasons that people are sick and go to the doctor. Anxiety disorders are the most common of the psychiatric illnesses in the United States, with approximately 30% of the population experiencing anxiety-related symptoms in their lifetime (Kessler et al., 2005). Eighteen percent of the U.S. population have been diagnosed with anxiety disorder.

According to the U.S. Centers for Disease Control and Prevention (2010), 9.1% of the population meet the criteria for current depression, including 4.1% who meet the criteria for major depression. A report from the World Health Organization tells us that depression has become the second most burdensome disease in the world—it causes more lost time and money than any other condition except heart disease (Ferrari et al., 2013).

Anxiety and depression are generally inextricable disorders—each often occurring with the other. About 58% of patients with lifetime major depressive disorder have anxiety disorder, while 48% of patients with generalized anxiety disorder also experience comorbid depression (Lieberman, 2009). Patients who suffer from both seem to have more severe, chronic types of anxiety. These patients also have more social and work challenges, as well as greater rates of alcoholism and substance abuse. Most unfortunate, patients with both are less likely to benefit from conventional care (Lydiard 2004). While the *Diagnostic and Statistical Manual of Mental Disorders*, version 5 (American Psychiatric Association, 2013) does not acknowledge "anxious depression" as a distinct diagnosis, it is a very common presentation of mood disorder. In holistic circles, many practitioners consider anxiety and depression a continuum, where certain stressors, as well as sleep, environmental, and lifestyle factors, will help decide whether a particular degree of anxiety, depression, or both may manifest.

Despite decades of drug dominance, many patients are now realizing that they prefer something else—possibly to avoid toxicity of these drugs, or maybe because they realize their medication is not fixing the problem. In 2007, over 38% of adults sought out some kind of natural or CAM support in the United States (Barnes, Bloom, & Nahin, 2008), a significant increase from the previous decade. In many cases, this CAM support may involve an anxious person going to the health food store to find a mineral, such as magnesium, to help with sleep. Or possibly a person with depression might try a supplement like tryptophan to lift mood. Other people may start regular acupuncture treatments or yoga therapy. Or they may visit a naturopathic doctor like myself, who may individualize lifestyle changes, recommend specific supplementation, and organize a holistic plan.

You have probably noticed this interest in CAM with your own clients—more and more are asking about this vitamin or that diet. Thus, a basic working knowledge of available CAM modalities and their efficacy is becoming an essential part of health care education. A general natural medicine knowledge base is becoming essential for any health care practitioner who wants to communicate and participate effectively in a health care strategy with his or her client.

## DEFINING ALTERNATIVE AND CAM MEDICINE

Before exploring how to assess your clients for various lifestyle and internal factors that may be contributing to their anxiety and depression, and the holistic approaches you can recommend, let's first get clear on some basic terms.

### Alternative Medicine

The term *alternative medicine* refers to various medical and health care systems, modalities, and recommendations that are not presently considered to be part of the typical conventional medical model. These remedies are called "alternative" because they are used in place of conventional medical care. When defining alternative care, the key here is understanding that, by definition, "alternative medicine" *replaces* mainstream medical protocol.

### Complementary and Alternative Medicine

Instead, I prefer to employ the term *complementary and alternative medicine* (CAM). CAM is a system that employs alternative modalities *alongside* conventional care. It does not necessarily replace conventional care but, rather, keeps all methods of care in mind when creating a plan of action for a particular patient (National Center for Complementary and Alternative Medicine, 2013a). In my experience, neither conventional nor alternative methods are superior. I prefer CAM because it is not mutually exclusive and allows the opportunity to use whichever treatment might be best for a patient at a given time. Using both conventional and alternative medicines together is termed *integrative medicine*.

CAM practitioners may be physicians of conventional medicine (e.g., medical doctors and osteopathic physicians) or physicians of naturopathic medicine like myself. Also considered part of the CAM world are nutritionists, herbalists, Chinese medicine and acupuncture practitioners, chiropractors, energetic healers, and so forth. Therapists who work with standard psychotherapy along other modalities such as yoga would also be under the CAM umbrella.

CAM therapies may incorporate nutrient therapies, botanical medicines, Native American healing, dietary changes, Ayurvedic medicine (ancient medicine from India), energy healing, hypnosis, acupuncture, spinal manipulation, animal-assisted therapy, physical medicines, and many other types of therapies.

## Holistic Medicine

CAM and integrative medicine are, at their best, a type of holistic care. Holistic medicine is a system of medicine that fully appreciates the multiple factors that affect a person's health. It considers each person to be a unified whole. This contrasts the biomedical approach of fragmenting the body into parts and specialties such as a nervous system, digestive system, hormonal system, and so forth. For example, when you have a stomach problem, you see a gastroenterologist. If you have skin issues, you see a dermatologist. In contrast, a holistic practitioner may recommend focusing on supporting the digestive tract to help the skin issues.

Biomedicine too often does not consider how tweaking one body system may affect the whole person. Let's take the common example of reflux, a condition affecting 60 million Americans every month. Common conventional treatment includes a proton pump inhibitor drug such as Nexium, which may help decrease symptoms and avoid discomfort. However, in the long term, such treatments can cause poor nutrient absorption, which leads to body deficiencies and risk of osteoporotic fracture (Fraser et al., 2013). A CAM and integrative approach may consider a drug like this in the short term only if really needed for symptom reduction or to heal a dangerous ulcer. In the meantime, a CAM approach will work on the underlying factors, such as balancing a patient's stress response, changing diet, modifying meal timing, improving sleeping habits, and using herbs and nutrients to heal the digestive tract lining—treatments I find work extremely well in practically all cases.

As the word *reflux* does not tell us why a person is having digestive discomfort; so too, the words *anxiety* and *depression* do not really tell us much about the underlying causes of a person's mood issues. When we hear of people with anxiety and/or depression, we know they are involved in an experience where they do not feel like at their best and are likely challenged to function optimally in their life. But we don't know why. Holistic medicine seeks the reason why and to help adjust various factors, such as sleep, movement, digestion, psychology, and spirit, as well as nutrient and supplement intake, to help the body balance itself.

## YOUR QUICK GUIDE TO CAM

In the following chapters, I detail the holistic approach to anxiety and depression. Along the way, I attempt to provide clinical stories along with the most up-to-date research and recommendations for practice. This book is designed for the busy mental health professional looking for a go-to primer about natural health care for anxiety and depression. As a busy clinician, you probably do not have the time to cull and synthesize the reams of research available on natural medicines efficacy and safety for depression and anxiety.

This book will do the work for you, streamlining the information into an easily accessible read. The appendices include summarizing charts and easy steps that you, as the mental health professional, can quickly refer to again and again for help in guiding patients through the new holistic medicine world. Instead of offering the whole kitchen sink when it comes to CAM recommendations, this book uses my decade of clinical experience and almost 20 years of research to help distill the most salient underlying factors and treatment options.

As the interest in CAM and natural medicine grows, a therapist who can speak knowledgeably about integrative care will be of more value to the anxious or depressed client. Whether you are looking to integrate yourself or your practice or are simply searching for the most current evidence-based recommendations on the principles and practice of natural and integrative medicine care for anxiety and depression, this book provides the foundation necessary to navigate this exciting approach to treatment. This book also provides the best available resources to further explore holistic care. For up-to-date research on natural medicines, please visit my website at www.drpeterbongiorno.com and join me on Facebook and Twitter (@drbongiorno). Also, please feel free to subscribe to my clinic newsletter at www.InnerSourceHealth.com.

## SAFETY FIRST

Groucho Marx once said, "Be open minded—but not so open-minded that your brains fall out." Please remember that while we focus on natural medicine and holistic remedies, patient safety is always paramount. The "complementary" aspect of this approach reminds us that sometimes drugs can also be a friend to the patient, and using natural therapies instead of needed urgent care can cause harm. Any good clinician considers risk and benefits with any treatment option and should choose safety first.

In cases where patients are severely impaired (e.g., patients with severe depression, suicidal ideation, or completely debilitating anxiety), first-line therapy may need to include medication and sometimes hospitalization for monitoring. In these cases, I recommend using pharmaceutical support to help a patient stabilize.

Once the patient is stable, then consideration of holistic options to work on the underlying factors can begin. While I typically prefer to have patients use natural care, if a patient can't even muster the umph to get out of bed, it is doubtful he or she will, say, go to the local health food store to buy salmon and kale and cook it up. Nor is it likely the patient will start exercising. Holistic options can be considered adjunctive in severe cases, but not necessarily as a first-line therapy in place of possibly quicker-acting drugs for urgent care needs. We must be realistic and keep patient safety in mind at all times.

## THE HEALING POWER OF NATURE

I am thrilled that you are reading this book. Together, I believe we are advancing the future vision of mental health care. My sincere hope is that this work will impart insight and greater recognition into what naturopathic doctors refer to as the *vis medicatrix naturae* (Latin for "healing power of nature"), as well as bring awareness that the body truly has the innate wisdom to heal. It is my sincerest hope that this guide brings great value to you personally and to your practice. Even more, I hope it inspires your clients' natural healing processes to move forward.

# Holistic Solutions for Anxiety & Depression in Therapy

# ONE

# Are Holistic Approaches
# Right for Your Client?

A friend is one to whom one may pour out the contents of one's heart, chaff and grain together, knowing that gentle hands will take and sift it, keep what is worth keeping, and with a breath of kindness, blow the rest away.

—George Elliot

Before diving head first into exploring complementary and alternative medicine (CAM), we first need to decide if holistic care is the right choice right now. Good practitioners use their knowledge and experience to help guide their clients to decide which path is worth taking and which do not make sense at that time. This chapter should help you answer that question in regards to holistic care. It gives some statistics about anxiety and depression and describes how to broach the idea of complementary care. It presents some basic clinical questions you may want to ask your client in order to determine whether natural and integrative medicines are appropriate. It will also help to identify safety issues that may suggest the need for medication, or contraindications that would suggest that, at the moment, it may be best to avoid holistic or more integrative care in order to focus on conventional biomedicine.

## IS THERE RESEARCH TO SUPPORT CAM FOR MOOD?

As a system, holistic care research is in its infancy. Cooley et al. (2009) looked for the first time at naturopathic care for subjects with moderate to severe anxiety. Eighty-one patients, randomized by age and gender, received either naturopathic care or standardized psychotherapy over 12 weeks. The naturopathic care group received a holistic plan of dietary counseling, deep breathing relaxation techniques, a standard multivitamin, and the botanical ashwagandha (*Withania somnifera*; 300 mg twice a day). The psychotherapy group received psychotherapy, matched deep breathing relaxation techniques, and a placebo. The primary outcome measure was the Beck Anxiety Inventory; secondary outcome measures included the Short Form 36, Fatigue Symptom Inventory, and Measure Yourself Medical Outcomes Profile to measure anxiety, mental health, and quality of life respectively. Final Beck scores decreased by 56.5 percent in the naturopathic medicine group and 30.5 percent in the psychotherapy group, with significant differences benefiting the naturopathic group regarding mental health, concentration, fatigue, social functioning, vitality, and overall quality of life. No serious adverse reactions were observed in either group.

Both groups in the Cooley et al. (2009) study saw significant advantages in moderate and severe cases of depression. I highlight this study to support the notion that holistic and CAM models like naturopathic medicine should be considered in virtually every case of mood disorder care. In the treatment of mood disorders there is established significant superiority in combining psychotherapy and pharmacologic intervention over using either alone (Furukawa, Watanabe, & Churchill, 2007). By adding a holistic medicine system such as naturopathic care or CAM to a team care approach, which includes the therapist and psychiatrist, I believe we can greatly increase the efficacy of treatment.

Many studies look at single aspects of holistic care, such as an herb, a dietary change, an exercise regimen, and so on. Many of these are reviewed in the following chapters. Few studies like that of Cooley et al. (2009) look at multiple changes in holistic care as a paradigm. While more studies are needed, my 10 years of clinical experience working as a naturopathic physician alongside fellow therapists, psychologists, and psychiatrists tells me that a team care approach utilizing the best among these medicines is more powerful than any single one alone. This is the future model of mental health care.

## WHY USE CAM?

There are a multitude of pharmaceutical treatments in conventional care for anxiety and depression. Depending on the patient, the efficacy of these drugs for reducing symptoms will vary from very effective to making conditions worse. In any situation, however, these drug treatments do not really address the multiple underlying causes of these conditions.

There's an old saying in natural medicine circles: "If you are driving in your car, and the check engine light comes on, you can either cover it up with electric tape so you don't see the light, or you can stop the car, check under the hood, and fix the problem." Well, if you are in a dangerous driving situation where you cannot stop, and the light is glaring in your eyes, not allowing you to safely see the road, sometimes you need that electrical tape as an urgent care measure. In this urgent care situation, covering up the "symptom" can be a lifesaver until you get to a place you can stop. Then when you are in safer and calmer place (and ideally a place you know a good mechanic), you can stop, check under the hood, and try to figure out the problem—maybe it's a crack in the engine block, maybe you simply forgot to add oil for the last 8 years. . . . However, if you are not in that acutely dangerous situation, it is best not to use the electric tape to cover up the problem. Instead, it makes the most sense to fix the underlying cause of the red light symptom.

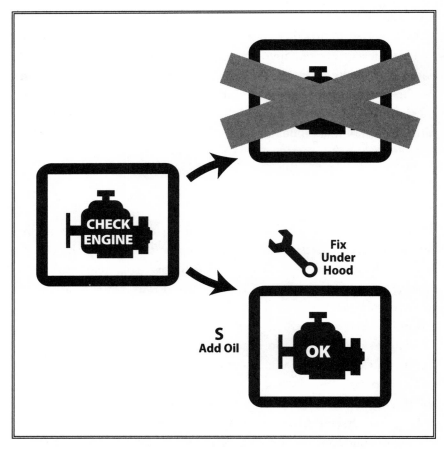

Figure. 1.1. Ignore the light or check your engine?

## Antidepressant Safety Concerns

The analogy above is that conventional biomedicine typically covers up the red light symptom and rarely addresses the underlying problem under the hood. Meta-analysis has shown that, in cases of depression, drugs do not work any better than placebo in mild to moderate cases (Fournier et al., 2010)—the major reason these millions of prescriptions are written. Even more startling, these drugs carry with them an increase in all-cause mortality, an increased likelihood many other problems, and side effects that impair quality of life. For example, antidepressants show a 32 percent increased risk for all-cause mortality, including a 45 percent increased risk for stroke (Smoller et al., 2009) in postmenopausal women. A comprehensive review of all the available published and unpublished controlled clinical trials of antidepressants in children and adolescents led the FDA to issue a public warning ( U.S. Food and Drug Administration 2004) about an increased risk of suicidal thoughts or attempts in children and adolescents treated with SSRI (selective serotonin reuptake inhibitor) antidepressants.

## Antianxiety Medication Safety Concerns

Efficacy for antianxiety medications is much higher than for antidepressants, with clear benefit in the short term, but these medications, like antidepressants, are fraught with side effects. According to Belleville (2010), people who use antianxiety medication have a 36 percent increased mortality risk. Even more, we have known for decades that long-term efficacy of antianxiety medication has not been shown (Committee on the Review of Medicines, 1980). Addiction to antianxiety medications is also another problem, as drug-induced changes in brain function lead to need for higher dosage, withdrawal symptoms, and greater disability (Mugathan et al., 2011). To sum up, antianxiety medications can help in the short term but pose clear dangers of addiction, likelihood of withdrawal problems, and increased risk of death.

## Medication Withdrawal

The experience of "discontinuation syndrome" (the medical term for what really is withdrawal) is a major challenge for both antidepressant and antianxiety medications. Symptoms include depression, anxiety, confusion, irritability, dizziness, lack of coordination, sleeping problems, crying spells, and blurry vision. And these symptoms herald a larger concern, for research shows that withdrawal itself evokes a major behavioral stress response (Harvey, McEwen, & Stein, 2003) and can cause significant neurologic damage through pathways that create nervous system overexcitement. Thus, the system we are trying to help can end up more damaged and unable to work in the long term.

As clinicians, we have all witnessed patients who have, unfortunately, stopped their own medications cold turkey, or could not get a hold of a refill in time—they are not happy people. Jean Paul Sartre's famous existential play *No Exit* features three characters with a fear of the unknown. They have a group dynamic of perpetual anxiety, which leaves them with no ability to flee their situation. In many ways, anxious and depressed patients given these medications too often have a sense of not being able to ever stop medication and flee, without serious withdrawal effects. This takes their power away, leaving them feeling trapped. Holistic care can help bring a sense of power and control back into their lives.

## Psychotherapy Benefits

While I am likely preaching to the choir on this one, I do want to note that psychotherapy has clearly been shown to be at least as beneficial as drugs in most cases (Cuijpers et al., 2013). Instead of suppressing symptoms, psychotherapy helps the underlying cause, by addressing the fundamental thinking that contributes to anxiety and depression. These thoughts and negative messaging prompt the primitive center of the brain known as the hypothalamus to overexcite the hypothalamic-pituitary-adrenal (HPA) axis. Short-term upregulation (increased activity) of the HPA axis can ready the body and help flee danger, and it is hoped, in the process, learn to protect against future danger. However, sufferers of anxiety and depression often have long-term upregulation, which leads to chronic symptoms of anxiety and depression and even increases risks for many diseases, such as cardiovascular illness, autoimmune disease, and bone loss. In the case of depression, research clearly shows that relapse rates with psychotherapy are much lower than with antidepressants (31 percent vs. 76 percent, respectively) (Hollon et al., 2005). Chapter 3 discusses dysregulation of the HPA axis.

## TOP FIVE PRINCIPLES OF HOLISTIC CARE

As discussed in the introduction, holistic medicine strives to look at the individual as a whole, not just separate body systems. The overarching tenets holistic care keeps in mind are as follows:

1. The body has the innate capacity to heal itself when given the opportunity to do so.
2. The body is an integrated whole, where an imbalance in one system will affect the rest of the body.
3. Symptoms (e.g. anxiety, depression, or pain) are calls to work on the basics of health: diet, sleep, exercise, psychology and spirit, digestion, and nutrient status.
4. The clinician's job is to identify the factors that are inhibiting the body's healing capacity and to formulate treatment to remove these.
5. Medication and/or surgery should be employed only in times of urgent need. Otherwise, a clinician should strive to use treatments that are more natural to the body and help it heal itself.

## HOW TO DECIDE WHEN HOLISTIC CARE IS APPROPRIATE FOR YOUR CLIENT

As touched on in the introduction of this book, the first order of business when working with someone with a health condition is safety. As a naturopathic doctor, I do believe modern biomedicine is wildly overused and in most cases does not address the underlying issues. Having said this, modern medicine is exceptional in urgent care situations and should be considered first-line therapy in cases where a client cannot reasonably work on the underlying cause through more natural modalities.

As an analogy, no matter how skilled a therapist you are, if a patient is too depressed to get out of bed to visit your office for psychotherapy work, your care can't possibly help. If medication can help get a patient out of bed to come to see you, then it makes common sense to work with the medication. While antidepressants are not very effective in mild to moderate depression, they do show efficacy in severe cases (Fournier et al., 2010), and should still be considered-first line therapy in these instances, for the safety of the client.

Natural medicines can be very effective and powerful, but they do take time to work, and often multiple changes in diet and lifestyle are needed to create an overall effect. As a matter of client safety and practicality, clients should be assessed for the need for pharmaceutical medications as first-line therapy:

1. Is there immediate and acute concern of patient harm to self or others, such as suicidal ideation or planning, history of harming self and others, or threats to do so? It is a key for any first and subsequent intake that the practitioner ask about suicidal ideation:

   *"Have you ever considered, or are you considering, suicide, or have you thought that it would be better if you weren't around? If yes: Have you ever devised a plan or do you have a plan to do this?"*

   *"Have you ever considered, or are you considering, doing harm to someone else? If yes: Have you ever devised a plan or do you have a plan to do this?"*

2. Is the anxious or depressed client not able to function in a capacity necessary to perform basic functions (e.g., going to and being effective at work) and is thus unable to feed or house himself or herself or dependents? An example of this may be a single parent whose responsibility is to take care of his children but he cannot leave his bed and, as a result, is placing the children in jeopardy.

If threat of immediate harm is suspected in either of these considerations, then medication and supervision of the patient may be needed and should be considered to first to stabilize your client. Two possible exceptions are cases of pregnancy and breast-feeding, which should be treated on a case-by-case basis.

If no threat of immediate harm is suspected, then the following questions will help assess whether holistic care should be first-line therapy:

1. *Does your mood stop you from taking care of yourself where you do not bathe or eat regularly?*
2. *Does your mood stop you from going to work and doing the basic things you need to do for yourself?*
3. *If you have children or people who depend on you, does your mood stop you from taking proper care of them?*
4. *Would you prefer trying natural methods to help balance your emotions?*

If your client answers yes to any of questions 1–3, then conventional medication should be first-line therapy, with natural medicine as an adjunct when possible. If the answer to question 4 is no, then it is much less likely that holistic therapies will be of value to this particular client, and you may want to focus on conventional care, for patient preference is an important predictor of effective care.

If medications are needed help stabilize the patient, natural medicine therapies that address lifestyle and psychology/spirit, as well as nutrient and supplemental therapies, can then be considered for the longer term. Chapter 7 reviews how to make recommendations and design treatment plans to support a patient using medication.

When using pharmaceutical medications, team management by the patient's prescribing doctor, therapist, and CAM provider (naturopathic doctor or other holistic practitioner) as a core team will afford the best overall care and allow the comanagement needed to consider future discontinuation of medications when appropriate. This possibility will be more appropriately realized once other lifestyle, psychological, physiologic, and nutrient factors are successfully addressed.

As described in the introduction, the team-care approach of a prescribing doctor (psychiatrist or psychopharmacologist), therapist, and holistic practitioner is the best of all worlds regarding optimal patient care. Once a decision is made that the patient does not meet the criteria outlined above that necessitates first-line pharmaceutical intervention, in team-care fashion, holistically minded recommendations should begin, while remaining vigilant to changes in the client's condition that could lead him or her to fulfilling the above criteria at a later time, necessitating pharmaceutical support.

According to David Mischoulon, a Harvard psychiatrist well known for researching nutrient therapies for emotional illness, the best candidates for natural remedies are those who are "mildly symptomatic, those who have failed multiple trials or are highly intolerant of side effects, and for those patients already on numerous medications, where the drug reactions due to polypharmacy may be significant" (Mischoulon & Rosenbaum, 2002).

While efficacy rates for antianxiety medications are high, the introduction discussed how the risk-to-benefit ratio is often too high, and healing the underlying causes is not addressed. The vast majority of patients treated for depression are actually seen in outpatient general practice settings, and most of these patients do not meet the diagnostic criteria for severe major depression. Most depressed patients who visit primary care physicians have milder forms of the illness ("Mild depression," 2003). For clients with these milder forms of depression, watchful waiting without active pharmacologic treatment may represent the most appropriate option because minor depression responds to both nonspecific support and active treatment (Oxman & Sengupta, 2002).

This time of "watchful waiting" is also a clear cue for employing holistic assessment and intervention. Under the direction of many conventional practitioners, these patients are needlessly treated with drugs. From a naturopathic perspective, it is regretful that so many of these patients are treated with medications as a first-line therapeutic option in lieu of psychotherapy and holistic care. In these scenarios, holistic care would probably do the most good by intervening with more natural options, while keeping common sense in mind: medications can be implemented as a last resort if the patient's condition does become severe.

## NOTE ABOUT PATIENT PREFERENCES

All practitioners working with anxiety and depression should note that, overall, patients generally do their best with the treatment they choose and believe in, whatever it may be. The practitioner should always keep in mind the importance of working with modalities preferred by the patient for best results and most rapid improvement. In one study, 315 patients with mood disorder who were treatment naïve and interested in receiving care were asked whether they preferred medications, psychotherapy, or both. Among these people, 15 percent preferred medication alone, 24 percent preferred solely psychotherapy, and 60 percent preferred both therapies (holistic care was not a choice in this study). Then these subjects went on to receive care that was randomly chosen for them. Those who received their preferred treatment clearly experienced the quickest results—no matter what the treatment was (Lin et al., 2005). It is likely that patients who visit a holistic practitioner are going to prefer the natural approach and will find benefit from working with their therapy of choice alone. As care givers, we should remember this.

As a holistic practitioner, I have a strong passion for natural medicine. It is my bias and tendency to desire natural medicine care for all my patients. But in truth, if this is not their wish or interest, it may not be to their benefit anyway, and I have learned to check ego at the door and help the patient find what he or she is looking for, even if it doesn't include my help.

## WHEN TO AVOID HOLISTIC CARE

When properly prescribed, holistic medicines have minimal risk and toxicity, and potentially powerful results. Holistic care is contraindicated only if conventional urgent care is needed, or if the client does not prefer it. However, there are some contraindications to specific vitamins and herbs, which are also discussed in this book.

# TWO

# Assessing Contributing Lifestyle Factors

Like an old gold-panning prospector, you must resign yourself
to digging up a lot of sand from which you will later patiently
wash out a few minute particles of gold ore."
                                        —Dorothy Bryant

OK, great. Now we are moving into the reasons you are reading this
book: to identify the underlying causes of anxiety and depression. Understanding the underlying causes helps the holistic practitioner pair treatments that are well researched, effective, and safe, as well as individualized
to your client. As a naturopathic physician, I am most excited about
understanding the underlying causes, for this understanding is the key to
creating the best plan. In the alternative medicine world, there are so
many treatment solutions: diets to follow, herbs, vitamins, detoxifica-
tions . . . the list is endless. It is seemingly impossible choose among them
all. As a result, holistic care can become a guessing game to the tune of
"this herb didn't work, now let's try this vitamin." This shot-in-the-dark
approach ends up frustrating both the patient and the practitioner.

Getting the lay of the land and understanding in depth the details of
a client's life will help to ultimately ferret out underlying issues and make
sense of it all, in order to make the best choices.

Anxiety and depression are typically not caused by one factor. If
there were only one cause, modern medicine would already have a drug
or procedure to fix it. As you are probably already aware, anxiety and
depression stem from multiple factors. This chapter discusses the most

important lifestyle factors, to help you organize them in your mind and ferret out which are the most salient for your client's needs.

### Case Study: Garrett's Reflux and Anxiety

*A few years ago, I had a patient named Garrett who was referred by a clinical social worker colleague. Garrett was a 33-year-old journalist and a busy guy. He taught in a respected school for journalism and worked on his own freelance assignments. About three years ago he started having incredible anxiety. He was placed on a daily dose of Lexapro to "keep it under control," while also using Xanax as needed (usually once or twice a week) when things "became overwhelming." He started therapy work about 6 months prior. During our first visit, I learned that Garrett also had stomach reflux and mild intermittent pain for the past 5 years that was controlled with Nexium. When I asked Garrett about his day, I learned he slept about 5 hours a night, claiming "I am good with that, I don't need more." He also told me he had to stop exercising when he took his teaching position due to time constraints.*

*At the first visit, we decided to hone in on sleep. Over the following months we were able to adjust his schedule to increase his sleep time. He found that with the increased sleep, he felt more motivated to exercise. Interestingly, he also was able to stop his Nexium, without having a return of reflux symptoms. This is likely because the increased sleep gave his digestive tract more time to heal. Within two months on the new plan, he stopped using his Xanax. Within 6 months, he weaned off the Lexapro. I believe that, combined with the psychotherapy he was doing, the adjustment to sleep helped his digestion. Better digestion helped his neurotransmitters balance. And the exercise helped burn excess stress hormones. All these helped him create mood balance.*

## SLEEP

All animals (including human animals) require sleep. Studies on human sleep deprivation show how inadequate sleep function increases risk of viral illness, weight gain, problems with blood sugar imbalance, slowed cognition, and increased brain inflammation consistent with problematic mood. For instance, Cohen et al. (2009) showed having that less than 7 hours of sleep each night raises the risk of contracting respiratory viral illness by 300 percent compared with those who had 8 or more hours of sleep.

Despite the importance of sleep, most of us are not getting enough. People are sleeping, on average, 20 percent less than we did 100 years ago. For people predisposed to anxiety and depression, sleeping problems will make mood worse. Sleep challenges typically precede and occur concomitantly with mood challenges. Insomnia is a well-known symptom of depression (Ringdahl, Pereira, & Delzell, 2004) and often heralds its onset or recurrence (Ford & Kamerow, 1989; Buysse et al., 1997). Sleep disturbances are highly prevalent in anxiety disorders (Staner, 2003); an estimated 90 percent of depressed patients have insomnia, and about half the population is losing sleep due to anxiety and stress.

The underlying cause of sleep disorder is different for each person. Typically, there is no one underlying cause. Instead, a few unbalancing factors are typically at play at the same time. Unless a person has an exceedingly rare condition called fatal familial insomnia, people with insomnia can usually fix their sleep patterns with individualized holistic care. We will go over some of these care options.

### "I Am a Night Owl" and "I Can't Get to Sleep"

Do you have clients with anxiety or depression who tell you they are "exhausted during the day and then wake up at night'—and that's often when they feel their best? Some will often say, "I have always been a night owl."

Inappropriate exposure to bright light and excessive stress can create disruptions in sleep patterns and can cause a condition called delayed sleep phase syndrome (DSPS). While not well known, this is actually a fairly common cause of insomnia. In the brain, the hormone melatonin is secreted by the pineal gland as the darkness of night approaches. Melatonin is a powerful antioxidant known to help our body detoxify and strengthen the immune system. Melatonin tells the body to prepare for sleep by lowering body temperature and inducing drowsiness.

The ability melatonin to be released at the right time is a key for optimal mood. When it is not, your client may end up with a circadian rhythm disorder. Characteristic symptoms of this often undiagnosed problem include sleep onset insomnia ("I can't get sleep at night") and waking up multiple times throughout the night, or waking too early in the morning. Generally people with DSPS feel more alert at night than in the morning—these are the self-proclaimed "night owls." Many suffer then from inability to wake up early enough to get their day going— these people want to keep sleeping, and then once they are up, they experience immeasurable and sometimes debilitating fatigue during the day. By the time night rolls around, they get a "second wind" that keeps the bad sleep cycle going. The prevalence of depression and personality disorders in people with DSPS is very high (Smits & Pandi-Perumal, 2005). Up to 10 percent of high school students have DSPS and suffer chronic sleep deprivation because their schedule dictates they go to sleep earlier.

### *"I Can't Stay Asleep" or "I Wake Up Way Too Early"*

Many patients with anxiety and depression will complain that they cannot stay asleep, even if they fall asleep well. Some will also complain about waking up early (around 3 a.m. to 5 a.m.) and feeling wide awake. They will get up and feel fine for a few hours and then slip into great fatigue for the rest of the day.

REM (rapid eye movement) sleep is a component of the last stage of sleep that occurs in both animals and people. Known as "dream sleep," this part of sleep tends to be a very light and active. People with anxiety and depression tend to have much more REM sleep and less deep sleep than normal. Newborns spend about 80 percent of their sleep in REM, but adults normally should not experience more than 25 percent sleep as REM. In REM sleep, the brain is processing. Because brain processing activity is similar to the type experienced in waking moments, the more REM sleep a person experiences, the less refreshing the sleep will be.

Sleep studies of patients with anxiety and depression have shown that patients tend to enter REM sleep unusually early and have an extended first REM phase along with a loss of later deeper phases of sleep. These are the patients who report that they cannot stay asleep and complain of early morning awakenings. Consistent imbalanced REM sleep is predictive of developing symptoms of anxiety disorders. Researchers looking at the sleep patterns of depressed patients found that they indeed have increased REM sleep in proportion to slow-wave non-REM sleep (Berger et al., 1983), and depressed patients who were purposefully deprived of REM stage sleep showed improved mood (Vogel et al., 1980).

### *"I Snore a Lot"*

Some patients (or, more often, their sleeping partners) will complain about snoring. While only about 6 percent of the general population struggle with a type of disturbed sleep known as sleep apnea where there are irregular breathing cessations of breathing throughout the night, 20 percent of people with depression have sleep apnea. So, especially for your clients with depression, you may want to keep this in the back of your mind. It is best to speak with a sleep specialist or pulmonologist to properly diagnose this condition. Natural methods to treat this include melatonin (see p. 20), avoiding food sensitivities (discussed in Chapter 3), and weight loss. If these are not effective, it is worth considering a continuous positive air pressure (CPAP) machine or possibly surgical procedures to help open the airway. Patients who have hypertension or are falling asleep during the day may need to consider the CPAP or surgery sooner for safety reasons (Milleron, et al., 2004).

### Questions to Ask about Sleep:

*How many hours of sleep do you get each night?*
*What time do you go to bed, and what time do you wake up?*
*Are you a "night owl"?*
*Do you have trouble falling asleep?*
*Do you wake up many times at night?*

*Do you wake up too early in the morning?*
*Do you wake up refreshed?*
*Do you or your spouse think you snore a lot?*

## Steps to Improve Sleep

Now you have asked the right questions, and assessed the symptoms of sleep. So let's talk about some ideas to reintroduce healthful sleeping patterns. For patients with anxiety and depression with sleep challenges, I recommend working on sleep first, before addressing anything else. Assuring healthful sleep is probably the best first step toward long-term healing of anxiety and depression. I recommend the following eight steps to help get sleep back on track.

*1. Get to bed before midnight (and ideally no later than 10:30 p.m.)*
There's an old Chinese medicine proverb that says "one hour before midnight is worth two hours after midnight." While the ancient Chinese did not know about endocrinology (the study of hormones), this suggestion makes physiologic sense for it encourages people to be in a still, dark place at a time when onset of melatonin release allows for optimal sleep and circadian regulation. Melatonin is the master hormone that tells your body it is time to go to sleep.

Melatonin release in the adult begins at about 10 p.m. (Smits & Pandi-Perumal, 2005). The right bedtime optimizes its release. Later bedtimes will suppress melatonin and encourage stress hormone activity. Unless nocturnal, the only animals that stay up past dark are in danger or need food. Humans who stay up late also experience a stress response that will encourage poor sleep, DSPS, and excess REM sleep.

If your client generally goes to bed later than midnight and wants to make a positive change, I recommend backing up bedtime by 15 minutes every week, possibly to settle in at a 10:30 to 11:00 p.m. bedtime at the latest. Supplemental melatonin can be used if needed to help (see more about melatonin with step 7 below and in Chapter 4).

### 2. Create an evening ritual

I recommend my patients start dimming the lights by 9:00 to 9:30 p.m. and shut down the TV and computer. My computer has an application called f.lux which is a free downloadable program that changes the screen light to a less melatonin-suppressing amber hue in the early evening, which will help curb melatonin suppression while still using the computer in the early evening. Sipping a calming tea such as chamomile or lavender is also smart choice at this time. It is best to make a small cup and sip slowly. This way the bladder does not fill and cause wakefulness during the night. As people create their own healthy sleep rituals, they will find comfort in consistency, and their body will learn to calm in preparation for sleep.

### 3. Lower the lights 30 minutes before bed

Avoid using any bright lights at this time. This includes shutting any computer and e-mail work, texting, tablet computers, and so forth. Bright light suggests to the body that it is daylight, which suppresses the release of melatonin. Reading calming literature using a lamp with an orange light bulb is also helpful to avoid melatonin suppression.

### 4. Keep the room dark and cool

Melatonin, human growth hormone, and other hormones are needed for repair and detoxification. These are suppressed when the room is too bright and too warm. If your client can see their hand when held one foot in front of the face, then the room has too much light. Consider covering all light sources (like cable boxes, clocks) and keep the cell phone charging in another room. I also recommend using completely occlusive blinds. Some of my patients install automatic openers that open the blinds gradually at the right time in the morning to assure a slow introduction of light. Keeping the temperature around 68° F assures optimal melatonin secretion.

### 5. Ask about food and blood sugar

Occasionally, eating too late and having too much food in the stomach can inhibit the natural ability to fall asleep. I have noticed certain patients are also quite sensitive to individual foods (common ones are wine, spicy foods, and dairy products), which can keep them up.

Alternately, when people have low blood sugar before bed, it can be equally hard to fall asleep. When blood sugar is low, this signals our animal brain to go hunt for food and trigger the release of stress hormones. If this is suspected, eating a small amount of protein and carbohydrate together (e.g., a little turkey with an apple slice, or nut butter with a rice cracker) right before bed can be helpful.

### 6. Journal before bed

Many of us lead very hectic lives and often do not have one quiet moment during the day until the moment we decide to go to bed. At this time, the brain gets us alone and says, "OK, I've got you. Let's go over some things," and wants to start processing lots of things, over and over. This is the moment all the thoughts flood in at one time: family problems, relationship issues, job stress, financial worries, worries about nuclear war, and so on. These come at us at once and become overwhelming. Placed in stress mode, the brain and body cannot shut off.

In these cases, it is a valuable practice to pause for a minute right before bed and jot down a to-do list for the next day, and/or write down the top issues that are of concern, and then fold over the paper and put it to the side, to "let go" of them until the next day. As a clinician, you may find it valuable to review this written list with your client, to see what comes up during those nighttime hours. Walt Whitman said: "I do not think until I read what I write." Although jotting them down may not fix the issues of concern, it can help create some balance by processing them before going to sleep.

### 7. Natural Remedies for Sleep, If Needed

I encourage patients to try the above steps for two weeks and see if sleeping improves. If it does not balance out completely, then natural medicines can be amazing to finish the job. Here are the top natural remedies I will typically use.

## Magnesium

Magnesium deficiency is common and is associated with chronic inflammatory stress (Nielsen, Johnson, & Zeng, 2010). Deficiency will increase dysfunction in the brain's biological clock areas of the suprachiasmatic nuclei and pineal gland (Durlach, 2002) and disorganize sleep patterns (Murck, 2013). This nontoxic mineral has been shown helpful in clinical trials for sleep efficiency, sleep duration, sleep onset latency, and early morning awakening (Abbasi et al., 2012).

Dosing is usually in the range of 400–500 mg/day. Many patients will take 250 mg twice a day, with the last dose right before bed. I often recommend the magnesium glycinate form, for glycine is an amino acid known for its own calming effect. While there is no known toxicity associated with magnesium, some sensitive individuals can have loose bowel movements with extra magnesium intake. In this case, the dose needs to be scaled back.

## Melatonin

Studies from the 1980s have shown that low or delayed melatonin levels can contribute to depression (Beck-Friis et al., 1984) and anxiety (Toffol et al., 2014). A powerful antioxidant, it protects brain and nervous tissue (Garcia et al., 1997). As a supplement, it was originally known to fix jet lag and is now known to help fight cancer (Al-Omary, 2013) and may even increase efficacy of chemotherapy (Lissoni, 2007).

Melatonin supplements are sold in dosages from 0.5 mg up to 20 mg. Regular (non-time-released) melatonin is best to help calm the body and let it know when it is time to fall asleep. Time-released (also known as sustained released) melatonin can be used for trouble falling asleep that occurs with difficulty staying asleep. Melatonin is quite safe and nonaddictive and is even used with children. A typical adult dose is 1–3 mg a half hour before the desired bedtime. Studies with DSPS have used very low melatonin doses of 0.125 mg in the late afternoon and evening, each dose 4 hours apart (e.g., at 4 p.m. and again at 8 p.m.). If your client finds using a single before-bedtime dose is not working, then try the low doses given at 4 and 8 p.m. Adolescents with DSPS have been given doses of 0.3–5 mg (Alldredge et al., 2012) to help retrain normal sleeping patterns. If a client is having trouble staying asleep, but not falling asleep, time-released melatonin in doses of 3–6 mg may help to keep a person from waking during the night.

While melatonin has no toxicity in the doses described above, it is best to scale it back if the patient feels groggy in the morning after use. Some research suggests that elevated melatonin levels are associated with exacerbations in nocturnal asthma, so melatonin should be avoided in someone who has nighttime asthmatic symptoms (Sutherland et al., 2003).

*Melatonin versus sleep medications*

Studies comparing hypnotic medication with melatonin found that melatonin caused no postural instability in seniors, whereas zolpidem (Ambien) impaired stability and caused body sway, a strong risk factor for falling (Otmani et al., 2012). Two studies comparing melatonin with Ambien found that melatonin had sleep benefits without the next-day cognitive, attention, psychomotor, or driving impairments reported with the zolpidem (Wesensten et al., 2005; Otmani et al., 2008). In my practice, it is common to use both melatonin, and sleep medications like zolpidem, especially when the sleep drugs stop working. While most research combining melatonin and zolpidem show no negative interactions, some research with extended-release zolpidem (Ambien CR) showed increased psychomotor impairments (Otmani et al., 2008). As a precaution, it is best to start on low doses of melatonin (around 1mg) and increase as needed until desired effect is achieved, while monitoring for daytime sleepiness and any impairment.

*Natural food sources of melatonin*

Oats (*Avena sativa*) are known to have a calming effect on the body and contain very small amounts melatonin. However, to get the same amount of melatonin that is found in a supplement pill, one would need to eat about 20 bowls of oats. Montmorency tart cherries, ginger, tomatoes, bananas, and barley also contain very minute amounts of melatonin (Iowa State University Extension and Outreach, 2009). One study of tart cherry juice found a modest effect on sleep (Pigeon et al., 2010), and it might work well for mild insomnia issues.

## L-Tryptophan

L-Tryptophan is a naturally derived amino acid that serves as a precursor to serotonin. Depletion of tryptophan contributes to generalized anxiety and panic attacks (Klaassen et al., 1998), and L-tryptophan levels are significantly lower in depressed subjects than in normal controls (Maes et al., 1997c). Low levels of tryptophan do not allow the body to manufacture enough serotonin. Lowered levels of serotonin can be a reason for poor sleep, especially for staying asleep.

Dosage at bedtime is usually 500–1,000 mg, while some patients may need up to 2,500 mg. For best absorption to the brain, it is best to take with a slice of simple carbohydrate (like an apple slice), because the carbohydrate will increase insulin levels, and insulin will promote tryptophan absorption into the brain.

Although most conventional psychiatrists are afraid to mix natural medicines like tryptophan with conventional medication, one 8-week randomized controlled trial of 30 patients with major depression found that combining 20 mg fluoxetine (Prozac) with 2 g tryptophan daily at the outset of treatment for major depressive disorder appeared to be a safe protocol that had both a rapid antidepressant effect and a protective effect on slow-wave sleep (Levitan et al., 2000).

Please note that several Internet sites state that L-tryptophan is unsafe due to past history of eosinophilia myalgia syndrome, a condition contracted by several people in the 1980s after ingesting tryptophan supplements, which led to the death of 30 people. This tragic event occurred because the company making the supplement had no quality controls and allowed the introduction of fatal bacteria. These deaths had nothing to do with tryptophan itself. Please see more about the use of tryptophan in Chapter 4.

## Valerian

Valerian is the best-studied herbal medicine for sleep. The root word *valere* comes from the Latin term for "good health." Please note that valerian has no relationship to Valium, except for the fact that both names share the same first three letters. Valerian is especially helpful for people who focus stress in their gut ("nervous stomach") and when there is a strong anxiety component accompanying inability to sleep. This herb has constituents that act to inhibit sympathetic nervous system neurons by enhancing levels of gamma-aminobutyric acid (GABA), a brain-calming neurotransmitter. The sympathetic nervous system activates the stress response in our body, sometimes called the "flight-or-flight" response.

A meta-analysis of 18 randomized controlled clinical trials suggests benefit using valerian (Fernández-San-Martín et al., 2010). In one randomized, triple-blind, controlled trial of 100 postmenopausal women, 530 mg of concentrated valerian extract given twice a day for 4 weeks resulted in better sleep quality compared with placebo. While most studies report positive effects, one randomized trial did not find benefit, although this study was in a small group of 16 women and used suboptimal dosing of 300 mg once a day before bed (Taibi et al., 2009). It is possible that using higher doses typically recommended may have showed benefit.

Valerian can also help with staying asleep when trying to wean off anxiety medications. In rat studies, valerian has been shown to help alleviate withdrawal syndrome resulting from the removal of diazepam (Valium) following prolonged periods of administration (Andreatini & Leite, 1994), while not showing any toxic effects (Tufik et al., 1994). A team out of Brazil had a similar notion when they prescribed valerian (100 mg three times a day, with 80 percent didrovaltrate, 15 percent valtrate, and 5 percent acelvaltrate from valerian root) to help patients with insomnia tolerate withdrawal from benzodiazepines. These 19 patients (averaging 43 years of age) were using benzodiazepines every night for an average of 7 years but still had poor sleep and were matched to 18 control subjects. Electroencephalogram patterns were studied during sleep while still on the benzodiazepines, and then for 2 weeks after while taking either valerian or placebo. The patients taking valerian reported significantly better subjective sleep quality than those on placebo after benzodiazepine withdrawal, despite the presence of a few withdrawal side effects from the medications. At the end of 2 weeks, there was a significant decrease in nighttime waking time after sleep onset in valerian subjects compared with placebo subjects. Nonetheless, valerian-treated patients did show increased alpha waves (corresponding to more difficulty falling asleep) as well as longer blocks of sleep latency than did control subjects. Despite subjective improvement, sleep data showed that valerian did not actually produce faster sleep onset, which was likely due to the medication withdrawal hyperarousal (a state where the withdrawal of the medication keeps the patient in a more awake state). The authors concluded that, overall, valerian was well tolerated and had a positive effect on withdrawal from benzodiazepine use, with no interactions between the two (Poyares et al., 2002).

Typical dosage of valerian is 450–600 mg about 2 hours before bedtime. Patients with daily anxiety or needing more sleep support may add an early afternoon dose. In many cases, valerian works best when taken over a few weeks rather than acutely. While safety has been shown in trials of children (Francis & Dempster, 2002) and in the senior population, it has not been evaluated in pregnancy. The active components of valerian may increase benzodiazepine activity and should be monitored by a physician if used with these medications.

### Supplements in combination?

While any of the above supplements can be of value alone, CAM practitioners typically combine some of these for even better results. For example, one double-blind study from Italy used 5 mg melatonin and

225 mg magnesium taken 1 hour before bedtime. Results showed significant improvements in sleep scores, as well as quality sleep, and alertness the following morning (Rondanelli et al., 2011). Very often I will start by recommending one supplement at a time and then add others after a few days if the one supplement does not create the full effect.

### Final Note: Cognitive Behavioral Therapy and Sleep

As of this writing, there is a near-completed study of 66 depressed patients showing that almost 90 percent of these patients (whether on an antidepressant or placebo) who worked with cognitive behavior therapy for insomnia twice a week found depression resolved in 8 weeks of treatment using either an antidepressant drug or a placebo pill—almost twice the rate of those who did not have cognitive behavior therapy. This particular therapy focuses on establishing healthy sleep rituals, which include keeping proper and consistent sleep times, avoiding daytime napping, and not reading, eating, or watching TV in bed (Carey, 2013).

## FOOD

If you have a dog with anxiousness, inflammation, digestive issues, or virtually any problem, when you bring the dog to a veterinarian, what is the first thing the vet asks? "What are you feeding this dog?" This is because the vet is trained to know that what the animal ingests will affect its health considerably.

Although a tenet virtually ignored by modern medicine until very recently, it stands to reason that what your client ingests is going to affect the body in a substantial way. Poor diet will increase the likelihood of a disease to which someone may be predisposed. Conversely, eating better leads to better mental health. This section discusses the benefits of good nutrition and then identifies some specific food choices particularly unhealthy for those with anxiety and depression.

## Healthy Dietary Choices for Best Mood

More and more studies are showing that healthy food intake prevents both anxiety and depression and blocks the ravages on the body that occur with mental illness (Antonogeorgos et al., 2012). One landmark five-year study out of Spain looked at the lives and eating patterns of 10,000 people. Those people who followed a Mediterranean diet were 50 percent less likely to develop anxiety or depression. The study specifically found that intake of fruits, nuts, beans, and olive oil supported mood best (Sánchez-Villegas et al., 2009a).

Other studies regarding the Mediterranean diet have also shown that the endothelial linings (inner lining of blood vessels) of these subjects were much healthier and predisposed them to lower rates of cardiovascular disease. Even more, further studies by the same group found that those people who ate in this healthy way also had higher levels of brain-derived neurotrophic factor (BDNF), a protein secreted by the nervous system that is critical for growth, repair, and survival of healthy brain and nervous system cells (Sánchez-Villegas et al., 2011). BDNF has been shown to be low in individuals with depression (Yoshimura et al., 2010) or with anxiety (Suliman, Hemmings, & Seedat, 2013).

Dr. Miguel Angel Martinez-Gonzalez, the senior author of this series of studies, offered his understanding of Mediterranean diet advantage: "The membranes of our neurons (nerve cells) are composed of fat, so the quality of fat that you are eating definitely has an influence on the quality of the neuron membranes, and the body's synthesis of neurotransmitters is dependent on the vitamins you're eating" (Rabin, 2009).

### Components of a Mediterranean Diet:

1. High amounts of monounsaturated fats and low amounts of saturated fats
2. High intake of legumes
3. High fish intake
4. High intake of whole-grain cereals and breads

5. High intake of fruits and nuts
6. High intake of vegetables
7. Moderate alcohol intake
8. Moderate intake of milk and dairy products
9. Low intake of meat and meat products

A recent cross-sectional study by Davison & Kaplan (2012) looked closely at the foods and nutrient intakes of 97 people with confirmed mood disorders, examining intake of fats, carbohydrates, and proteins, as well as vitamins and minerals. They evaluated these patients using Global Assessment of Functioning (GAF) scores, as well as the Hamilton Depression Rating Scale and the Young Mania Rating Scale. Significant correlations were found between GAF scores and energy (kilocalories), carbohydrates, fiber, and total fat. Also correlated were intakes of linoleic acid (an omega-6 fatty acid, discussed in Chapter 4), riboflavin, niacin, folic acid, vitamins B6 and B12, pantothenic acid, calcium, phosphorus, potassium, iron, magnesium, and zinc. The study showed higher levels of mental function associated with a higher intake of nutrients. When dietary supplement use was added to the nutrient intakes from food, GAF scores remained positively correlated with all dietary minerals, suggesting that supplementation, along with healthy foods, can play a role in helping mood disorder. (Chapters 4 and 6 discuss supplementation further.)

Often, patients and fellow practitioners alike will ask me my opinion on which is the best diet. While I think this question is best answered by understanding each patient case and possible food sensitivities, if I did not know the individual, or his or her history, I would recommend the Mediterranean diet. Although no one diet is completely perfect for every individual due to possible allergies and sensitivities, there is reason to believe the Mediterranean diet may far surpass the benefits of other choices for those with mood problems. While no one diet is 100 percent effective and healthy for every person, the Mediterranean diet has often been considered one of the most healthful for many different people and conditions, and the research seems to back up this bold statement.

## Some Specifically Healthy Foods

So, what should your client with depression or anxiety be eating? This next section is going to go over some basics about diet to help make some healthful and emotionally supportive choices.

### Protein sources

The Centers for Disease Control and Prevention suggests at least one-third of the population is obese (Ogden et al., 2012). Despite our over-eating, many people actually are not getting enough protein. Our population tends to eat copious amounts of high-carbohydrate foods but not enough quality protein. Low protein intake is a problem especially for people inclined to have mood issues, for two reasons. One is that proteins break down to amino acids, which are the building blocks of neurotransmitters, our molecules of emotion. The second reason is that it is very challenging to regulate blood sugar with insufficient protein—and blood sugar dysregulation is an important factor in both anxiety and depression (more about blood sugar further below). Pregnant women who ate a vegetarian diet typically low in protein had a 25 percent greater likelihood for high levels of anxiety symptom (Vaz Jdos, et al. 2013), likely due to low protein levels. Excess protein can also be a problem: too much protein can actually suppress central nervous system serotonin levels, which will negatively affect mood.

So, how much protein should your clients be getting? To help understand how much protein a person generally needs, you can use the formula

[weight (lb)/2.2 lb] × 0.8 g = grams of protein you need per day.

For example, a 120-pound person will require about 44 g protein. (Note that elite athletes should multiply by 1.2 g instead of 0.8 g; a person with kidney disease may need to decrease protein intake below the formula's recommendation.)

The healthiest protein sources are beans, raw nuts and seeds, tofu, fish and natural poultry, and grass-fed meats.

*Fish and healthy oils*

There is ample evidence showing correlations between low seafood consumption and higher rates of mood disorder. Conversely, solid research also tells us that higher intake of fish may help prevent and treat anxiety and depression.

Seafood intake is shown to lower both anxiety and depression. One study showed that the likelihood of anxiety was 43 percent higher for those who rarely or never ate dark and oily fish compared with those that ate it one to three times a week or more (Vaz et al., 2013). A thorough review spanning 13 countries demonstrated that there is an inverse relationship between intake of fish and depression (Hibbeln, 1998).

There are two main types of healthy omega-3 fatty acids in fish: eicosapentanoic acid (EPA) and docosahexanoic acid (DHA). It is believed that these substances help balance inflammation in the body and brain and lower the likelihood of mood disorder. These omega-3 fats are especially high in wild salmon, striped bass, mackerel, rainbow trout, halibut, and sardines. While science is still trying to understand whether EPA or DHA is more important, it is clear that individuals with anxiety and depression who eat less fish show marked depletions in omega-3 fatty acids in blood cell fats compared with people who do not have these mood disorders (Jacka et al., 2013), and these lower levels correlate with more anxious and depressive states.

The standard American diet (with the apt acronym "SAD") tends to be quite low in healthy omega-3 fish oil and high in omega-6 oils. Omega-6 fatty acids are found in saturated fats and red meats. It is well established that diets with high omega-6 to omega-3 ratios increase the risk of heart disease, as well as contribute to mood problems. Swedish researchers looked at senior patients and found that depressive symptoms and markers of inflammation increased with higher ratios of omega-6 to omega-3 fatty acids. They concluded that diets with high ratios can increase the risk of not only cardiovascular disease but also depression (Kotani et al., 2006).

Because the brain and nervous system are made of mostly fats and water, it stands to reason that healthful dietary fats are crucial for the mood of your clients. While we focus on the omega-3 fats, healthy oils such as cold-pressed extra virgin olive oil (which consist healthy omega-9 fats or oleic acids) and flax oils are also highly recommended. Organic and natural foods and wild fishes are preferred due to the lower levels of pesticides, neurotoxins, and metals that may play a role in some mood illnesses.

Below is a list of recommendations by the National Resources Defense Council (2013) for how often different types of fish should be eaten, based on their average mercury content.

### Fish Consumption Recommendations
### Based on Mercury Content:

Low mercury, OK to eat two to three times a week:

Anchovies

Catfish

Flounder

Herring

Rainbow trout

Salmon

Sardines

Scallops

Shrimp

Sole

Tilapia

Moderate mercury, eat once or twice a month:

Cod fish

Snapper

High mercury, try to avoid or eat rarely:

Halibut

Lobster

Mackerel

Sea bass

Tuna

## Probiotic foods

Amazing new research is emerging regarding the role of the microbiome of the digestive tract lining. The microbiome refers to the healthful bacteria, or "good germs," that line our digestive tracts. As will be discussed in Chapter 3, the digestive tract is an important player in best mood, and good bacteria is an important part of healthy digestion. Probiotics not only are known to help the digestion but also are key factors in obesity, hormonal balance, healthy kidney function, and much more.

Medical research is uncovering the mechanism of probiotics in mood. These healthy germs boost mood in two important ways: they generate a brain-calming neurotransmitter called gamma-aminobutyric acid (GABA), and they enhance the brain receptors for GABA. GABA is calming amino acid, known to calm areas of the brain that are overactive in anxiety and panic.

Bravo et al. (2011), working with mice, showed those mice that ingested probiotics were, in general, more chilled out than the control mice. The probiotics-fed mice had lower levels of corticosterone in response to stress—corticosterone is the mouse version of the human stress hormone cortisol. High levels of cortisol are common in both anxiety and depression. These mice were fed a broth either with the probiotic strain *Lactobacillus rhamnosus* or without these bacteria. The lactobacillus-fed animals showed significantly fewer stress, anxiety and depression-related behaviors than those fed with just broth.

Human studies have also corroborated these mouse findings. Messaoudi et al. (2011), in a double-blind, placebo-controlled, randomized parallel group study, learned that giving humans specific strains of *Lactobacillus* and *Bifidobacterium* for 30 days yielded beneficial psychological effects, including lowered depression, less anger, hostility, and anxiety, and better problem solving, compared with the placebo group.

While a healthy microbiome will contribute to good mood, an unhealthy one full of *Candida albicans* (yeast), and all the toxins associated with it, may also contribute to mood disorder. Presence of yeast will alter the ability to absorb nutrients and push hypersensitivity reactions

31

to toxin by-products, which translates to inflammation in the body. Inflammation will greatly contribute to depression, anxiety, and poor mental function (Rucklidge, 2013).

Unhealthy microbiome → yeast buildup → toxic by-products → hypersensitivity reactions → inflammation → mood problems (anxiety and depression)

While Messaoudi et al. (2011) gave a supplement, there are also many wonderful natural foods full of probiotics. These include natto (a traditional Japanese fermented food), kimchi (Korean-style fermented vegetables), yogurt, kefir, tempeh, fermented milk (e.g., buttermilk), miso, and nonbaked cheeses (e.g., aged cheese). Sauerkraut is also a good probiotic source, however, store-bought sauerkraut has less of the healthy probiotics due to pasteurization and preservative content, so obtaining freshly made versions may be best.

### Crunchy vegetables

Notice how most people get pleasure from crunchy foods—the idea that someone "can't eat just one"? There's a scientific reason why we go for these. It's because crunching makes people feel happier (when they are doing the crunching themselves—not so much when someone right next to you is the cruncher). Hoch et al. (2013) used enhanced MRI technology with rats given either regular chow or crunchy snacks to figure out the reasons behind "hedonic hyperphagia" (which means eating to excess for pleasure). He found that crunchy snacks activate many more brain reward centers than the noncrunchy chow. Other research suggests that the crunching sound allows pleasure centers to release more endorphins. Because crunchy food calms, this can be used to help anxiety.

That said, when people eat too many calories from junky-crunchy foods, they tend to feel even worse. So, instead of unhealthy chips and cookies, we will want to recommend healthful crunch foods, such a carrots, celery, and peppers. Also, a number of healthy low-temperature-baked snacks, such as flax meal crackers and high-bran-fiber crackers, can also do the job. Nuts are great, too, but should be raw (see below for why).

### Ideas for Healthy Crunch Foods:

Baby carrots

Dried crunchy vegetables: peas, carrots, peppers, etc.

Celery with raw almond butter or natural peanut butter

Raw nuts and seeds: almonds, walnuts, cashews, pumpkin seeds, sunflower seeds, etc.

Baked crackers made out of flax

Bran- and whole-grain-fiber crackers

Raw food crunch snacks: dried kale or veggie 'chips', etc.

*Raw nuts*

Raw nuts have been eaten by health-conscious people for millennia. Besides their crunchiness, which can help calm the brain, nuts are chock full of healthy fatty acids and oils, as well as protein and minerals. Nuts have been studied for their ability to lower inflammation in the body as well. Salas-Salvadó et al. (2008) looked at levels of inflammatory markers in people who ate nuts regularly. These people had lower levels of C-reactive protein (CRP), which is a protein found in the blood when inflammation is high. This marker is strongly correlated with cardiovascular disease and is likely a better predictor of heart and blood vessel problems than cholesterol. Other inflammation markers, such as the immune system component interleukin-6 (IL-6) and vascular adhesion factors (which make blood vessel walls sticky) were also lower. CRP and IL-6 are typically quite high in people who have anxiety (Vogelzangs et al., 2013) and depression (Howren, Lamkin, & Suls, 2009). Salas-Salvadó et al. (2008) believed the benefit in nuts is probably due to both the healthy fatty acids and high magnesium levels.

Healthy raw nuts include almonds, Brazil nuts, chestnuts, and cashews. Heating the nuts can damage the oils, making them go rancid and rendering them unhealthful for the brain and body. If you prefer the taste of roasted nuts, you can try mixing two or three parts raw to one part roasted, to keep the majority of your intake as intact uncooked fat.

### Salt intake

While many of us take in too much salt through processed foods, a number of people who eat "healthy" may actually restrict their salt intake too much. Clinical and experimental observations in animal and human studies suggest that low sodium intake can induce behavioral characteristics that are quite similar to psychological depression, as well as modify brain regions for motivation and reward specifically geared to salt intake over other pleasures (Morris, Na, & Johnson, 2008). Salt intake should be in moderation, unless a person is a salt-sensitive hypertensive, in which case it should be avoided.

## Foods to Avoid

As healthy foods can help support a health nervous system and good mood, poor-quality foods will work against the best health of your client. This discussion about food started with foods that are healthy, for this is the best place to start. With most patients, often it is not effective to begin by focusing on what they should not eat. I have learned that if we start with foods "to avoid," patients will feel deprived and sometimes angry, and they may have the opposite reaction, eating even more of the "unhealthy" foods as a way to gain a sense of control or as a type of backlash reaction.

As such, it is best to start by having your client add foods that are healthful. For example, if a client eats fast foods three times a day, a movement it the right direction might be to suggest he or she eat a rib of celery between breakfast and lunch and an apple between lunch and dinner. As the patient accomplishes these small tasks, then you can add others (e.g., a cup of greens with dinner and a glass of water in the morning). In my experience, as patients feel healthier and more empowered, eventually the unhealthy foods start to decrease without the sense of being deprived.

Also, it is important to check patient taste preferences. Research shows that the brain reacts similarly to both something morally violating and a taste that is unpleasant, so among the healthy foods, pick ones that the patient finds palatable—unpleasant tastes may exacerbate negative mood.

### High glycemic foods

Sugary foods (juices, cakes, cookies, candy) and simple carbohydrate foods (breads, pasta, rice) are known as high glycemic foods. These foods contain higher levels of easily absorbed sugar, which triggers any disease to which someone may be predisposed, and contributes in the long term to diabetes, dementia, heart disease, and cancer.

Specific to mood disorder, high consumption of sugars and carbohydrates causes depletion of important minerals, such as magnesium (Barbagallo & Resnick, 1994; Pennington, 2000). Minerals are important cofactors for the production of neurotransmitters and help minimize the effect of toxic burden (see more about minerals in Chapter 4).

High-glycemic foods also trigger release of excess insulin. Insulin drives inflammation. Brain inflammation contributes to mood problems. Higher insulin levels also will drop blood sugar below normal values, making someone hungry. Hunger and hypoglycemia (low blood sugar) are primitive signals known to set off the stress response in a person. In people who are predisposed, anxiety and depression can be common segues to this stress response.

### Unhealthy fats

Which foods are most damaging to mood? In contrast to the benefit of healthy fats, hydrogenated oils, highly heated vegetable oil, fried foods, and non-grass-fed animal-based saturated fats are best avoided. While the healthy fats keep nervous system membranes fluid and calm inflammatory pathways in the body, unhealthy fats will replace the good fats in cell membranes and make them rigid, not allowing toxins to clear or nutrients to get in. Immune system cell membranes that lack fluidity also contribute to inflammation.

*Foods additives*

Food additives such as artificial colors, glutamate, and artificial sweeteners have all been linked to mood problems. While there are strict FDA guidelines for food additives, the safety of these not been rigorously proven, with most studies being conducted by the companies that produce them.

**Artificial colors.** Color additives have been linked to conduct and mood disorders (Schab & Trinh, 2004) and attention issues in children. A study by Kamel and El-lethey (2011) in animals showed that those taking in both low and high doses of tartrazine (as FD&C Yellow no. 5) exhibited increased hyperactivity, with significant promotion of anxiety responses. Depression responses were also greatly heightened compared with animals not exposed to tartrazine. The authors concluded that the study "points to the hazardous impact of tartrazine on public health." Human studies have also linked anxiety to these chemicals (Rowe & Rowe, 1994). Tartrazine is used in colored foods, candies, and even medications used for mood.

**Glutamate.** Glutamate is an excitatory neurotransmitter our brain produces in small physiologic amounts as a by-product of everyday cell metabolism. Monosodium glutamate (MSG) is the salt form of glutamate. While this compound does occur naturally in some foods (including hydrolyzed vegetable protein, yeasts, soy extracts, protein isolates, cheese, and tomatoes), the additive MSG is used in high amounts primarily to enhance taste. While the FDA considers the additive MSG as to be "generally recognized as safe" (GRAS), it can be toxic to the brain and mood. In fact, excess glutamate is more cytotoxic to neurons than is cyanide (Mark et al., 2001), and studies show that levels of glutamate in patients with depression are significantly higher than in healthy people (Kim et al., 1982). Many people react to Chinese food, which often has a large amount of added MSG—these people probably have a larger stores of glutamate already and/or are not able to detoxify it. While the brain uses a very sophisticated system to remove glutamate, inflammation and heavy metal burden can decrease its ability to remove it. People with anxiety and depression should avoid taking it in altogether.

***Artificial sweeteners.*** Artificial sweeteners (e.g., saccharin, aspartame, sucralose, acesulfame potassium) are also known to possess toxic effects on the nervous system and may directly assault the neurotransmitters of mood. A study by Yokogoshi et al. (1984) revealed that aspartame may contribute to abnormal balance in the neurotransmitter serotonin. Anxiety relief has been reported in numerous cases by removing ingestion of aspartame, with recurrence upon reexposure (Roberts, 1988). One large study (Butchko et al., 2002) did find aspartame as "safe" with "no unresolved questions regarding its safety"; it should be noted this study was funded by the NutraSweet Company.

## Coffee and Green Tea

As the most-used psychoactive drug of all time, coffee is an interesting case. Studies show some wonderful positive health effects for coffee. It can decrease a prediabetic's risk for developing diabetes, lower incidence of bile tract and liver cancer, and even help prevent heart attacks after a meal. In fact, a review of larger epidemiologic studies (Bhatti et al., 2013) shows regular coffee consumption to reduce mortality, both for all-cause and for cardiovascular deaths. Coffee is associated with lower risk of dementia and Alzheimer's Disease, with the lowest risk (a 65% decrease) was found in people who drank 3 to 5 cups per day from midlife onward (Eskelinen et al., 2009). In addition, coffee intake is associated with lower rates of heart failure, stroke, diabetes mellitus, and some cancers.

As far as mood is concerned, coffee can be both beneficial and harmful. So what about your client? As with many questions in holistic medicine, the answer here is, "It depends on the individual."

The positive mood effects of coffee lie in caffeine's ability to increase a sense of euphoria, as well as increase sense of energy—likely by helping the brain produce dopamine in the brain's prefrontal cortex, an area important for mood regulation. In a 10-year cohort study of more than 50,000 older women, investigators found that, compared with those who drank 1 cup or less of caffeinated coffee per week, those who drank two to three cups per day had a 15 percent decreased risk for depression, and those who drank four cups or more had a 20 percent decreased risk (Lucas et al., 2011). For people predisposed to depression, daily intake may make good sense.

However, there is a threshold for coffee's benefit. Tanskanen et al. (2000) found that, although the risk for suicide decreased progressively for those consuming up to seven cups of coffee per day, the risk started increasing when consumption exceeded eight cups a day. Also noteworthy is that decaffeinated coffee, caffeinated tea, and chocolate did not have positive effects.

Whether coffee is best for your client really depends on his or her particular situation. Long-term coffee use can contribute to "burnout" in people who are already depleted and deficient. Also, caffeine at high doses can encourage loss of minerals, such as magnesium, which is an important cofactor in brain neurotransmitters. Coffee may also contribute to fluctuations in blood sugar, which can raise anxiety levels. Caffeine-sensitive individuals may see more insomnia. As discussed above, poor sleep will promote both anxiety and depression in predisposed individuals.

Coffee and green tea research out of Japan was also very positive for depression support. In a study of 537 people by Pham (2014), among the green tea drinkers, those drinking two to three cups a day were 41 percent less depressed than those who drank one cup or less. Among coffee drinkers, those who drank more than one cup per day had a 26 percent lower chance of becoming depressed, and those drinking more than two cups had a 40 percent decreased risk. In both groups, higher caffeine correlated with lower depression risk.

Originally used by the Chinese over 4,700 years ago, green tea's first well-known use was by monks, who used it to attain a state of "relaxed wakefulness" while meditating. While the caffeine content is likely responsible for this effect, two other components may account for the relaxation effect. Studies in animals suggest that the green tea polyphenol epigallocatechin gallate can induce anxiolytic (anxiety relieving) activity via interaction with brain GABA receptors (Vignes et al., 2006)—receptors that are exploited with anxiety-relieving drugs like alprazolam (Xanax). Green tea also has theanine, a naturally occurring amino acid that has anxiety-improving and blood-pressure-lowering effects, even in people who had high blood pressure increases in response to stress (Yoto et al., 2012b).

It seems that coffee is beneficial for those susceptible to low mood, low motivation, and depression, but it can often be disruptive for people with anxiety and should probably be avoided in anyone who is osteoporotic or has a tendency for insomnia. Green tea can be helpful for both anxiety and depression, but I would caution its use in people with anxiety who are especially caffeine sensitive.

### Healthful Foods to Increase:
Mediterranean diet
Fish
Raw nuts and seeds
Probiotic foods
Crunchy vegetables

### Foods to Avoid:
High glycemic foods (sugary foods and simple carbohydrates).
Unhealthy saturated fats
Foods additives: MSG, dyes, FDA colors, artificial sweeteners

**Coffee:** best for depressive mood, avoid with anxiety and insomnia

**Green tea:** OK for depression and in anxiety patients who are not caffeine sensitive

## EXERCISE

Known since the times of Hippocrates as a mood balancer, exercise protects the brain areas needed for stable mood. Experts believe it may be the most effective treatment for both anxiety and depression. Exercise has been shown to reduce anxiety and depression and to slash negative mood, while simultaneously improving self-esteem and even memory (Callaghan, 2004; Coventry et al., 2013).

## How Does Exercise Help Anxiety and Depression?

There seem to be a few physiologic effects at play regarding the mood benefits of regular exercise. Among them, exercise increases the production of brain-derived neurotrophic factor (BDNF), an important central nervous system molecule. BDNF plays a strong role in building nerve cells (called neurogenesis), as well as helping the nervous system repair damage and communicate. These roles are critical for mood (Cotman & Berchtold, 2002). Exercise has also been shown to maintain the brain's hippocampus, an area vital to mood, spatial relationships, and memory. A study of 120 older adults with dementia by Erickson et al. (2011) showed the after 1 year, subjects who performed moderate-intensity aerobic exercise 3 days a week increased hippocampal volume by 2 percent—and effectively reversed any age-related loss in brain volume. Expected brain loss was seen in the group who did not exercise aerobically, but instead did only stretching and toning work.

## Evidence for Exercise in Anxiety and Depression

Exercise has been studied head to head against leading antidepressant and antianxiety medications and has shown to be quite effective. One randomized controlled trial of 156 adults compared exercise with the antidepressant sertraline (Zoloft). Exercise took a little longer to help but worked just as well as the drug in the long run and had significantly lower relapse rates (8 percent vs. 31 percent) than subjects in the medication group (Babyak, 2000). A second randomized controlled trial looked at patients at least 50 years of age with depression. These volunteers were recommended either exercise or antidepressant medications. Again, there was quicker improvement in the drug group, but after 16 weeks, exercise provided equal benefits (Blumenthal et al., 1999).

Exercise seems to have clear benefits for anxiety states as well. Because of the flood of the stress hormone cortisol (discussed further in relation to the hypothalamic-pituitary-adrenal axis in Chapter 3), the brain's hippocampus shrinks in people who are chronically anxious (Sapolsky, 2001). Animal studies have shown us how exercise can actually reverse this shrinkage (van Praag, Kempermann, & Gage, 1999). As discussed above, human studies also show the same benefit. Exercise helps create new brain cells but can also help calm them when they are overexcited. Mouse studies by Schoenfield et al. (2013) suggest that regular exercise not only grows new neurons but also creates more cells that release gamma-aminobutyric acid (GABA), a brain-calming neurotransmitter. GABA is discussed in the supplement section of Chapter 4.

As a side note, the benefits of exercise do not seem to hold if an animal is sleep deprived (Zielinski et al., 2013) so it may be important to create a strong sleep schedule first and not dip into needed sleep time in order to exercise.

## How to Get Started with Exercise

For clients that are new to exercise, I generally recommend they start slow in order to avoid injury and increase enjoyment. An excellent way to get moving would include being outside in nature if possible, in green areas among the trees, and in the sunlight. Jogging, walking, and tai chi are all wonderful. If your client has joint or weight-bearing limitations, swimming or an elliptical trainer might be gentler. A few of my patients who can't walk or move their legs use a tabletop arm pedal exerciser.

For anyone who would like to replicate the hippocampus-building study by Santarelli et al. (2003), it is described below.

### Hippocampal Growth Exercise
### (four out of seven days each week):
1. Low-intensity warm-up on a treadmill or stationary bicycle for 5 minutes
2. Stretching for 5 minutes
3. Aerobic training for 40 minutes: choose among stationary

bike, treadmill running, Stairmaster climbing, or training with an elliptical

4. Cool down and stretching for 10 minutes

## SUNLIGHT

Hippocrates, the father of medicine, also recognized that people with mood challenges needed plenty of sunlight. Three ways healthful exposure to sunlight can help mood is by keeping healthful levels of serotonin, balancing circadian rhythm, and building up vitamin D stores. John Denver sang "Sunlight on my shoulders makes me happy." While I am not sure he ran a clinical trial on this, he did seem to have a clear understanding of sunlight's benefit on mood.

### The Yin and Yang of Light

When the eye is exposed to sunlight, the brain's center area called the hypothalamus is activated. The hypothalamus houses our body clock

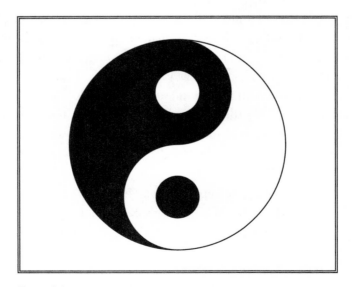

Figure 2.1.

and is also the nexus for our nervous system, immune system, and endocrine system. Balanced exposures to light and darkness are key to creating circadian rhythms consistent with a healthy body and good mood. Traditional Chinese medicine (TCM) is based on the notion of balancing our "yin and yang." Yin represents darkness and nighttime, while yang represents light and daytime. In TCM, one cannot have health unless you have balance between yin and yang. The discussion above on sleep mentioned the essential role darkness plays for our circadian health. This section discusses the benefits of light.

## The Connection between Serotonin and Light

Serotonin levels are known to increase with brighter light, and not surprisingly, research sampling the jugular vein blood of 101 men suggests that serotonin levels are at their lowest in the winter. Even more, the rate of serotonin production depended on how long a person was exposed to light, as well as the light intensity (Lambert et al., 2002). Other studies have also shown how serotonin transporters, which will bind up and inactivate serotonin, are more plentiful in the brain during dark periods (Praschak-Rieder et al., 2008). Darkness sends a signal to our bodies to stay "low."

## Sunlight and Circadian Rhythm

Our modern world is full of ways to block the sun. During the day we work indoors, we wear clothes, and we travel in vehicles that block the sun. Air pollution has particles that block healthful sun exposure. Even more, modern medicine has all but scared us into blocking the last bit of sunlight we might accidentally receive by telling us to use sunblock. It is possible that increased rates of anxiety and depression may correlate with the lack of outdoor activity and sun exposure of modern society.

Limited access to sunlight, especially in the morning hours, does little to support our circadian rhythm. Healthful normal circadian rhythms reveal high morning cortisol (an adrenal stress hormone), which generally decreases as the day goes on. Lowest levels are in the evening, when melatonin is secreted into our system to help us sleep (see figure 2.2a). Patients with depression and anxiety are known to have strong dysregulation of this system and often will have low levels of cortisol in the morning and higher levels at night (see figure 2.2b). Unusual cortisol patterning points to a dysregulation of the hypothalamic-pituitary-adrenal (HPA) axis, which plays a central role in the pathophysiology of anxiety and depressive disorders. This is discussed further in chapter 3.

Mood disorder has been clearly associated with delayed releases of melatonin much later than normal, which can happen when cortisol is too high at night and/or we go to bed too late. Conversely, people who are "morning types" often experience earlier evening sleep onset and earlier waking. And, those who wake earlier are more likely to get out and have morning bright light exposure, decreased morning melatonin secretion duration, more healthful circadian rhythms, and better mood.

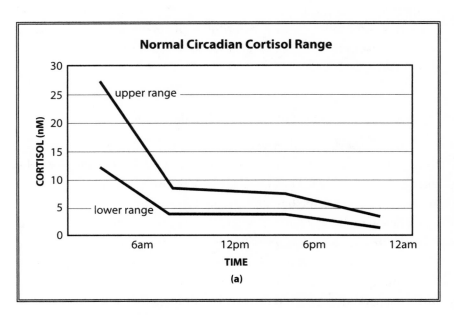

Figure 2.2a. Normal circadian rhythm.

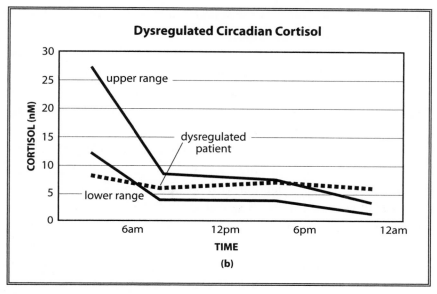

Figure 2.2b. Dysregulated circadian rhythm.

## Sunlight and Vitamin D

Low vitamin D levels have strong associations with increases in risk of death from cancer, heart disease and respiratory disease (Schöttker et al., 2013). While the goal is to reduce skin cancer deaths, fear of the sun may actually be causing more deaths from all other disease, as well as contributing to mood problems.

The components of sunlight are visible light, ultraviolet radiation, and infrared radiation. The two ultraviolet wavelengths are ultraviolet A (UVA; 320–400 nm) and ultraviolet B (UVB; 290–320 nm). Besides sunlight's ability to suppress of daytime melatonin, which creates a healthful circadian rhythm of this hormone (as discussed above), another likely mechanism toward healthful mood is sunlight's production of vitamin D through exposure to UVB rays. Ultraviolet light helps the skin transform a chemical called cutaneous 7-dehydrocholesterol into vitamin D3.

Feldman et al. (2004) investigated the relation of exposure of skin to ultraviolet light and mood. Over a period of 6 weeks, frequent tanners used two different tanning beds that were identical except that one had ultraviolet light filtered out. Even though they could not tell which one had the ultraviolet light, participants reported they were more relaxed and less anxious after exposure to the bed with ultraviolet light. When allowed to freely choose which bed to use, 11 of 12 participants chose the one with ultraviolet light.

A study of 198 multiple sclerosis patients over 2.3 year period found that sunlight exposure, and not vitamin D levels, was best correlated with mood and fatigue symptoms (Knippenberg et al., 2014), suggesting that overall time in the sun is probably more important than taking a supplement to get levels up. (Chapter 4 discusses vitamin D supplementation.)

While the ability of UVB to make vitamin D may be important, sunlight's infrared wavelengths may play a separate and distinct role in mood. Animal research shows that the amount of time before an animal will "give up" and become depressed after continuous stress is increased significantly after 4 weeks of exposure to infrared irradiation, suggesting that application of infrared irradiation has antidepressant effect (Tsai, Hsiao, & Wang, 2007). In my office, I often combine acupuncture treatments with the use of an infrared device called a Teding Diancibo Pu (TDP) lamp, heating body parts such as the abdomen or lower back with far-infrared heat. Patients tell me that this TDP application helps them feel very "calm," "secure," and "nourished," as well as warmer, during their acupuncture session.

## SPENDING TIME IN NATURE

The premise of naturopathic medicine includes the principle that "nature heals." In Chinese medicine, healing occurs by rebalancing your body's energy with the energy around you. One way we can help encourage our clients' healing and balance for both physical and mental health is by recommending time in nature.

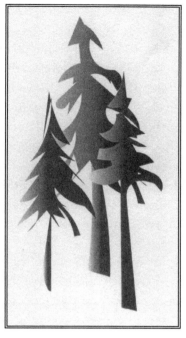

Figure 2.3.

One fascinating medical outcome study by Ulrich, Lundén, and Eltinge (1993) compared the recovery from gall bladder surgery among patients who had a bedside window view of either trees or a brick building wall and those with no nature view. Those with the nature view had shorter hospital stays and suffered fewer minor postsurgical complications, such as persistent headache or nausea. Furthermore, patients with the view of trees were more frequently reported by hospital staff as "in good spirits." Those in the wall view group elicited far more negative evaluations, including "the patient is upset" and "patient needs much encouragement." Even more impressive, the patients with tree view needed far fewer doses of strong narcotic pain drugs.

In Japan, there is a practice called Shinrin-yoku (forest bathing), which is known for its health benefits, including mental health and support of the immune system. Forest bathing involves visiting a forest for relaxation and breathing in the air, which has molecules given off by the trees. A 2007 paper from Nippon Medical School looked at 12 healthy males 37–55 years of age who took a three-day and two-night trip through nature while researchers took blood and urine samples at various intervals. On the first day, subjects walked for two hours in the afternoon in a forest field. On the second day, they walked for two hours in the morning and afternoon, respectively, in two different forest fields. Blood was sampled on the second and third days. Natural killer cells and other intracellular anticancer proteins were significantly higher (about 50%) on the forest bathing days than before. Moreover, levels of natural killer cells stayed elevated for 30 days after the trip. In addition, the study found that levels of the stress hormone adrenaline, which the body releases in response to anxiety, had dropped after forest bathing trips (Li et al., 2007).

Factors from the plant kingdom that may provide beneficial physiologic effects include the aroma of plants, as well as such various factors as temperature, humidity, light intensity, wind, and oxygen concentrations. It is suggested that the natural aromatherapy found in the forest in the forms of antimicrobial organic compounds called phytoncides may signal the brain to help release immune-related compounds. Other corroborating studies in seniors have found that forest exposure helps lower cortisol, blood pressure, heart rate, and inflammation, while enhancing parasympathetic activity (Mao et al., 2012). Parasympathetic activity refers to the relaxation response of the autonomic nervous system and is sometimes called the "rest and digest" response.

## A Multimodal Mood Study

Brown et al. (2001) published what I think may be one of my favorite studies of all time. This study looked at 112 women with mild or moderate depression. The study asked the women to walk outside during daylight hours for 20 minutes 5 out of 7 days and to take a multiple vitamin (which included vitamin B1 50 mg, some vitamin B2 and vitamin B6, folic acid 400 µg, vitamin D 400 IU, and 200 µg selenium). A control group did not do any walking and received a placebo vitamin. Eighty-five percent of the walking group showed less depression, better all-around mood, and greater self-esteem and well-being. That result is better than any antidepressant medication result to date.

I think this study is special because it heralds the course of future medical studies: a paradigm of multiple interventions designed to support whole-body healing using nature and vitamins. It employed a few gentle, natural treatments together in synergy. In contrast, most conventional research looks only at the (usually suppressive) effects of one chemical drug in the body. In my opinion, this multimodal study moves closer toward the naturopathic tenet of supporting the body's own healing process instead of covering a symptom with a drug. This tenet is at the heart of the best that holistic medicine can offer patients with anxiety and depression.

### Two Ways to Get into the Light: Nature Cure and a Light Box

Probably the simplest nature cure therapy is to get out into nature. Encouraging clients to take an early morning walk outside or sitting or moving in the park is a great start. When the weather is amenable, it is healthful to try to get at least 50 percent of the body exposed to the sun for 10–20 minutes a day. One journal reports that 12 min of exposure of 50 percent of body skin to noontime sun on a clear day is equivalent to oral intake of 3,000 IU vitamin D3 (Garland et al., 2007). For most people, this will not cause damage but will start the vitamin D process. It is a good rule to get out of the sun if one starts to see the skin turning pink or red. Any fair-skinned people or those with personal or family history of skin cancer may need to check with their doctor first and consider vitamin D supplementation or a phototherapy light box.

A second step, if needed, would be phototherapy, or light box therapy. While this is most often used in depressive illness and seasonal affective disorder, many of my patients with anxiety and insomnia patients who have imbalanced cortisol patterns (where cortisol is up at night, and low during the day) tend to see benefit as well. Typical light box therapy uses a 10,000-lux full-spectrum white light for at least 30 minutes every morning. Smaller-power light boxes do not seem to provide the same benefit.

### Bringing the Outside In: Pictures of Plants and Houseplants

The benefits of the outdoor environment discussed above are created by the presence of plant life. Studies are also showing the benefit of bringing plants indoors to create a calming and healing indoor environment. Studies at Texas A&M in the 1980s looked at 160 heart recovery patients who were shown pictures of nature (e.g., trees and water or forests), an abstract picture, or a blank white field. The patients who viewed the scene of trees and water were significantly less anxious postoperatively and were able to more quickly get off the strong narcotic pain drugs and use moderate strength analgesics. Interestingly, the more modern-style abstract picture dominated by rectilinear forms produced higher patient anxiety than control conditions with no picture at all (Ulrich, 1984).

Houseplants are shown to be quite calming as well. One unique study by Koga et al., in 2013 found that men who touched a houseplant (devil's ivy) for two minutes had a more serene sense and psychological calm. Stressed-activated areas of the brain had reduced blood flow and metabolism when the men interacted with the foliage. The authors suggested that most houseplants with soft and smooth leaves would have a similar effect. A study by Lohr, Pearson-Mims & Goodwin, 1996 showed that people who work in a windowless computer room with plants have clear drops in blood pressure over those in the same room without the plants. Finally, in a study by Park and Mattson (2009) of 90 hemorrhoidectomy patients, patients who were given house plants and flowers in the postoperative room enjoyed lower blood pressure, less pain, and less fatigue and anxiety than those in the nonplant rooms. These patients also had higher satisfaction levels, saying the plants "brightened up the room environment" and "reduced stress," and they believed the hospital staff appeared more caring.

## HYDROTHERAPY

Mankind used to spend much more time outdoors, exposing ourselves to variations of temperature in certain geographic regions, especially when submerged in water. Hydrotherapy (also known as water therapy) may be defined as the application of water for the maintenance of health or the treatment of disease (Barry & Lewis, 2006). Hydrotherapy has been employed since ancient times as a way to balance the body and mind. According to Hippocrates, water therapy "allays lassitude."

Therapeutic water therapy applies water at temperatures above or below the body temperature—and this can help change our physiology and mood. When humans take a cold swim, once over the initial shock of the cold, it is usually very invigorating. This is because wet and cold causes our surface vessels to vasoconstrict (tighten up), making blood move from the surface of your body to the core, as a means to conserve heat. It not only conserves heat but also reflexively bathes the brain and vital organs in fresh blood, as well as gently detoxifying the body. Throughout our millions of years of evolution, primates have endured physiologic stressors like temporary cold and heat temperature changes as a part of daily life. Hydrotherapy is designed to take advantage of the natural body reaction. It has been theorized that brief changes in body temperature like a cold swim or warm bathing could help brain function.

Medical research has supported the use of hot and cold baths as well. Decreases in cortisol levels have been reported with water bathing (Toda et al., 2006), likely because the affinity of the serotonin transporter increases (Marazziti et al., 2007). Warm footbaths have been shown to induce relaxation by decreasing both sympathetic nervous function and serum cortisol levels (Yamamoto et al., 2008).

While used extensively for hundreds of years as a part German water cure, relatively little clinical research has been done to study hydrotherapy for mood. One study suggests that patients with anxiety can benefit from the mechanisms of hydrotherapy. Balneotherapy (using water baths for healing) was compared with paroxetine (Paxil), a leading selective serotonin reuptake inhibitor, by Dubois et al. (2010). In a randomized 8-week multimember study, 117 of 237 patients with generalized anxiety disorder were assigned randomly to balneotherapy, and the remainder to paroxetine. The balneotherapy treatment consisted of weekly medical visits and daily bath treatments using natural mineral waters (containing sodium, calcium, magnesium, and sulfates) for 21 days. Every morning, patients were immersed in a bubbling bath (37°C for 10 min). Next, they took a shower with a firm massage-like pressure targeting the abdominal, paravertebral, and cervicobrachial regions (for 3 min), and then their legs as well as cervicoscapular and paravertebral areas were massaged under water (10 min). Sounds nicer than taking a drug for sure! The mean change in HAM-A scores showed an improvement in both groups, with a clearly superior result of the water therapy compared with the effect of the drug. Sustained response rates were also significantly higher in the hydrotherapy group (respectively, 19 percent vs. 7 percent, and 51 percent vs. 28 percent). The water therapy was found to be safe and without side effects as well.

One group of researchers suggest that hydrotherapy may be useful to treat cancer and chronic fatigue (Schevchuk & Radoja, 2007) and depression (Schevchuk, 2008). For the treatment of depression, it is suggested that cold exposure therapies may be the best choice. Because the density of cold receptors (the structures that sense cold) in the skin is thought to be 3–10 times higher than that of warm receptors (Iggo & Iggo, 1971), the simultaneous firing of all skin-based cold receptors caused by jumping into cold water may result in a positive therapeutic effect. Lowering the temperature of the brain is known to have neuroprotective and therapeutic effects and can relieve inflammation (Arrica & Bissonette, 2007), a known mechanism in depressive illness (see Chapter 4 for more on inflammation). In addition, exposure to cold has been shown to activate the sympathetic nervous system, increase blood levels and brain release of norepinephrine (Jedema et al., 2001), and help increase production of beta-endorphin, a "feel good" molecule that gives a sense of well-being (Vaswani, Richard, & Tejwani, 1988).

It has also been analogized that cold hydrotherapy may have a mechanism similar to that of electric shock therapy, another proven antidepressant treatment that has long been used to treat drug-resistant forms of depression. These effects may well help depressed patients, especially those who do well with increased release of norepinephrine, such as patients who respond well to duloxetine, or other serotonin-norepinephrine reuptake inhibitors that help increase the neurotransmitter norepinephrine.

I recommend patients with depression to use brief whole-body exposure to cold water in the form of a cold shower. Patients can start a shower at a comfortable warm temperature and slowly cool the water over a 5-minute period down to 68°F, at which point you can sustain for 2–3 minutes, using a thermometer to check the temperature. This can be performed once or twice a day and may be continued for weeks to several months (Shevchuk, 2008). Although mild cold stress seems to help the brain work better, animal research has shown that extreme cold stress may actually impair cognitive function (Mahoney et al., 2007)— suggesting too cold is not good.

## ELECTRONICS USE: TELEVISION, COMPUTER, AND CELL PHONE

While sunlight, trees, and water represent being outside, use of technology usually means being cooped up inside. For most of us, electronics are an important part of our everyday life. Whether it's the television, computer, tablet, or cell phone, we rely on these little sources of bright light to organize our schedule, give us information, and keep us connected with friends and loved ones. While these can be an indisputably helpful part of life, for those predisposed to mental health challenges these can also cultivate poorer mood.

## The Brain on TV

T. S. Eliot said, "The remarkable thing about television is that it permits several million people to laugh at the same joke and still feel lonely." Television's role in influencing the mental and physical state of our society has been profound. Most people seem to enjoy coming home at night and turning on the TV. Like any opiate, it is a way for many to "get away" from the stress of our day. And, in fact, in the short term TV seems to have a relaxing effect. Studies using functional MRI during TV viewing have determined that humorous television programming can activate the insular cortex and amygdala, which are brain areas activated and needed for balanced mood (Moran et al., 2004).

Unfortunately, longer-term use of TV seems to create problems; for instance, watching television over 2 hours per day and eating while watching television are each associated with obesity (Johnson et al., 2006). In our country, two-thirds are overweight or obese (Ogden et al., 2012), and obesity is a leading cause of a lower life expectancy, cardiovascular disease, cancer, and diabetes. Even more, it is setting us up for mood disorder early: each extra daily hour of television watching among children is associated with an 8 percent increase in developing depressive symptoms by young adulthood (Primack, et al., 2009). Television time is also taking us away from more healthful activities: although many people report "lack of time" as a major barrier to doing regular exercise, the average American adult spends over 4 hours each day watching television.

Analysis of over 30 years of U.S. national data shows that spending time watching television may contribute to viewers' happiness in the moment, but the longer-term effects are not good. In a study by Robinson and Martin (2008), participants reported that on a scale from 0 (dislike) to 10 (greatly enjoy), TV watching was nearly an 8. Despite these high marks, it seems that the enjoyment from TV was very short lasting, and eventually gave way to discontent. Unhappy people reported watching 25 hours of television a week, compared with 19 hours for happy people—a 30 percent difference (but still quite an alarming number). These results held even after taking into account education, income, age, and marital status. These data from nearly 30,000 adults led Robinson and Martin (2008) to conclude that

> TV doesn't really seem to satisfy people over the long haul the way that social involvement or reading a newspaper does. We looked at eight to ten activities that happy people engage in, and for each one, the people who did the activities more—visiting others, going to church, all those things—were more happy. TV was the one activity that showed a negative relationship. Unhappy people did it more, and happy people did it less. The data suggest to us that the TV habit may offer short-run pleasure at the expense of long-term malaise.

In short, happy people do not watch a lot of TV.

## Computer Blues and Benefits

Computer use has expanded greatly in the last few decades, allowing amazing rates of computation, animation, and socialization. Computers are unlike other interactions humans have in the sense that computers respond very quickly and create expectation regarding interaction with our environment that may have profound implications on the function of our HPA axis.

Mandal (2012) found that participants who used the computer in the form of computer games for more than 33 hours a week have 15 percent more anxiety and 20 percent more depression, based on responses to the Depression Anxiety Stress Scale questionnaire, compared with those who spent 21 hours a week. Both groups also exhibited stress, anxiety, and depression way above normal levels overall. Mandal postulated that the gamers developed inappropriate coping skills that rely on distraction to deal with challenges. A study by Becker, Alzahabi, and Hopwood (2013) also suggests that using multiple forms of media simultaneously, such as playing a computer game or using a cell phone while watching TV, is correlated with higher levels of anxiety and depression.

Computers and media can also aid those with anxiety and depression. A few high-quality studies have suggested that online cognitive behavioral therapy (CBT) may hold great promise (Boschert, 2011). In a meta-analysis of 1,746 patients with depression, social phobia, panic disorders, and anxiety, those who used online CBT showed about a 50 percent improvement (Andrews et al., 2010), which is pretty good result for a single medical therapy. I was most struck by a comment by Dr. Gavin Andrews, a psychiatry professor from Australia who headed the study: "There was no hint of relapse reported in any study, which is just foreign to my experience. Depression is supposed to be a relapsing and recurring disorder. What on earth is it doing just disappearing after someone does CBT over the Web? This is not what any of us were trained for (Andrews et al., 2010)."

A study by D'Mello (2011) recounted the experience of 26 patients hospitalized for severe depression from an adult in-patient psychiatry unit. These subjects' mood states improved significantly after using one 60-minute computer-assisted CBT session. It is pretty astounding that only one session could have any effect at all, for severely depressed patients from an in-patient ward are the toughest to treat.

## Social Media and Cell Phones

A study by Starr & Davila (2009) of teenage girls looked at the amount of combined time 83 girls spent texting, using social media, and talking on the cell phone to discuss the problems in their lives. Those girls who spent more time discussing their problems this way were more likely to have anxiety and depression. A study by Merlo & Stone (2007) of 183 people revealed that those with more anxiety had clearly more cell phone dependence and overuse. Using the Cellular Technologies Addiction Scale and the State-Trait Anxiety Inventory, most subjects did not self-report dependence symptoms (e.g., compulsion for phone use and emotional attachment to the phone) or abuse (personal problems from cell phone overuse). However, anxiety did correlate with use and dependence results. For people predisposed to anxiety traits, the phone might encourage these. For example, someone with social phobia might avoid real-life contact by using the phone, and obsessive-compulsive traits may manifest by someone using his or her phone to check things repeatedly.

# THREE

# Assessing Contributing Internal Factors

Chapter 2 discussed lifestyle and environmental factors that are key players in mood. This Chapter discusses what goes on inside the body. Anxiety and depression can be a symptom of the imbalances in our physiology. This Chapter will help bring awareness to the basics of the physiology that greatly influence mood and explain what is going on "under the hood," so to speak, and how to assess contributing factors from a person's physiology.

### Case Study: Sandra

*Referred by a psychotherapist colleague, Sandra was a 55-year-old suffering from bouts of depression and anxiety for the past two years. Two psychiatrists told her she had "menopausal depression" and shuffled her through a few different medications, of which the latest was Zoloft when she came to see me. Her psychotherapist knew her children's health issues were a strong part of her mood but referred her to me for a holistic assessment. While the Zoloft seemed to help the anxiety, the depression was no better. After taking her history, I learned her digestive system had been problematic for the last 10 years, with hallmark symptoms of irritable bowel syndrome, including bouts of mostly constipation and occasional diarrhea. Her blood work revealed a low normal thyroid function, which was followed up to reveal mildly positive thyroid antibodies, meaning her immune system was slowly beating up her thyroid gland. These levels were not enough to alarm her conventional doctor but suggested to me that it was a factor in her digestive and mood issues. She was positive for C-*

*reactive protein, suggesting there was a lot of inflammation in her body. Her hormonal panels were relatively normal for a woman her age.*

*Understanding her symptoms and seeing these blood tests were very helpful to create a plan that worked. We decided she should avoid all gluten and dairy products and consume an anti-inflammation diet comprising healthy lean proteins, fish, vegetables, and healthy oils. She also consumed some healthy fibers, such as flax meal. I also put her on some St. John's wort and fish oil to support both her digestion and mood, as a well as a selenium supplement to support thyroid. Within 8 weeks, Sandra's depression all but disappeared, and her anxiety was reduced greatly (some anxiety is occasionally spurred by stressors with her children). By four months, she weaned off the St. John's wort and hasn't needed it since. In Sandra's case, it was not menopause or even hormonal issues causing her mood issues; instead, it centered on digestion and inflammation affecting her thyroid and brain neurotransmitters. Working on her digestion, thyroid, and inflammation ultimately helped her rebalance.*

## BLOOD AND SALIVA TESTING

While no one or two lab tests are diagnostic of anxiety or depression, from a holistic perspective there are many tests that can help a holistic clinician care for a patient's best mood by explaining some aspects of physiology that may be contributing to the underlying causes of the mood issues. It is true that a single test never cured anything by itself, but using lab testing wisely can help the holistic practitioner understand, in part, how to create and individualize a holistic treatment plan.

### Fasting Blood Sugar and Hemoglobin A1C

Blood sugar levels play a major role in mood regulation. Poor control with too many lows or highs will contribute to both anxiety and depression. Research with diabetic patients suggests that good blood sugar control supports healthy mood and good judgment (Cox et al., 2001). While many people can have transient mood problems if they haven't eaten, some people with a regular tendency toward low blood sugar known as hypoglycemia are known to be at greater risk for depression. A study by Dowdy et al. (2008) evaluated lung injury patients in an intensive care unit and noticed that subjects who had low blood sugar (<60 ng; normal is 80–100 ng) were at a 360 percent increase risk of depression 3 months later. Case studies dating back to the 1930s have shown the relationship between low blood sugar and anxiety.

The hormone insulin is responsible for helping move sugar from the blood into the body's cells. High levels of insulin can be a sign of insulin resistance, a situation where the body no longer responds to insulin. An association between anxiety and insulin resistance has been established, and insulin resistance is a known factor in future cardiovascular disease as well (Narita et al., 2008). If blood sugar is imbalanced, and your client would like to check further into the role insulin may play, then he or she may want to have their physician run a fasting serum insulin or a glucose tolerance test.

While low blood sugar can cause mood issues, it is also true that regular hyperglycemia (high blood sugar) can also contribute to anxiety and depression. Studies of diabetic patients are clear that high blood sugar episodes will deteriorate mood, cause cognitive difficultly, and most notably, increase sadness and anxiety (Sommerfield, Deary, & Frier, 2004). People with hyperglycemia or high insulin levels are also predisposed to depression. A study in adults in their late twenties and early thirties showed that when blood sugar or insulin was too high, the chances of getting depressed was 50–100 percent greater (Pearson et al., 2010).

Besides laboratory blood tests, it can be of value for the clients themselves to use a home glucose meter (purchased at any pharmacy) to check blood sugar throughout the day for two nonconsecutive days. This will help describe daily levels in real life. Daily blood sugars can be measured at the following times:

First thing in the morning upon waking
Right before breakfast

One and a half hours after breakfast
Right before lunch
One and a half hours after lunch
Right before dinner
One and a half hours after dinner
Before bedtime

Fasting blood sugar is considered ideal between 75–96 ng/mL. Values below 60 are considered too low. Values between 109 and 120 are considered prediabetic, and numbers above 120 are considered diabetic. Hemoglobin A1C indicates the level of damage sugars are making in the body. When blood sugar, in the form of glucose, comes in contact with body tissue proteins in the presence of normal body heat, these tissues actually crust, the way bread gets crusty when toasted. HgbA1C is a 3-month-long indicator of blood sugar levels and gives a better idea of whether levels have been too high over time. A level of <5.7 percent is generally regarded as normal; 5.7–6.4 percent is considered prediabetic, and >6.4 percent is considered diabetic.

## How to Balance Blood Sugar

For both low and high blood sugar, it is important to eat small, frequent meals, at least every 2–3 hours. It is best to pick foods and snacks that have good protein sources with a little healthy carbohydrate (e.g., almond butter on an apple slice), as opposed to simple carbohydrate foods (e.g., a cookie), because simple carbohydrates and sugar will spike blood sugar, which spikes insulin. Insulin then drops blood sugar even lower than when it started, creating a negative cycle.

**Ideas for good blood sugar control:**
1. Eat a healthy protein source in the morning (e.g., boiled or poached eggs, fish, or a protein shake with berries). People who eat breakfast are known to be happier and less stressed (Benton & Brock, 2010).
2. Eat small meals/snacks every 2–3 hours.

3. Every meal should include protein sources (e.g., fish, grass-fed meats, eggs) and some healthy fat (e.g., avocado, nut oils, fish oil, olive oil). Some examples include apple or celery with almond butter, raw nut and seed mix with dark chocolate chips and some organic raisins, or carrots and hummus.
4. Reduce or eliminate simple carbohydrates (e.g., cakes, cookies, and breads).
5. Proper sleep, exercise, and stress management are also important for best blood sugar control.
6. Supplemental chromium (200–600 µg/day) and 1 tsp of cinnamon a day can also help balance blood sugar (see Chapter 4).

## Blood Chemistry Panel

A blood chemistry panel takes a snapshot of events with the liver and kidneys and reports blood levels of calcium, protein, and electrolytes. Abnormalities with any of these related organ systems can contribute to mood changes and should be followed up with a physician.

### Cholesterol (lipid panel)

While most conventional physicians are concerned when cholesterol levels are too high, there may be value in checking into these to make sure they are not too low, for low cholesterol is associated with both anxiety states and depression (Suarez, 1999).

Cholesterol is important for the function of the receptors in the brain that recognize serotonin. Cholesterol is also the precursor (building block) to all steroid hormones, including glucocorticoids (for blood sugar regulation), mineralocorticoids (which maintain mineral balance and blood pressure regulation), and sex hormones (Harvey & Chompe 2005, pp. 235–238). Cholesterol levels in the central nervous system can be abnormally low in many people with mood disorders.

**Statin drug–mood connection.** In the United States, over 250 million prescriptions were written for cholesterol-lowering drugs known as statins in 2011 (Ledford, 2013). Statin medications are one of the most prescribed drug class on the planet and have increased in use substantially since the medical community lowered the threshold for high cholesterol a few years back. Despite common use of these drugs, a meta-analysis of 11 randomized controlled trials suggests that statins do not reduce the risk of cardiovascular events in people without preexisting heart disease (Ray et al., 2010). Mounting medical research is suggesting that these drugs may be harming our mood, too.

Statins work by blocking a key enzyme involved in the body's production of cholesterol. Lab tests by Shrivastava et al. (2010) using human serotonin receptors revealed how statin medications disturb the structure and function of a cell's serotonin receptor, making it unable to react to serotonin. When cells treated with mevastatin were given cholesterol, they came back to normal and responded to serotonin. According to the investigators of this study, these results show how the effect of long-term cholesterol depletion in the brain can unbalance neurotransmitters, thus triggering depression or anxiety.

Other studies have also suggested that statin medications deplete mood-supportive polyunsaturated fatty acids in the brain as well (Hibbeln et al., 1997). Low levels of total cholesterol postpartum (after child birth) have been associated with anxiety and depression (Troisi et al., 2002). Low cholesterol levels are also suggested to correlate with higher likelihood of relapse in people who have already suffered from depression (Steffens, McQuoid, & Krishnan, 2003).

A review by While and Keen (2012) found conflicting information regarding whether statins adversely effect mood. My sense is these drugs may not negatively effect everyone's mood, but clients predisposed to mood disorder (likely almost all the people you work with) may be better off without these drugs unless they already have documented heart disease.

***HDL cholesterol can help elevate mood.*** Low levels of high-density lipoprotein (HDL—the "good cholesterol") are a known risk factor in cardiovascular disease. HDL carries bad cholesterol away from the artery walls and plays a role in toxin removal as well. HDL cholesterol levels are often low in major depression patients and even lower in people who think about suicide. Maes et al. (1997a), looking at HDL levels and mood, concluded that HDL cholesterol can be used as a marker for major depression and suicidal behavior. No correlations with low HDL and anxiety are known.

***How to treat low HDL.*** If HDL cholesterol levels are in the low range (usually <40 mg/dL for men and <50 mg/dL for women), holistic recommendations such as stopping smoking (Dwyer et al., 1998), exercise (Hata & Nakajima, 2000), and intake of fish oil (Peterson et al., 2002), as well as moderate alcohol consumption (one to two drinks a day; Ellison et al., 2004), are all known to help naturally increase HDL cholesterol levels. Foods that can help include oranges, dark chocolate, extra virgin olive oil, and hibiscus and black teas. The fiber supplement beta-glucan can also raise good cholesterol levels.

*Homocysteine*

Derived from sulfur and methionine, homocysteine in high levels is directly related to depression. It is a well-known marker of inflammation and an independent risk factor for cardiovascular disease (Sun et al., 2009), and it may be a more accurate marker of cardiovascular risk than cholesterol. In a large study of 3,752 men 70 or more years of age, an increase in plasma homocysteine was associated with a significantly increased risk of depression. Research shows that approximately 45–55 percent of patients with depression develop significantly elevated serum homocysteine. There is evidence suggesting that lower levels of homocysteine may decrease the incidence of depression in the elderly (Almeida, 2008). B vitamin treatment of celiac patients with high homocysteine lowered homocysteine, which correlated with significant improvement in well-being, most notably anxiety and depressed mood (Hallert et al., 2009).

Homocysteinemia may have anxiogenic effects, too (Hrnčić et al., 2013). High homocysteine in the blood causes a decrease in S-adenosylmethionine (SAMe), a compound made out of the amino acid

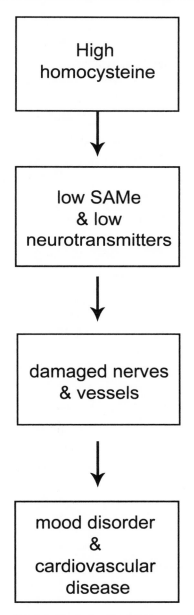

Figure 3.1. Implications of high homocysteine.

methionine that has been shown to specifically help depression. (SAMe is discussed in Chapter 4.) Having inadequate amounts of SAMe impairs your body's ability to make brain neurotransmitters. There is a strong correlation between high homocysteine and trauma of the endothelium (inner lining) of the blood vessels, leading to atherosclerosis and cardiovascular disease. High homocysteine will also activate N-methyl-D-aspartate (NMDA) receptors in the brain. This activation will lead to higher glutamate levels in the brain, negatively affects neuronal structure, and increases oxidative stress in the brain, encouraging mood disorders (Karakula et al., 2009). This may explain the link between cardiovascular disease and depressive disorders.

***How to address high homocysteine.*** While it is unclear whether using natural therapies such as B vitamins and folic acid is really useful to lower homocysteine and ultimately protect against cardiovascular illness (Wang et al., 2007; Ebbing et al., 2008), the study by Hallert et al. (2009) described above does suggest a clear benefit for anxiety and depression.

For anyone with high homocysteine I will typically recommend the following:

- *B-complex with folate:* B complex dosage should include about 40 mg vitamin B6, 1.2 mg B12 in the methylcobalamin form, and 2 g folate (in the form of L-methyltetrahydrofolate) daily.
- *Betaine (also called trimethylglycine):* 3,600 mg every day (Olthof & Verhoef, 2005).

### C-Reactive protein

Similar to homocysteine, C-reactive protein (CRP) levels increase when the immune system is in an inflamed state. Inflammation in the brain is a contributing factor to mood disorders and cardiovascular illness. High CRP levels have been shown to be related to generalized anxiety disorder (Copeland et al., 2012b) as well as depression in both men (Danner et al., 2003) and women (Cizza et al., 2009). Episodes of depression also are predictive of higher CRP levels (Copeland et al., 2012a).

***How to Address high CRP.*** Exercise in the form of interval training, an aerobic training using high intensity interspersed with lower intensity, has been shown to be effective in lowering CRP and blood pressure in patients with hypertension. Lamina and Okoye (2012) looked at 245 males with mild to moderate high blood pressure. Half of these men performed 8 weeks of interval training programs between 45 and 60 minutes, at intensities of 60–79 percent of heart rate reserve. The control group remained sedentary during this period and did not find the benefits in blood pressure or CRP that the active group enjoyed.

Reduce the intake of highly cooked food. Chemicals called advanced glycation end-products (appropriately called AGEs) from foods that are cooked at high temperatures will increase CRP levels (Uribarri et al., 2005). For instance, a study on potato chip eating revealed eating those delicious little chips for 4 weeks increased both the oxidation of LDL and CRP levels (Naruszewicz et al., 2009). Eating more raw foods, and minimally cooked foods (e.g., using boiling, poaching, and slow cooking) is best.

Because the majority of the immune system is in the digestive tract, eating plenty of fiber, especially in the form psyllium husk, will help douse the CRP fire by whisking it away with a bowel movement. Studies of using 28 g fiber a day, either as a psyllium supplement or in a high-fiber diet, showed clear CRP-lowering benefits in patients whose total fiber intake was only around 12 g a day (King et al., 2007). One teaspoon of psyllium husk as about 5 g fiber and can be mixed in 8 ounces of water, in the morning and evening, with the remaining 18 g satisfied by eating good-quality fruits, vegetables, and flax meal throughout the day.

CRP can also be lowered by taking fish oil and vitamin C. Patients with end-stage renal disease given 2 g of fish oil supplements showed significant lowering of CRP versus the control group (Bowden et al., 2009). I usually recommend 1 teaspoon of a high-quality, molecularly distilled fish muscle oil a day for balancing inflammation in the body.

In a randomized trial of 396 healthy nonsmokers, Block et al. (2008) found that, among participants with CRP indicative of elevated cardiovascular risk, 1,000 mg vitamin C reduced the median CRP by 25.3 percent versus placebo. Taking 500 mg vitamin C two or three times a day should be effective in lowering CRP.

### Complete blood count and iron panel

A complete blood count (CBC) records the numbers of red and white blood cells. An iron panel looks at the amount of iron available in the blood (serum iron) and how much is stored (ferritin). Red blood cells carry oxygen throughout the body to keep all tissues alive and energy up. Iron forms the center of the hemoglobin molecule and helps carry oxygen. The term "anemia" applies to anyone who has low red blood cell number or volume, low hemoglobin, or low serum iron or ferritin.

With anemia, fatigue and mood problems are quite common for not enough oxygen gets to the various parts of the body, which enhances the stress response. If a person is anemic and they are predisposed to anxiety or depression, these will more likely manifest (Bokemeyer & Foubert, 2004). The lassitude can be debilitating and has been shown to contribute to lost work, decreased physical and emotional well-being, and interference with clear thought.

Verdon et al. (2003) looked at a total of 134 very fatigued women, most of whom had low ferritin. Half of the group received iron supplementation every day for 4 weeks, and the other received a placebo. The level of fatigue after 1 month decreased 29 percent in the iron group versus only 13 percent in the placebo group. Although the iron group benefit was double that in the controls, not all the women improved, likely because other issues beyond iron were also at play—possibly digestive issues, sleep, blood sugar issues, and so forth. It may be a good to time to mention that the purpose of this book is to underscore how multiple factors can contribute to mood issues. Fatigue caused by low iron may just be one of many contributing factors. The study by Verdon et al. (2003) suggests that for 29 percent of the women in the treatment group, iron was likely the sole issue, but for the other 70 percent, other factors still needed addressing. Nevertheless, getting 30 percent improvement with the simple recommendation of iron was pretty good.

Any cases of anemia should be worked up by a physician—especially when it happens in men and nonmenstruating women, for blood loss elsewhere in the body or bone marrow issues may need to be addressed. If the cause is simply low intake or absorption of iron or B12 (which helps build red blood cells), then a supplement is appropriate. One study on anemic schoolchildren found that giving a multiple vitamin with iron increased hemoglobin and reduced anxiety (Zhang et al., 2013).

For iron-deficient anemia I usually recommend a patient start with the following:

1. *Check CRP levels,* for those with high CRP are at increase anemia risk—suggesting inflammation may be a causative factor (Eisele et al., 2013).
2. *Check nutrient intake* for adequate amounts of iron and B12. This may be especially challenging in the vegetarian and raw food population.
3. If intake is adequate, *consider working on digestive health* (see next section) for better absorption of nutrients.
4. *Take an iron supplement,* starting 25 mg/day with food and increasing to 25 mg three times a day with food. I usually use the gentler iron succinate or iron fumarate forms, which are easier on the stomach and tend to cause less constipation. Also, it is helpful to take about 500 mg vitamin C with the iron for best absorption. With some cases of anemia I recommend the herbs nettles and yellow dock for supporting and absorption effects. Food sources of iron include grass-fed beef, dark turkey meat, dark leafy greens, and using an iron skillet for cooking.
5. *Vitamin B12:* A patient can ask his or her doctor for B12 shots or can start with a methylcobalamin lozenge, using 1,000 µg once a day. Sublingual lozenges or shots tend to help increase B12 levels more effectively over capsules or tablets.

*Thyroid panel (TSH, T3, T4)*

Abnormal thyroid function is quite common in modern society. According to the American Academy of Clinical Endocrinologists (AACE), 1 in 10 Americans suffers from thyroid disease, and almost half of these remain undiagnosed (AACE, 2002). Environmental medicine experts suspect the heavy metal pollution and radioactive by-products from nuclear power plants may be increasing the incidence of many thyroid diseases, (Levnin et al., 2013) for heavy metals may mimic the effect of iodine in the body and block its function. Overactive thyroid symptoms include anxiety, sweating, fast heartbeat, weight loss, diarrhea, and greasy skin. Low thyroid symptoms may include low mood, weight gain, slowed thinking and memory problems, feeling cold, and constipation. Often, low thyroid can be an early or even first symptom of oncoming depression (Davis & Tremont, 2007).

In a normally functioning thyroid (euthyroid) state, thyroid-stimulating hormone (TSH) is produced in the brain's pituitary and tells the thyroid gland to make thyroid hormone. The thyroid makes mostly thyroxine (known as T4), which gets converted to a more active thyroid hormone called tri-iodothyronine (also called T3). The T4 and T3 float around in the blood stream, and the brain samples this to decide how much TSH is needed at that moment. This amazing thyroid feedback loop allows the brain to keep thyroid hormone in balance.

If TSH is greater than 2.5 µIU/mL, or less than 0.5 µIU/mL, I usually recommend patients run what is called a thyroid antibody panel and check thyroid stimulating immunoglobulin levels. These blood tests will help decide if the thyroid is malfunctioning because the immune system is attacking it. The AACE has been lowering the threshold of TSH because the group of people used to create normal ranges likely had many with undiagnosed thyroid disease. The AACE acknowledges that with subclinical hypothyroidism, treatment with thyroid hormone should keep TSH levels below the 3.0 µIU/mL threshold (Baskin et al., 2002).

***How to Work with Thyroid Issues.*** If any urgent issues, consider conventional care. Of course, it is prudent to visit an endocrinologist and consider thyroid hormone replacement, especially in cases of severe symptoms. Excess thyroid hormone can cause exophthalmos, a condi-

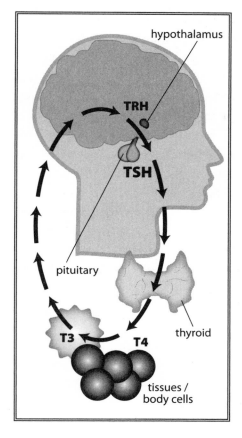

Figure 3.2. The thyroid feedback loop.

tion where the eyes can bulge from the sockets, and can also cause a racing heart and severe anxiety. This needs conventional treatment for safest results. For cases of low thyroid, pharmaceutical thyroid replacement such as thyroxine is a reasonable choice while working on the underlying conditions: the drug thyroxine, while synthetic, is actual "bioidentical" in the sense that it is the same exact molecule that the body produces, so when dosed appropriately, it does not tend to have negative side effects, promote cancers, or cause other problems that secondary metabolites from other synthetic hormones like hormone replacement estrogens and progestins can cause.

*If there are autoimmune thyroid issues, start anti-inflammatory work:*

From a holistic perspective, if there is an autoimmune thyroid condition, it is best to focus on digestive and anti-inflammatory work suggested later in this chapter to help calm the inflammation. I have seen a number of autoimmune thyroid cases resolve simply with the elimination of gluten from the diet alone. The literature suggests a correlation between gluten reactions and thyroid autoimmunity (Hakanen et al., 2001; Akçay & Akçay , 2003), although a recent study of 27 celiac patients with thyroid disease did not see antibodies resolve on a gluten-free diet after 1 year (Metso et al., 2012), suggesting that other foods/sensitivities may also play a role in a number of people. Selenium supplementation at 200 µg daily has been show to help reduce levels thyroid autoantibodies (Zhu et al., 2012).

*If there is hypothyroidism with no autoimmune issues, consider natural thyroid supports:* If there is no autoimmune condition and a patient's TSH is above 2.2 and T4 is low, while T3 is in the normal range, consider the following:

- Work on managing stress, for stress decreases function of the hypothalamic pituitary thyroid axis (Tsigos & Chrousos, 2002).
- Eat extra kelp and seaweed every day.
- Take 300 mg tyrosine per day.

Also consider natural thyroid hormone. Work with a naturopathic physician or other holistic physician to start on a low dose of natural thyroid replacement. Brands include Armour Thyroid or Nature-Throid, which are made from dried pig thyroid. Most standard endocrinologists do not prefer natural replacement, stating that it is not well standardized from batch to batch. This is based on old studies from the 1970s, before newer techniques were available to keep consistency. My experience suggests that patients have done quite well on it. Holistic practitioners generally prefer natural thyroid hormone for it contains thyroid gland, which includes not only active T4 but also T3 and other lesser known thyroid hormones that may have a role in supporting the thyroid system. If using natural thyroid replacement, the doctor should check pulse and symptoms before starting, and recheck once a week to see how the pateint feels, as well take blood tests every few weeks to recheck thyroid levels. If natural thyroid replacement is not helping the patient feel better, you can also try the synthetic thyroid replacement thyroxine (T4). Synthetic thyroid is actually bio-identical, for it is the same molecule our body makes, and is generally without side effects when used at the proper dose. With any thyroid replacement, the clinician should watch for excess signs of palpitations and heart racing, increased temperature, excessive sweating, and/or weight loss. Some patients fare better with natural thyroid, while others are more compatible with synthetic thyroid. As such, both should remain as options.

*If T3 is low, consider working with a prescription for Cytomel:* Cytomel is pure active T3. Usual starting dose is 5 µg in the morning, increasing by 5 µg every 3 days until symptoms improve. It is best not to take more than 60 µg total if the patient is over 55 years of age, or 125 µg if younger. Reasons to discontinue or lower dose include racing heart, excess sweating, shakiness, anxiety, or fast-paced thought patterns.

### Parathyroid (PTH)

The parathyroid glands are four little pea-sized organs placed directly in the midst of the thyroid gland. Primary hyperparathyroidism (an over-functioning parathyroid gland) will show a high PTH number on blood tests. This high PTH is frequently accompanied by high blood calcium and a reflexive vitamin D deficiency. High PTH can cause digestive issues and bone problems, as well as many mood symptoms, including anxiety, obsession-compulsion, interpersonal sensitivity, depression, hostility, and psychoticism. Low vitamin D can contribute to depression and poor mood. Depressive disorders and anxiety can normalize after treatment of hyperparathyroidism (Peterson, 1968; Watson & Marx, 2002; Solomon, Schaaf, & Smallridge, 1994), which may include surgical removal of one or two of the four glands. While PTH is not routinely checked, it is worth checking if vitamin D is consistently low, especially if supplementation doesn't bring it up in a timely manner.

*DHEA and DHEA sulfate*

Considered a "neurosteroid," dehydroepiandrosterone (DHEA) and DHEA sulfate are molecules produced by the adrenal gland and somewhat related to testosterone. Low levels have been related depression severity (Goodyer et al., 2000), anxiety, and even schizophrenia (Strouss et al., 2003).

DHEA may protect against the adverse effects of stress, especially the ravages of the stress hormone cortisol. Like exercise, DHEA can increase neuronal growth in the hippocampus and will protect new nervous tissue from getting destroyed by stress hormones (Karishma & Herbert, 2002). Levels naturally decrease with age, and with it, physical health and mood may be affected. Unfortunately, DHEA is known to decline with psychological challenge and stress (Wang et al., 2009).

Supplemental DHEA has been clinically assessed for safety and effectiveness. A study by Alhaj, Massey, and McAllister-Williams (2006) treated 24 healthy young men with a 7-day course of high-dose oral DHEA (150 mg twice a day) in a placebo-controlled double-blind, randomized, crossover study. Researchers found that memory was significantly improved after taking DHEA. DHEA was shown to encourage hippocampal activation and early differential activation and neuronal recruitment of the anterior cingulate cortex, and to decrease evening cortisol levels. Reduced function of the anterior cingulate cortex can contribute to behavioral disorders, including diminished self-awareness, depression, and aberrant social behavior (Devinsky, Morrell, & Vogt, 1995).

DHEA seems to be supportive to balance anxiety. A randomized, double-blind controlled study giving heroin addicts 100 mg for one year to help with withdrawal found statistically significant improvement in the severity of withdrawal symptoms and in depression and anxiety scores, while the control groups deteriorated in all measures, suggesting that DHEA might benefit this particular population (Maayan et al., 2008).

Studies of adolescent girls with adrenal insufficiency caused by brain malfunction found 25 mg DHEA helped improve anxiety scores (Binder et al., 2009), although another analysis in adrenal-deficient women found benefit for depression and quality of life but not for anxiety (Alkatib et al., 2009).

A number of studies report the benefit of DHEA supplementation for its antidepressant effects (Gallagher et al., 2008). Specifically, DHEA may be effective for midlife-onset minor and major depression. One placebo-controlled, randomized trial of a double-blind, crossover treatment study looked at 23 men and 23 women 45–65 years of age with midlife-onset major or minor depression. These patients were randomized to either 6 weeks of DHEA therapy, using 90 mg every day for 3 weeks and then a whopping 450 mg every day for 3 weeks, or 6 weeks of placebo followed by 6 weeks of the other treatment. The subjects did not receive any other antidepressant medications during the study. DHEA treatment for 6 weeks was associated with improvement in both primary outcome measures compared with both baseline and 6 weeks of placebo. After DHEA treatment, 23 subjects had a 50 percent or greater reduction in depression rating scores, as did 13 subjects after placebo treatments. The treatment with DHEA was well tolerated. The response to DHEA did not seem to differ between men and women. Larger doses did not seem to confer any additional benefit (Schmidt et al., 2005).

***How to work with low DHEA.*** Work on stress—stress lowers hypothalamic-pituitary-adrenal (HPA) axis function and will imbalance DHEA status. Although supplementation is discussed next, in most cases stress is the culprit, and dealing with this will help in the long term. Of course, working with psychotherapy is a must. Also consider yoga, meditation, and other relaxation work.

For supplementation, DHEA is available as over-the-counter hormonal therapy. When needed, taking DHEA appears to reduce stress hormone concentrations and can improve mood. Though many studies have used 50–450 mg given every day in divided doses, in my opinion it is best to first check blood levels. If low, or low-normal, start with 5–10 mg every day for women and 10–25 mg for men. When beginning supplementation please check blood levels every 2–3 weeks. If mood does not improve, and/or the level of hormone does not increase, then you increase in increments of 5–10 mg while continuing to monitor with blood tests. The only known food source for DHEA is from the wild yam, but these levels are too low for any clinical effect (Araghiniknam et al., 1996).

**Cautions with DHEA.** DHEA levels should always be checked before starting supplementation. Taking too much may cause problems by increasing levels of other hormones like testosterone and estrogen. I am especially concerned with the effect of too much DHEA in women, due to the theoretical potential to exacerbate or initiate hormone-responsive tumors. While I do not find women complaining of side effects often, the most commonly reported side effects in the literature include male hormone-like skin effects such as greasy skin and hair, acne, scalp itching, hair loss, and facial and body hair (especially along the midline of the lower abdomen) (Wiebke, 2006). Men with prostate cancer or benign prostatic hyperplasia (BPH) should check with their doctor before starting DHEA.

*Serum testosterone: Free and total testosterone*

Testosterone is the hormone most associated with being male. However, both men and women need it to keep up a good mood. Low testosterone levels may cause flattened mood, anxiousness, low sex drive, loss of motivation, fatigue, and general loss of well-being in both women (Davis 2002) and men (Carnahan & Perry, 2004). Testosterone administration in 15 females resulted in reports of reductions in unconscious fears in a placebo-controlled, double-blind crossover trial (van Honk, Peper, & Schutter (2005)).

Low testosterone is often underdiagnosed due to the nonspecific symptoms that may appear identical to clinical depression or anxiety states and should be tested in anyone with these symptoms. Testosterone replacement has also been shown to help cases of drug-resistant depression helping antidepressant medication work (see Chapter 6).

I have observed that males with low testosterone often (but not always) have a bit of belly fat around their middle that is "hard to lose," along with low mood, or irritable mood (the "curmudgeonly" type of fellow). Please consider having your client check testosterone, and if it is low, have him talk to his doctor about taking a small amount and monitor mood, while checking for levels monthly. The occasional female may also fit this picture, although not as often.

***What to do if testosterone is low.*** For testosterone replacement, oral, short- and long-acting parenteral, and transdermal patch and gel formulations are all available. Transdermal patches are a better choice because oral prescriptions that go through the liver at first pass can cause the liver to send out a binding protein (called sex hormone binding globulin), which can lower the availability of a number of hormones and create imbalances in thyroid, reproductive, and adrenal function.

As a note, it has been shown that serotonin reuptake inhibitors (SSRIs), the most commonly prescribed antidepressant medication, can cause infertility by lowering testosterone and sperm levels. So, if a depressed man with normal serotonin and low testosterone is given an SSRI, it is possible to make his depression even worse.

***Cautions with testosterone.*** Too much testosterone can cause excess body and facial hair, as well as acne. Testosterone replacement is thought in some studies to exacerbate prostate cancer risk, while others suggest low testosterone may increase risk as well. Recent studies also suggest giving extra testosterone in senior men may increase cardiovascular risk up to 30 percent (Vigen et al., 2013). Testosterone replacement should be regularly monitored by a doctor using blood tests and by checking for clinical excess signs and may be best avoided if there is heart disease risk.

*Serum estrogen and progesterone*

Low levels of estrogen have long been considered a factor in mood disorder. Estrogen is the predominant female hormone known for its ability to affect the levels of serotonin in the brain, by changing the ability of nerve cells to recognize this important mood transmitter, as well as lowering levels of an enzyme called monoamine oxidase, which breaks down serotonin (Carrasco et al., 2004).

While some menopausal patients using estrogen report reduction in mood symptoms (Miller et al., 2002), the majority show no benefit (Demetrio et al., 2011). One study in 115 seniors older than 70 years showed no benefit when given a 20-week course of high-dose estrogen to help cognitive function, mood, or quality of life (Almeida et al., 2006), and another in 417 women 60–80 years of age given 2 years of low-dose transdermal (skin patch) estradiol also did not see any improvement (Yaffe et al., 2006). Women taking the high-dose therapy also had double the adverse events versus the placebo group.

Like testosterone therapy, estrogen replacement therapy may actually improve the effects of conventional antidepressants (Schnedier et al., 2001), which is discussed further in Chapter 6.

The research on progesterone replacement suggests that it may block estrogen effects and actually support breakdown of serotonin in the brain. Optimal levels of progesterone are known to help calm the brain, improve sleep, and improve libido.

Progesterone treatment given without estrogen, such as the synthetic drug depot medroxyprogesterone acetate (Depo-Provera) has been shown to worsen depression in women who already have a tendency toward or clinical signs of depression (Jelovsek, 2009; Fraser & Lobo, 1999). However, other research does not corroborate this. One study looking at the birth control implant levonorgestrel (Norplant), another synthetic progesterone, showed the depression scores of the women most depressed actually improved during the study period (Westoff et al., 1998). While a number of preclinical and animal studies data suggest a positive antianxiety effect of progesterone (Auger & Forbes-Lorman, 2008), very few studies have been conducted reviewing the effects on mood. One study of 176 postmenopausal women found that taking oral micronized progesterone (a natural form of hormone replacement) resulted in significant improvement in vasomotor symptoms, somatic complaints, and anxiety and depressive symptoms over using the synthetic form of medroxyprogesterone acetate (Fitzpatrick, Pace, & Wiita, 2000).

The take-away from these studies of hormones is that hormonal replacement may help if given to the right person, but more than likely, it is only one piece of the puzzle. This is the reason it is important to address foods, lifestyle, sleep, exercise, and nutritional supplementation to create a CAM approach that will work for the depressed or anxious patient.

***If estrogen and/or progesterone is low:*** As a point of caution, the use of any hormones, synthetic or natural, should not be taken lightly, and should done with the care of a knowledgeable practitioner. Often, I will not recommend these unless other more basic care is addressed first (e.g., balancing the diet, exercise, sleep, work). It has been my experience that, in most cases, when these basics are addressed, women do not necessarily need hormones, or lower doses can achieve desired results.

If it is decided to consider replacement therapy, I recommend considering natural hormone replacement therapy instead of conventional synthetic hormones. Although much less research is available for natural therapies, it is likely that they will have fewer side effects due to the body's ability to recognize these compounds over their synthetic sisters. The above study by Fitzpatrick, Pace, & Wiita, (2000) also suggests the effect may be better as well.

If estrogen is going to be used, it is a good idea to also use some progesterone to protect the tissues in the body that may be susceptible to cancer risk (e.g., breast and uterus). Progesterone itself may be most useful in cases where there is much anxiety with the depression. For cases of insomnia, I would also recommend using a nighttime oral dose of micronized progesterone, which is helpful to potentiate gamma-aminobutyric acid (GABA) in the brain, an effect elicited by benzodiazepines (Babalonis et al., 2011).

Compounding pharmacies are the best source for natural hormones and will formulate these specific to the needs of the patient. These are usually prepared as oral preparations, transdermal creams, suppositories, or subdermal pellets and can include estrogen, progesterone, testosterone, and DHEA individually dosed.

### Celiac panel

Parallel to the massively increased consumption of gluten and grain products, there has been a dramatic rise in the past 50 years in the incidence of celiac disease, an inflammatory reaction to the gluten component of wheat or spelt grain. According to a National Institutes of Health panel, celiac disease is considerably underdiagnosed, with estimates suggesting about 1 in 100 persons is affected (U.S. Department of Health and Human Services, 2004).

There is a correlation between overt gluten allergy (celiac disease) or gluten sensitivity and mood disorder in adults (Jackson et al., 2012) and behavioral issues in children (Hernanz & Polanco, 1991). In addition, people with the undiagnosed disease have a 4-fold increased risk of death (Rubio-Tapia et al., 2009).

A celiac panel comprises four different tests: anti-gliadin antibody IgG, anti-gliadin antibody IgM, tissue transglutamase, and secretory IgA. Although not a perfect test, it has typically an 80–90 percent accuracy (Fasano & Catassi, 2001). The gold-standard test for Celiac disease is biopsy of the small intestine's jejunum. For the blood test, it is helpful to be eating gluten products regularly a few weeks before the test, otherwise the antibodies may not be found in a patient who is truly celiac.

**What to do if celiac positive:** Simply stated, it is best to avoid all gluten proteins, which occur in wheat, rye, barlely, and spelt. Gut linings can heal in 3–6 months. There are naturopathic herbs, such as geranium and marshmallow, that can also aid in healing. In my clinical experience, mood issues can improve within as little as 2 weeks. Most other grains, like rice, quinoa, amaranth, millet, and wild rice, are perfectly fine to eat. Oats are fine if the manufacturer assures they are processed away from other wheat and gluten products. For patients with severe depression, it is best to slowly lower gluten intake, for completely avoiding it at one time can induce a withdrawal effect and contribute to even worse mood. Like any drug we are addicted to, gluten can also cause an ugly withdrawal when removed too fast.

### Serum carnitine

Serum carnitine is an amino acid cofactor that serves to help turns fats into energy. Carnitine also plays a neuroprotective role in mood by acting as an antioxidant and anti-inflammatory (Soczynska et al., 2008). L-Carnitine has been shown to help mood, fatigue, and depression in patients with cancer (Cruciani et al., 2006) and hepatic encephalopathy (Malaguarnera et al., 2011). While administration of carnitine in rats have shown antianxiety benefits (Levine et al., 2005), no trials have studied anxiety benefit in humans. Another form of carnitine called acetyl-L-carnitine (ALC) is similar in structure to the neurotransmitter acetylcholine and acts as a cholinergic neurotransmitter. ALC has also been shown to have epigenetic effects (see the section "Behavioral Epigenetics" below) on production of receptors in the hippocampus and prefrontal cortex, to contribute to a rapid antidepressant effect (Nasca et al., 2013). An MRI study in geriatric depressed patients found that imbalances in the prefrontal cortex were resolved using doses of ALC (Pettegrew et al., 2002). For senior patients, the ALC form may be best for supplementation.

In a randomized double-blind placebo-controlled trial in 82 patients with amyotrophic lateral sclerosis (ALS) taking the drug riluzole, patients taking 3 g ALC daily had a median survival of 45 months, versus 22 months for the placebo group—an astounding improvement in the treatment of ALS (Beghi et al., 2013).

**If carnitine is low:** I recommend starting with 500 mg L-carnitine twice a day, preferably away from food for best absorption. I also would recheck carnitine blood levels in 6 weeks to look for improvement. If there is no improvement, consider doses up to 3,000 mg/day while looking into digestive support (see the section "Digestive Health" below), to help absorb nutrients better. Levels of 3,000 mg/day have not shown any toxicity. Effective dosages of ALC in most clinical trials range from 1 to 3 g/ day, given in divided doses (Gaby, 2011). For cognitive issues with depression, ALC may be the better choice.

**L-Carnitine natural food sources.** As the word *carnitine* comes from the Latin word *carne*, which refers to meat, it is not surprising that the highest concentrations of this amino acid are in red meats. Other relatively higher amounts are found in dairy products, nuts, and seeds, and lesser amounts are found in beans, vegetables, and grains.

### Serum folic acid and vitamin B12

Known best for preventing the neurologic disorder spina bifida in newborns, folic acid also plays a key role in the production of the neurotransmitters dopamine, norepinephrine, and epinephrine (Stahl, 2008). Vitamin B12 is a cobalt-containing molecule is known to help support production of red blood cells, the manufacture of DNA and nervous tissue and to play a role in normalizing the SAMe and homocysteine pathways, as well as helping in the synthesis of serotonin. Both vitamin B12 and folic acid can help patients when antidepressants do not work on their own (see Chapter 6).

Low folate status is noted in about 33 percent of people with depression. Conversely, people with diets high in green vegetables full of folate tend to have high levels of folate in their blood and less major depression ( Coppen & Bolander-Gouaille, 2005).

Studies using B complex formulas that include 1,000–2,000 µg methylfolate and 260–420 µg vitamin B12 have found significant and more continuous improvements in depressive and anxiety symptoms in depressed patients compared with placebo, with improvements in Beck Depression and Anxiety Inventories (Lewis et al., 2013).

**Steps to take if folic acid and/or B12 is low:** Taking both folic acid (800 µg up to 15 mg daily) and oral vitamin B12 (1,000 µg daily) will help. B vitamins like folic acid and B12 are water soluble and generally safe. For folic acid, the methyltetrahydrofolate version is the most natural form. Regular "folic acid" should be avoided. Methylcobalamin is the preferred form of vitamin B12.

**If B12 and folic acid levels are normal:** If levels are normal but symptoms of anxiety or depression are present, it may still be prudent to supplement with extra B12 and folic acid, especially if medication treatments are not working (see Chapter 7). It is quite possible that some people may have deficiency in their body tissues while still showing reasonable levels in the blood. For example, some genetic research suggests that transporters which bring vitamin B12 to the central nervous system may not function well, leaving B12 levels higher in the blood but still deficient in the brain. Additionally, other lab abnormalities, including high homocysteine and low red blood cells, may be suggestive of B12 deficiency. Mutations in the *MTHFR* (methylenetetrahydrofolate reductase) gene also suggest the need for taking in extra methyltetrahydrofolate (see next section about the MTHFR gene tes).

**Dietary sources of folate and B vitamins.** Excellent sources of folate are spinach, asparagus, romaine lettuce, turnip greens, mustard greens, calf's liver, collard greens, kale, cauliflower, broccoli, parsley, lentils, and beets. And vegetable sources have the methyltetrahydrofolate form. Excellent sources of B12 are snapper and calf's liver; other sources include venison, shrimp, scallops, salmon, and beef. Vegetarian sources have significantly lower available B12, and the best of these are sea plants (e.g., kelp), algae (e.g., blue-green algae), brewer's yeast, tempeh, miso, and tofu.

### MTHFR gene test

There is a relatively new genetic test for the *MTHFR* gene that is gaining widespread attention in both the holistic and conventional medical world. *MTHFR* is found on the short arm of chromosome 1 codes for an enzyme (methyltetrahydrofolate reductase) needed to process folic acid into its most useful form, methyltetrahydrofolate (MTHF). If someone has a mutation in the *MTHFR* gene, it is usually best to supplement with extra folate. And the best form to take is MTHF, not regular folic acid. MTHF dosage is often 1–5 mg a day, which is much higher than what is found in a multiple vitamin or most prenatals. MTHF has a strong relationship to both anxiety and depression (Almeida et al., 2005). Studies in treatment-resistant depression dose up to 15 mg folic acid (Fava et al., 2010). More about MTHF for this use is discussed in Chapter 6.

### 25(OH)vitamin D or serum vitamin D

Well known for bone strength, vitamin D is a steroid molecule with receptors that recognize it all over the body. Vitamin D deficiency is implicated in autoimmunity, cardiovascular diseases, cancers, and chronic pain (Straube et al., 2009). One meta-analysis suggested that all causes of death might be lowered by giving supplemental vitamin D (Autier & Gandini, 2007).

Mice genetically altered to lack vitamin D receptors show greatly increased anxiety behavior (Kalueff et al., 2004). Vitamin D deficiency is linked to both anxiety and depression in people with fibromyalgia (Armstrong et al., 2007). One study of 1,000 older adults found mean levels of serum vitamin D were lower in those with minor depression and major depression compared with controls (Hoogendijk et al., 2008).

Low levels of vitamin D are likely involved in mood in several ways. Vitamin D affects nerve growth factor, which is important for brain and neuronal repair and growth (Wion et al., 1991). Vitamin D also helps production of serotonin, testosterone, and thyroid hormone (Stumpf, 1995). Hypothalamic brain centers are responsive to the presence of vitamin D, and low levels will affect the HPA axis as well, contributing to poor mood (Eyles et al., 2005).

Increased depressive symptoms are found in the adults born from women with low vitamin D while pregnant (O'Loan et al., 2007), suggesting that it may be possible to head off mood disorder in the next generation by checking vitamin D in prepregnant and pregnant women. Preventing mood disorder in the next generation would be the ultimate in preventive care!

Research demonstrates that dosages of 4,000 IU vitamin D per day in depressed patients tend to improve well-being (Vieth et al., 2004). A small study evaluated 44 healthy participants during the wintertime, when vitamin D levels are low. They were randomly assigned to 5 days of treatment with 400 or 800 IU of vitamin D3 or a placebo. Compared with placebo, both doses of the vitamin increased positive mood and decreased negative mood (Lansdowne & Provost, 1998). A Norwegian study of 441 overweight people measured serum 25-hydroxyvitamin D levels. Those with levels <40 nmol/L (16 mg/dL) were shown to be more depressed on the Beck Depression Inventory. These subjects were then given 20,000 IU, 40,000 IU, or placebo once a week. Those given 40,000 IU had a 33 percent reduction in depression scores, those given 20,000 IU had a 20 percent reduction, and the placebo group had a 5 percent decrease (Jordea et al., 2008). These results are modest and suggest that vitamin D plays a role, but deficiency may not be the sole cause of mood issues.

***Dosing vitamin D.*** Vitamin D ranges in the normal adult between 30 and 100 ng/mL. An ideal level of vitamin D is around 50, and in my experience very few patients come in with normal levels, unless they are already supplementing. Sunlight exposure is the method nature prescribed for humans to keep up vitamin D levels, as there are few food sources, and even eating large amounts are not enough to raise levels of vitamin D. Garland et al. (2007) reported that 12 min of exposure of 50 percent of body skin to noontime sun on a clear day is equivalent to oral intake of 3,000 IU vitamin D3.

As discussed in Chapter 2, some sun is very healthful. Unless there is a clear immediate skin cancer risk, remaining in the sun long enough to allow the skin to pink a bit (not burn) is enough to help convert vitamin D without allowing excessive radiation damage to skin cells.

If supplementing with vitamin D, I recommend 2,000 IU/day of vitamin D3 for every 10 ng/mL we are looking to increase. For example, if a patient is at 20 ng/mL, and we would ultimately like to achieve 50 ng/mL, then 6,000 IU/day is a reasonable dose, and we will recheck blood levels in 3 months to monitor.

*Food sources of vitamin D.* The best dietary source of vitamin D is fish. Much of the literature ascribes the mood benefit of fish to their essential fatty acids (Hibbeln, 1998), but vitamin D may also play a role. Eggs, butter, mushrooms, and parsley have small amounts of D.

*Vitamin D toxicity.* Vitamin D is a fat-soluble steroid molecule that can be toxic in high levels. Hypervitaminosis D may lead to high calcium in the blood, kidney issues, and excessive bone loss. It is not known what supplemental amount may be problematic. Likely, this number may vary from patient to patient, which is why it is best to run lab tests to check pre- and postsupplementation. Studies of patients given long-term treatment of 14,000 IU/day orally seemed to have no toxicity and did show significantly decreased depression relapse rates (Burton, 2009).

One study suggests hypervitaminosis may start at regular 20,000 IU/day dosing (Vieth, 1999), with other research suggesting blood levels should not exceed 100 ng/mL (Hollis & Wagner, 2004). One meta-analysis suggests that long-term ordinary dosages of 400–800 IU/day are not associated with adverse effects (Autier & Gandini, 2007).

Conflicting information spurs the question of which form of the supplement is better: vitamin D2 (ergocalciferol) or D3 (cholecalciferol). Plants manufacture vitamin D2, whereas vitamin D3 is synthesized by humans in the skin when it is exposed to ultraviolet B rays from sunlight. Clinically, I have used vitamin D3, which shows efficacy for raising blood levels, as well as improving mood. For patients not finding benefit with vitamin D3, vitamin D2 may be a consideration.

*One note about vitamin D tests.* Although there are a few forms of vitamin D in the body that can be tested, the test indicative of true vitamin D status is the 25-hydroxy(OH)vitamin D test, and it is the best test for making clinical decisions regarding dosing.

### Serum mercury

High mercury levels in the blood and body tissues can contribute to many nervous system disorders, mood disorders, and cardiovascular disease. I recommend running this test to see if there has been recent exposure to this deadly heavy metal. It may also be ordered to monitor those who are regularly exposed to mercury. In my practice over 10 years, I have seen six patients with depression and neurologic challenges who had high serum mercury due to high intake of tuna and sushi. Please note, this test does not tell you if you have had a long-term exposure to mercury that has accumulated in the body tissues over a long period of time.

In patients with sudden onset of depression with possible exposure, is worth checking mercury levels. I have also seen in middle-age and senior patients that the initiation of osteoporosis can release stored mercury and other heavy metals from bone into the body. This sudden release of these metals can contribute to mood challenges, nervous system changes, and high blood pressure. We will talk a little more about how to treat both acute and long-term mercury and other metal poisonings in the section on detoxification at the end of this chapter.

### Saliva Adrenal Function Testing

As discussed in Chapter 4, the function of the hypothalamic-pituitary-adrenal (HPA) axis is central to appearance and severity of both anxiety and depression. The saliva adrenal test asks the patient to donate saliva for a series of time points throughout the day, from which bioactive hormones such as cortisol, as well as DHEA and DHEA sulfate, are accurately measured. Generally stated, abnormal levels of cortisol and lower levels of DHEA may indicate a dysregulated HPA axis. This allows the CAM practitioner to correlate clinical symptomology with hormonal levels throughout the day, allowing for more specific use of lifestyle recommendations and supplementation. While saliva testing is not common in conventional medical care, salivary hormone testing is accurate and follows results found in plasma testing (Kumar et al., 2005).

## DIGESTIVE HEALTH

*"It's a gut feeling"*

*"There are butterflies in my stomach"*

*"The way to a man's heart is through his gut"*

*"My heart's in my stomach"*

How often have we heard about the association between one's feelings and the digestive tract? More than we can count—we see it in literature, art, and mass media. Nevertheless, modern psychiatry has still all but ignored the strong association between the gastrointestinal system and mood.

Naturopathic doctors have an old saying: "If you don't know what is wrong or what to treat, then treat the gut." Digestion is the default system to focus on for difficult-to-treat cases. For decades it had been observed by holistic practitioners that improved digestion can lead to better overall health, including mood. Modern science is starting to catch up to this concept.

Conventional biomedicine has relegated mood disorders solely to the realm of the psychiatrist. The preceding section touched on the realms of the hematologist, endocrinologist, neurologist, cardiologist, toxicologist, and nutritionist. This section discusses why the gastroenterologist should be getting involved, too.

Healthy digestion is critical for mood. Michael Gershon's book *The Second Brain* (1999) took a new perspective regarding the digestive system: not just as a means for nutrient absorption and elimination, but also as a neuroendocrine organ. He explained to a mass audience for the first time that lying within this organ system is a robust nervous and hormonal output that rivals production found in the central nervous and hormone systems themselves. Called the enteric nervous system ( *enteric* refers to the digestive tract), the gastrointestinal tract is the main source of neurotransmitters in the body. For example, one of the neurotransmitters, serotonin, is an amine that is produced from food sources of tryptophan in the digestive tract's ubiquitous enterochromaffin cells and enterochromaffin-like cells. Poor digestive function (often due to stress, poor diet, sleep problems, and toxins) creates inflammatory issues and lowers the ability to absorb tryptophan. In patients who have celiac disease, chronic inflammation leads to poor nutrient absorption (Mäki &

Collin, 1997). Additionally, irritating foods will spur the digestive tract to send copious amounts of serotonin into the digestive system as a protective mechanism, where it encourages fast motility as a means to empty out the gut. This is a likely cause of diarrhea in people who have mood disorders, poor diet, and/or accompanying high stress.

Evidence shows that bowel disorders are correlated with mood. In fact, 20 percent of patients with functional bowel disorders such as irritable bowel syndrome have diagnosable psychiatric illness (Agazzi et al., 2003). Almost one-third of patients with major depression are thought to have constipation, and patients with irritable bowel syndrome are more prone to both anxiety disorders and depression (Kabra & Nadkarni, 2013).

How often do you work with women who have self-esteem challenges? Well, bowel movements are intimately linked with feminine self-esteem, as well as being able to maintain a relationship. An interesting study by Emmanuel, Mason and Kamm (2001) compared 34 women 19–45 years of age who had significant constipation for at least five years with women who did not have constipation. The constipated group had poorer health scores, had difficulty forming close relationships, and described themselves as "less feminine." The constipated women also had reduced rectal blood flow, which was strongly associated with anxiety and depression, as well as negative body symptoms and impaired socialization. The authors concluded that a women's individual psychological makeup alters the function of the involuntary nerves that link the brain to the gut. Reduced activity of these nerves slows down gut function, resulting in constipation. Because it is known that most neurotransmitters needed for healthy mood are made in the digestive tract, slowed gut function likely plays a role in how a woman feels about herself and how she responds in a relationship.

## How to Avoid Constipation

Learning the importance of good bowel movements, it makes sense to help get things moving. I recommend patients move their bowels at least once each day. Although some medical texts cite three times a week as normal, I believe once a day is the minimum. Steps to create a healthy bowel movement include the following:

1. *Adequate hydration:* Besides helping absorption of important amino acids, water is the liquid that keeps things flowing throughout our body. If we do not have enough water, the body will steal it from the colonic contents, making us constipated. Sipped throughout the day, two liters (about 64 ounces) of pure, clean water is ideal for most people.

2. *Fiber intake:* About 25 g/day will go a long way for better mood. Add a plentiful amount of fruits and vegetables. If this is not enough, sometimes flax meal, psyllium, or organic dried prunes may do the trick. A study in senior patients using 7g twice a day of psyllium worked better, and helped 63 out of 92 (69%) patients wean off of more addictive and more expensive laxative prescriptions (Khaja et al., 2005)

3. *Stress reduction work:* Many of my patients will tell me when they are on vacation, they move their bowels every day. This suggests that stress is a major factor in shutting the bowels down and limiting rectal flow, as the above study illustrated. Whether it is acupuncture, meditation, yoga, or taking a vacation, regular stress reduction is important.

4. *Natural laxatives:* If the above steps are not enough, then natural supplements can help. Magnesium supplementation is gentle and can help the bowels move quicker: typical doses for laxative effect start at 400 mg and may move up to 1,000 mg. Magnesium oxide is the cheapest form of magnesium and may have the best stool-softening effect. Also, concentrated Epsom salt baths (made from magnesium sulfate) have a laxative effect by absorption through the mucosa in the anal area. High doses of vitamin C ($\geq$3 g/day) can also act to loosen stool. Magnesium and vitamin C can be used together.

If the above still are not enough, then laxative herbs like senna can be taken as a tea, or stronger forms come in pill can also help, but these herbs should be used sparingly and only in the short term (a few days), for the colon can start to rely on these and become resistant, creating a situation of more difficult constipation (Kinnunen et al., 1993).

## Steps to a Healthy Digestive Tract

So, if a client wants to start working on creating a healthy digestive tract in order to balance mood properly, these are the steps to consider:

1. *Fix constipation:* If a person is not having regular bowel movements, the above steps would be the first order of business to achieving healthful digestion
2. *Before-meal ritual—breathing and bitters:* A deep diaphragmatic breath or two before a meal is helpful to calm the body and bring circulation to the digestive system. Additionally, a little aperitif before a meal can be relaxing and stimulating to the digestive tract. Aperitifs (also called "digestifs") usually have a small amount of alcohol and bitter herbs like gentian. These act as digestives (increase digestive enzyme production) and cholerectics (stimulate of bile from the liver) to help prepare for protein and fat digestion. Those avoiding alcohol can add bitters like gentian and skullcap extract to warm water or seltzer and create the same healthful effect on digestion (Olivier & van Wyk, 2013).
3. *Chewing:* There's an old saying: "Nature castigates those who don't masticate." Well, the teeth are the hardest substance in our body and serve to pulverize food for best digestion. For physical digestion, birds have gizzards, which are made for grinding, and cows have multiple stomachs—but humans do not. We have to chew our food well.

   If we do not chew and chew well, even healthy foods will be more likely to spur inflammatory reactions in the body, for poorly broken down food particles will stimulate the gut immune system, which comprises about 70 percent of our total immune system, creating inflammation throughout the body. Also, lack of chewing means less digestion of carbohydrates—many patients with bowel disorders like Crohn's disease, ulcerative colitis, and small intestinal bowel overgrowth would improve if carbohydrates were broken down properly in the mouth as nature intended.

Decades prior, Americans usually chewed their food as many as twenty-five times before swallowing. Current reports state that American chews only ten times before swallowing (Kessler, 2009). Most people do not even chew that many. I personally know that, if I do not think about it, I will tend to chew things once or twice, and swallow it virtually whole.

I recommend taking reasonable-size bites and chewing 20 times, until the food is texturally unrecognizable. Taking a deep relaxing breath before starting to eat also helps to insure our system is ready to digestion.

4. *Choose Healthy Foods:* Generally, eating whole foods as prescribed by the Mediterranean diet is a great place to start (see Chapter 2 for more on this). Also, if the digestion is not strong, soups and slow-cooked foods may be easiest for the digestive tract to break down and assimilate.

5. *Relaxation and Psychological Work:* A robust digestive tract requires some calm. When an animal thinks a bear is going to attack, the primitive brain shunts all energy to the organs needed to fight or run (muscles, brain, heart, etc.). This is called the sympathetic response. Part of the sympathetic response is shutting down the organ systems not needed, like the digestive tract and reproductive system—their is no interest in eating or sex while running from a bear. Once the stressor has passed, then the animal returns to parasympathetic response, also known as "rest and digest." Here, digestion can resume.

Breathing, meditation, acupuncture, yoga, and tai chi can all help lower stress hormones and return to the parasympathetic mode. As you already know quite well, psychological counseling can help teach methods to lower reaction to situations that are not really life-threatening. This work is invaluable to creating a healthy gut.

## Inflammation, Leaky Gut, and Mood

The majority of the body's immune system is housed in digestive tract, where it is known as mucosa-associated lymphoid tissue and gut-associated lymphoid tissue. Stress and poor digestion leads to an activation of the inflammatory components of the immune system, which lead to inflammation. Ingestion of charred, fried and overly cooked foods create more advanced glycation end-products (AGEs; Uribarri et al., 2005), which will also increase inflammation in the body. Inflammation can travel to the brain and contribute to both anxiety and depressed mood. This is the reason why psychiatric problems are much more prevalent in patients with the intestinal inflammatory condition celiac disease (Jackson et al., 2012).

Significantly greater amounts of inflammation are present in people with anxiety (Vogelzangs et al., 2013) and depression (Dinan, 2009). Inflammatory markers such as C-reactive protein (CRP), interleukin-6 (IL-6), and tumor-necrosis factor-alpha are raised and correlate with brain changes as well as damage to other body tissues. Depending on a person's particular predisposition and individual genetics, this process will contribute to practically any health issue. In the brain and central nervous system, inflammation causes mood problems or may contribute to multiple sclerosis. In the blood vessels, inflammation will cause coronary artery disease. Skin inflammation manifests as eczema, psoriasis, and acne. Kidney and lung inflammation will cause lupus and other organ problems, while various tissue inflammations are known propagators of cancer. Nondescript global inflammation may manifest as fibromyalgia and chronic fatigue. Almost every disease has an inflammatory component. And it is likely that every inflammation has a digestive and stress component.

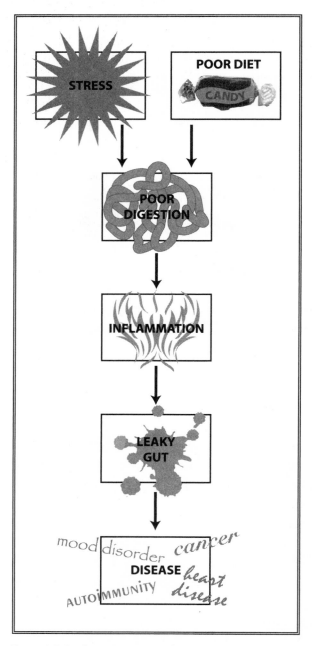

Figure 3.3. Leaky gut: genesis and implications.

The immune response in the digestive tract is known to lead to sick-ness behavior, including flu-like symptoms of fatigue, anxiety, and depression (Anisman & Merali, 2003). Part of my work at the National Institute of Mental Health in the 1990s was to elucidate which immune factors might be turned on in the brain when the body was inflamed. Up until the 1990s, the brain's immune system was not well described, and historically many people in medicine considered the brain to be without immune cells. In our work, we gave healthy Sprague-Dawley rats regular doses of a bacterial cell wall compound called lipopolysaccharide. The rat immune system "sees" this compound and prompts a strong inflammatory response. The inflamed animals showed "sickness behavior," including fatigue, anxiousness, low mood, low motivation, and other symptoms and signs that clearly correlate with both anxiety and depression (Wong et al., 1997).

*What is intestinal permeability/leaky gut exactly?*

For the past few decades, natural and CAM practitioners have referred to a concept called "leaky gut" as being a foundational connection between poor digestion and inflammation-derived disease process. Any foods to which a particular person is sensitive will spark immune-related responses in the digestion, eliciting inflammatory cascades throughout the body. Stress will also increase the likelihood of immune response by inhibiting proper enzymatic production, which allows macromolecules to reach the intestines without being properly broken down and provoke a greater inflammatory response.

The concept of leaky gut suggests that excess inflammation over a long period of time will significantly compromise both the structure and repair mechanisms of the digestive tract. Under this inflammatory fire, tight junctions known to hold digestive tract cells together begin to deteriorate. When these structures break down, material in the lumen of the gastrointestinal tract now has greater access to the blood stream. This is known by the more technical term of "gut permeability" or what many people simply call "leaky gut."

Particles that escape from the digestive tract will travel to the rest of the body and contribute to global inflammatory effects and eventually to disease. As discussed in the last section, if someone has a predisposition to disease, leaky gut and its accompanying inflammation will increase the likelihood this disease will manifest.

When there is leaky gut, the intestinal inflammation and leaked particles travel through the hepatic portal system, spur upregulation of hepatic Kupffer cells (immune cells in the liver), an trigger upregulation of brain microglia (immune cells in the brain). Inflammation in the brain will result in brain degeneration and poor mood. The likelihood of this cascade of events is far greater with leaky gut than if the intestines are intact (Maes et al., 2009).

While intestinal permeability/leaky gut is fairly well recognized in natural medicine and CAM circles, conventional biomedicine has spurned this concept, calling it laughable, unproven, and the work of pseudoscientists. In fact, the National Health Service of England (2013) echoes the sentiment of mainstream medicine regarding leaky gut:

> There is little evidence to support this theory. While it is true that certain factors can make the bowel more permeable, this probably does not lead to anything more than temporary mild inflammation of an area of the bowel. Some scientists and sceptics believe that people who promote "leaky gut syndrome" are either misguided and read too much into the theory, or are deliberately misleading the public to make money from the "treatments" they sell.

It also goes on to state: "Generally, it is wise to view 'holistic' and 'natural health' websites with skepticism—do not assume that the information they provide is correct or based on scientific fact or evidence."

Although standard in the conventional medical world, this opinion seems to fly in the face of medical research, as emerging information suggests leaky gut syndrome is indeed quite real and is a strong contributor to disease, including mood disorder (Maes, Kubera, & Leunis, 2008). Maes et al. (2008) looked at the serum concentrations of IgM and IgG antibodies in chronic fatigue patients. The presence of these antibodies is indicative of the presence of gram-negative enterobacteria in the blood—effectively serving as a marker of a leaky gut situation. Forty-one of these patients were given a leaky gut diet and prescribed natural anti-inflammatory and antioxidative supplements, such as glutamine, N-acetyl cysteine, and zinc. After an average of 10–14 months, 24 patients showed a significant clinical improvement or remission and normalization of the IgA and IgM responses.

Leaky gut has also been elucidated and implicated in other disorders, such has gall bladder and liver disease (Reyes et al., 2006; Hartmann et al., 2012), heart disease (Rogler & Rosano, 2014), kidney disease (Anders, Andersen, & Stecher, 2013), vascular problems (Hunt, 2012), type I diabetes (Vaarala, Atkinson, & Neu, 2008), and autoimmune disease (Fasano, 2012), to name a few.

### Food Allergy and Food Sensitivity (Food Intolerance)

Chapter 2 discussed the basics on good healthful diet for mood; this section explains the less straightforward notion of how food allergies and food sensitivities may be players in mental health via the mechanism of leaky gut and inflammation. Following the axiom "one man's food may be another man's poison," this section discusses working with this difficult concept.

Food allergy refers to an overt immune system response that results in creation of antibodies and may result in tissue swelling and even anaphylaxis. The most common food allergies are shellfish, nuts, fish, milk, peanuts, and eggs. Celiac disease is an allergy involving an autoimmune response to gluten (a protein present in wheat, rye, and barley). Food sensitivity or intolerance is a subtler response that occurs in the digestive tract, often occurring when foods are not well digested, and spur unwanted inflammatory reactions.

The nervous system is vulnerable to the ravages of food reaction. Neurologic manifestations in patients with established celiac disease have been reported since 1966. However, it was not until 30 years later that gluten sensitivity was shown to manifest not so much with digestive issues but instead solely as neurologic dysfunction, such as unexplained neuropathies and ataxia (uncoordinated muscle movements) (Hadjivassiliou et al., 2010). Mood issues are likely to be involved as well.

While celiac is an antibody-mediated disease affecting 1 percent of the population and is generally characterized by gastrointestinal complaints, gluten sensitivities are subtler in reaction, often without overt gastrointestinal problems, and will more likely manifest as extraintestinal neurologic and psychiatric symptoms. Sensitivities occur at six times the rate of celiac disease and occur without celiac's hallmark antibodies or villus breakdown (Jackson et al., 2012). Even more interesting, when gluten foods are withdrawn, patients with sensitivities enjoy even more improvement in gut symptoms than patients with celiac—75 percent versus 64 percent, respectively (Campanella et al., 2008).

### How to work on inflammation

There are various ways the body reveals increased levels of inflammation. These could be the presence of skin conditions (rashes, eczema, psoriasis, rosacea, etc.) or more internal (e.g., autoimmune conditions, cancers, cardiovascular disease, mental health issues, and inflammatory bowel diseases). Also, blood tests (such as high levels of Erythrocyte Sedimentation Rate, CRP, homocysteine, and/or autoimmune markers like Auto Nuclear Antibiodies, thyroid autoantibodies, or celiac antibodies) can point to inflammation.

Steps to start to balance inflammation in patients with anxiety and depression include the following:

1. *Meditation/relaxation/mind-body work* will help increase parasympathetic response and support circulation to the digestive tract (discussed in Chapter 5).
2. *Sleep work:* aim for 8 hours of sleep, getting to bed by 11 p.m. at the latest to help balance immune function (see Chapter 2).
3. *Exercise* at least three times a week for half an hour to help burn stress hormones and calm the nervous system, as well as build muscle to support insulin sensitivity, thus lowering insulin, which is pro-inflammatory (see Chapter 2).
4. *Food work:* focus on anti-inflammatory foods and the Mediterranean diet: fish, green vegetables, raw nuts and seeds, and

plenty of fiber. Avoid dairy, gluten and foods cooked at high temperatures (fried and charbroiled foods, etc.).

5. *Use supplements* to help lower inflammation and heal a leaky gut:

*Probiotics* are beneficial to heal the mucosal membrane (Barbara et al., 2012). Dosages will vary with preparation.

*Zinc:* studies on Crohn's patients have shown zinc supplementation can resolve permeability alterations in patients with Crohn's disease and help prevent relapse in remitted patients (Sturniolo, 2001). Typical dose is 15 mg twice a day of zinc carnosine.

*Curcumin* helps decrease inflammation and oxidative stress in the gut (Rapin & Wiernsperger, 2010). Dosage will depend on preparation and is best between meals. More about curcumin and turmeric in the botanicals section of Chapter 4.

*Glutamine* is a preferred fuel for digestive tract cells and helps with repair of the intestines (Hulsewe et al., 2004). Standard dosage is one teaspoon twice a day in liquid away from meals.

*Robert's formula* is an old naturopathic formula with anecdotal efficacy for healing the digestive tract, although no formal research has been done on this herbal combination. While there are variations, the standard formula usually includes *Althea, Echinacea, Ulmus, Geranium, Phytolacca, Hydrastis,* and cabbage powder. Cabbage is high in glutamine. Some versions also include niacinamide and pancreatic enzymes as well. This formula is typically dosed one or two capsules up to three times a day between meals.


## HYPOTHALAMIC-PITUITARY-ADRENAL AXIS

The HPA axis is composed of central parts of the brain (hypothalamus and pituitary) along with the adrenal glands, which sit on top of the kidneys. These vital structures act collectively as a nexus for the hormonal and nervous systems (known collectively as the neuroendocrine system) with the immune system. It is primarily among these structures that stress responses are coordinated. Impaired functioning of the HPA axis has been associated with several physical and psychiatric disorders, such as the metabolic syndrome (Bjorntorp & Rosmond, 2000), fibromyalgia, depression (Holsboer, 2000), and posttraumatic stress disorder (Yehuda, 1997).

Found deep in the center of the primitive brain, the hypothalamus is implicated in the pathogenesis of mood disorder. Postmortem studies reveal greatly altered levels of the neuropeptide corticotropin-releasing hormone (CRH; formerly called corticotropin releasing factor) in individuals with anxiety and depression (Meynen et al., 2007). CRH moderates the neuroendocrine, autonomic, and behavioral responses and is considered the main mediator of the response to stress.

Changes in the hypothalamus affect the amygdala, a brain area very much involved in the fear and emotional responses. The amygdala expresses high levels of CRH receptors in chronically stressed individuals, making it more reactive in times of stress. Stress-induced changes within the amygdala are a likely critical step in the pathophysiology in the development of chronic anxiety states. It is further proposed that such a change in the limbic neural circuitry (composed of the brain's hippocampus, hypothalamus, and thalamus) is involved in the transition from normal vigilance responses to hypervigilant pathologic anxiety, manifesting in panic and posttraumatic stress disorders (Shekhar et al., 2005).

The limbic system, made up of a number of brain structures including the hippocampus, hypothalamus, thalamus, cinglulate gyrus and amygdala. It is the area of the brain involved with emotion, behavior, motivation, and memory.

This chapter has already reviewed how the gut is a source of inflammation and that in inflamed digestive states, amino acid absorption is compromised and lower blood levels of tryptophan result. Lowered tryptophan will lead to a decrease in cerebral serotonin, which is linked to an increase in the HPA axis activity found in depression (Swaab, Bao, & Lucassen, 2005).

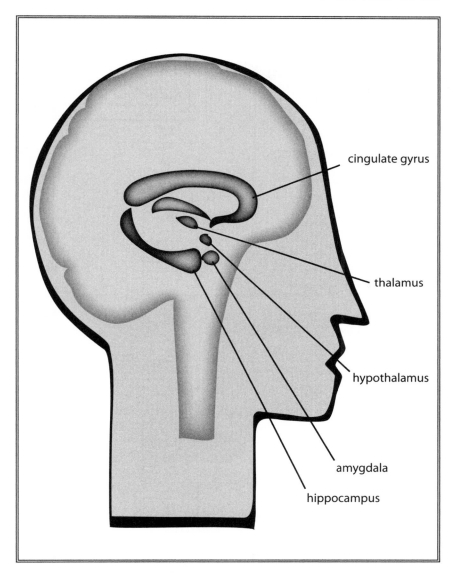

Figure 3.4. Areas of emotion: the limbic system.

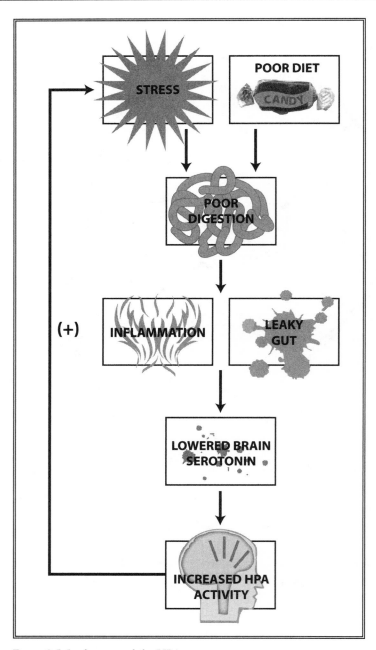

Figure 3.5. Leaky gut and the HPA.

There is overwhelming evidence to indicate that adaptation to chronic stress involves response from both the neuroendocrine and immune systems. Perceived emotional stress results in alterations of the HPA axis with changes in the release of cortisol, while at the same time altering both innate (nonspecific) and adaptive (antigen-specific) immune function.

In response to stress, the hypothalamus secretes corticotropin-releasing hormone (CRH). This stimulates the anterior lobe of the pituitary gland to secrete adrenocorticotropic hormone (ACTH). ACTH reaches the adrenal cortex initiating cortisol secretion into the bloodstream. Cortisol is the major glucocorticoid for mediating the stress response. Imbalances in adrenal production are seen in treatment-resistant depression, as evidenced by higher ratios of cortisol to dehydroepiandrosterone (DHEA) (Markopouloua et al., 2009).

Cortisol keeps blood sugar high by blocking insulin and inhibiting glucose uptake. Cortisol leads to increased heart action and blood flow. Cortisol also suppresses collagen synthesis (needed for youthful skin), osteoblast activity (needed for strong bones), hematopoiesis (production of red blood cells), protein synthesis, immune responses, and kidney function. As a result, those with high prolonged levels of cortisol can have thinning of skin, osteopenia and osteoporosis, low blood count, poor muscle growth, low immune response, and/or renal compromise. As a mediator of the stress system, chronically released cortisol alters physiologic processes and genetic expressions that ultimately cascade into fear and anxiety (Korte, 2001), as well as depressive states (De Kloet, 2004). Thus, chronic stress is not good, to say the least, for the body or the mind.

## Glucocorticoid Resistance and HPA Dysregulation Syndrome

The human animal is designed to withstand some stress, but not all the time. A little bit of stress can be good but should be followed by long periods of calm. For example, a cat is chased by a dog: the cat instinctively has a fear response and runs up a tree to safety. After some barking at the base of the tree, the dog gives up and leaves. The cat then returns to its home and relaxes. This is a acute and temporary response that saved the cat from harm. When the cat first perceived danger, CRH was produced in high amounts in the hypothalamus, which signals release of ACTH from the pituitary, which prompts release of catecholamines (epinephrine and norepinephrine) from the adrenal glands. The HPA axis is under negative feedback control from cortisol. This means higher levels of cortisol from the adrenal glands will feed back to the brain, prompting the brain to lower the CRH output. Cortisol is the primary regulator of the HPA axis, with negative feedback on ACTH and CRH, exerting its control of both the hypothalamus and the pituitary gland. Under normal short-term stressors, like the cat running up the tree, the HPA axis responds well to cortisol, which negatively feeds back to lower cortisol levels.

Let's now say the dog recruited all of his friends, and they took turns standing vigil at the base of the tree, barking and threatening the cat every time it moved, for days and days on end. With this kind of pro-longed stress, the cat adrenal glands keep pumping out cortisol and stress hormones chronically. High levels of cortisol create a situation where the HPA axis stops responding cortisol. This has been termed "glucocor-ticoid resistance syndrome."

This syndrome is similar to insulin resistance in the type II diabetic, where higher than normal levels of insulin result in the body no longer "listening" to insulin, prompting the production of more and more insulin from the pancreas. But instead of insulin, in this case of chronic stress the body does not recognize cortisol, which drives the adrenals to make more and more cortisol in an effort to be "heard." The prolonged stress response causes continuous cortisol synthesis and chronically elevated cortisol levels.

In this state of prolonged stress, increased cortisol levels are linked to metabolic syndrome (excess weight, blood pressure issues, high lipids, obesity), chronic fatigue syndrome, chronic inflammatory states, ner-vous system problems, cardiovascular disease, anxiety, insomnia, depres-sion, and more (Tsigos & Chrousos, 2002). This is referred to as the resistance phase of the stress adaptation syndrome. If allowed to persist, there is a significant increases to all of these diseases.

High levels of cortisol, as seen in chronic anxiety and depression, leads to loss of neurons and glial (brain immune) cells, atrophy of the brain's hippocampus and prefrontal cortex, and loss of molecules like brain-derived neurotropic factor (BDNF), which is needed for proper brain repair and maintenance. Anxiety behaviors and chronic stress will also lead to the final stage of the stress adaptation syndrome, which is exhaustion.

## HPA Dysregulation and "Adrenal Fatigue"

In the most extreme, this exhaustion phase may manifest as more acute and serious collapse of vital organ systems and functions. Most people do not experience full collapse. More commonly, you will see symptoms in your clients like extreme lassitude (often part of chronic fatigue syndrome), depression, and pale complexion. Sometimes, there is low blood pressure. Often, there is an inability of the adrenal gland to keep putting out adequate cortisol. In holistic circles, this is sometimes labeled "adrenal fatigue." In conventional biomedicine, "adrenal fatigue" is reserved for conditions like Addison's disease, where there is actually no output from the adrenal gland. Therefore, I prefer to use the term "HPA dysregulation syndrome."

Evidence of HPA alterations is found in the common symptoms of anxiety and depression. Hallmarks of early HPA dysregulation include fatigue and sleep disturbances, as well as diminished interest behaviors and appetite changes for women (Hollinrake et al., 2007), and may predispose to eating disorders as well. These symptoms are classic presentations of sickness behaviors orchestrated by the hypothalamus.

Besides the increased risk of metabolic syndrome, obesity, chronic fatigue, chronic inflammatory states, lipid oxidation, artery disease, anxiety, insomnia, and depression, it has been shown that hypothalamic-pituitary-thyroid (HPT) axis and the hypothalamic-pituitary-ovary/testicle axis are also in jeopardy of proper function. This is important to note, for

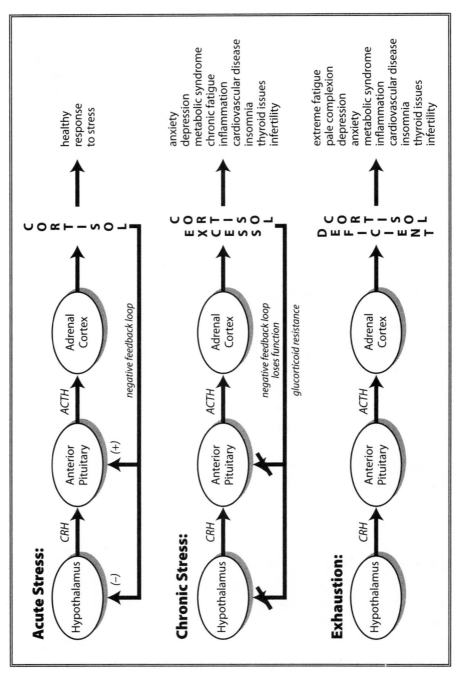

Figure 3.6. Three phases of the HPA: acute stress, chronic stress, and exhaustion.

chronic stress can be a main factor in both hypothyroidism and infertility.

### In Utero and Childhood Effects on the HPA Axis

While daily life stressors modulate current HPA activity, the prenatal environment and childhood experience may have far greater impact on the overall tone of the HPA axis. Like the volume setting on your stereo, events in utero set the baseline levels of the HPA axis and decide how "loud" or "soft" it will "play."

When a pregnant mother is under duress, the offspring will be more likely to sustain altered brain physiology and behavior changes with lifelong consequences, including predisposition to anxiety and depression.

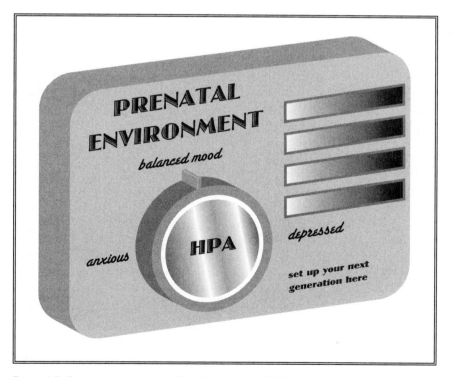

Figure 3.7. Events in utero control baseline levels of HPA.

Several animal studies have reported specific links between prenatal stress exposure and glucocorticoid resistance in offspring (Weinstock, 2005). Maternal anxiety or depression during pregnancy predicts HPA hyperactivity, as well as changes in cortisol, in infants and preadolescent children (Field, Hernandez-Reif, & Diego, 2006 O'Connor, 2005). Stressful maternal experiences will also alter genes expressed in the brain in a epigenetic fashion (meaning the genes themselves do not change, but whether they are expressed or not can change). Stress basically turns on the genes that will make the offspring more prone to mood disorder (Zucchi et al., 2013). Turning on and off the expression of genes that control HPA responsiveness is considered "epigenetic."

The first evidence in humans of an association between prenatal psychosocial stress exposure and subsequent alterations in the regulation of the HPA axis was found in a study of 31 healthy young adults whose mothers experienced severe stress during their pregnancy. These adults had much higher CRH and cortisol levels when experiencing stressors compared with controls (Entringer et al., 2009).

From a holistic standpoint, it should also be noted that emotional stressors, dietary imbalances like poor nourishment, low birth weight, maternal overeating, and high-fat diets will also contribute to HPA and mood disorders in the next generation. Increases in anxiety and decreases in learning capacity are found in mouse offspring whose pregnant moms ate a high-fat diet. These effects did not vastly change if the newborn pups were given a normal diet, suggesting that dietary imbalances before birth may not be fully reversible if the offspring eats a more balanced diet after being born (Bilbo & Tsang, 2010). This is an argument for teaching health basics like diet to women before and during pregnancy.

Of course, factors after birth will continue to affect HPA function. Victims of child abuse, those that experienced maternal separation as evidenced through parental loss in the 9/11 terrorist attacks (Pfeffer et al., 2007), and children exposed to the 1995 Oklahoma City bombing all displayed significant HPA dysregulation and predisposition to anxiety and depression (Pfefferbaum et al., 2012). Studies on rat pups reveal that overfeeding of neonates will also increase HPA hyperresponsiveness and predisposition to mood disorder (Spencer & Tilbrook, 2009).

Along with proper nutrition, mind-body modalities in the prenatal and childhood period may hold the greatest promise in balancing HPA axis function for the next generation. Pregnant women receive profound health benefits from mind-body therapies when used in conjunction with conventional prenatal care. In a meta-analysis, progressive muscle relaxation was the most common intervention used in pregnant women. Other positive studies employed a multimodal psychoeducation approach or a yoga and meditation intervention. Treatment group outcomes included higher birth weight, shorter labor, fewer instrument-assisted births, and reduced perceived maternal stress and anxiety (Beddoe & Lee, 2008).

## GENETICS AND BEHAVIORAL EPIGENETICS

Genes have a role, but they are not fate. There are definitely environmental factors involved also. This is a disease of gene and environmental interaction.

Both anxiety and depressive disorders are the result of variable and multiple complex interactions between genes and environmental influences. About 30–40 percent of the variance contributing to these disorders is heritable (Norrhom & Ressler, 2009). A person has a two- to threefold risk of depression if a first-degree relative has the disease and somewhat less risk if an aunt or uncle has it (Hyman & Greenberger, 2001.

Although some experts have postulated that a single gene may be responsible for anxiety and depression, no single gene has been shown to cause these disorders so far. The greater likelihood is that multiple genes combined with environment are involved.

The main area of genetic focus has been on hereditary genetic polymorphisms (variations) for the serotonin transporter (5-HTT) in the brain that may be triggered by stress. An association between these polymorphisms and mental disorders has been reported by some, but not all, investigators. The long allele (type or variation) of the *5-HTT* gene is associated with higher expression of brain 5-HTT, while the short allele is associated with reduced 5-HTT expression and function (Weizman & Weizman, 2000). People with a history of child abuse or other major life stressors who have the short allele for this transporter are about twice as likely to develop depression as those who have the long allele (Beers & Berkow, 1999, 1526). Similarly, in anxiety, individuals with one or two copies of the short *5-HTT* allele experience increased fear and anxiety-related behaviors and greater amygdala neuronal activity in response to fearful stimuli compared with individuals homozygous for the long allele (Hariri et al., 2002), and they also have greater startle response (Brocke et al., 2006).

A study by Caspi et al. (2003) strongly intimated that the reason some people bounce back after a stressful life event while others plunge into lasting despair was due to a functional polymorphism in the promoter region of the *5-HTT* gene. This research followed 847 people from birth to age 26 and found that those most likely to sink into depression after a stressful event (e.g., job loss, sexual abuse, bankruptcy) had the gene polymorphism. The authors suggested that individuals with one or two copies of the short *5-HTT* allele exhibited more depressive symptoms, diagnosable depression, and suicidality in relation to stressful life events than individuals homozygous for the long allele.

In a meta-analysis of all the studies relating to this gene polymorphism, Risch et al. (2009) looked at over 14,250 participants in 14 studies published from 2003 through early 2009 and found that stressful life events clearly increased the risk of depression. However, the short *5-HTT* allele did not show a relationship to increased risk for major depression, alone or in interaction with stressful life events. Risch et al. concluded that there is "no evidence of an association between the serotonin gene and the risk of depression," no matter what people's life experience was. This substantiates other research suggesting there is no relationship between serotonin and depression. Even more, the drug tianeptine (Coaxil), a serotonin reuptake enhancer, which works completely opposite of SSRIs by helping break down serotonin at faster rates, has been shown to be as effective as SSRIs in depression and more effective than some at lowering anxiety (Wagstaff, Ormrod, & Spencer, 2001).

Other candidate genes being considered as playing possible roles in anxiety and depression include those for the dopamine receptor D4 (*DRD4*) and catechol-O-methyltransferase (*COMT*). Dopamine is highly implicated in anxiety, depression, and attention-deficit challenges. The DRD4 receptor is a target for drugs that treat schizophrenia and Parkinson disease. Polymorphisms of the *DRD4* gene are associated with anxiety disorders, including obsessive compulsive, avoidant disorders and depression (Tochigi et al., 2006). The *COMT* gene is mostly considered in relationship to anxiety. It is involved with helping to breakdown dopamine. People who had variations in the *COMT* gene showed more anxiety when given personality tests and had higher startle responses when given uncomfortable scenes to watch. Generally, those with the *COMT* variation are higher-level thinkers, with higher levels of anxiety. It is possible that people with this genetic change may keep higher levels of dopamine, epinephrine, and other neurotransmitters around and are less able to take their attention away from unpleasant pictures and sounds (Montag et al., 2008).

## Behavioral Epigenetics: Proof That Holistic Medicine Makes Sense

Genetic variances may play a role in mood disorder, but it seems genes themselves are not the only determinants, and may not be even the main determinants, for anxiety and depression. Beyond the genes themselves, there lies an overarching contributing factor likely much more important.

Epigenetics is the study of gene expression caused by factors other than the hard-wired DNA sequences. The field of epigenetics clearly supports and helps explain the critical role that nutrition, diet, and environment play in mental and emotional health. For decades, biomedicine did not believe the important roles that lifestyle, stress, and foods play in health. It was thought you were dealt all your genetic cards at birth, and what was going to happen will happen, with no way to change your genes.

Then, studies from Hebrew University by Howard Cedar and Aharon Razin laid the foundation for understanding that molecules called methylators could play a role in whether certain genes were expressed or repressed. Methylators are molecules that bind to genes, locking and unlocking the genetic codes, in a process called methylation. Studies by Cedar and Razin (1994) found that methylation was altered by the foods we ate and by environmental factors, such as the level of human touch and nurture we received as children.

Today we know about 30 percent of genes are considered "household genes"—genes that turn on and off automatically and are not under environmental control. Eye color is an example of a household gene, for no matter what foods one eats, or how much one exercises, eye color will not change. However, the good news is that about 70 percent of genes are "luxury genes," meaning these genes may be turned on or off based on how we bathe our genes through choices in food, lifestyle, sleep, exercise, toxin burden, and even supplementation (Bland, 2002).

These lifestyle choices will turn up or down the volume of a gene, not unlike how you can turn the volume control on a radio speaker. Cedar and Rozin's work helped us understand this mechanism. Now we know healthy green vegetables are methyl donors, and this is a reason they can be so protective against cancer. In fact, a very large epidemiologic study in the United Kingdom suggests that cancer is about 40 or 45 percent (women or men, respectively) preventable by diet and lifestyle factors (Parkin., 2011). So, given the right foods, exercise, and so forth, we can "turn down" the expression of cancer genes up to 45 percent. There is no drug that can boast such a record. If there was, we would all be taking it.

The HPA section above discussed how experiences of trauma in a pregnant mother's past will predispose children to anxiety and depression. This is due to changes in methylation. So, epigenetic behavioral and psychological traits will also be passed on to the next generation without any changes to the genetic code itself.

Even the foods our grandmother ate while pregnant changed methylation patterns on our DNA, creating "scars" that can remain floating on top of our genetic code, modifying its expression. Methylation patterns placed by foods and traumatic events can even be passed from one generation to the next. For example, studies of rats show that a fatty diet during a grandmother's pregnancy will significantly increase breast cancer incidence in the grandchildren. In one study, 80 percent of the rats given breast-cancer-causing carcinogens that had two high-fat diet grandmothers developed breast tumors, versus only 30 percent who that grandmothers who ate healthful diets (De Assis et al., 2010).

In the early 1990s, Michael Meany and Moshe Szyf ushered in the concept of behavorial epigenetics. They postulated that not only could diets or toxins change genetic expression, but physical touch and stressful events could as well. By the 2000s their group was clearly outlining the epigenetic importance of touch in early life. Looking at rat pups, they found epigenetic changes in the glucocorticoid receptor with increased rates of gene methylation. Rat pups raised by inattentive mothers had lower levels of the receptor due to this lack of touch and caring, had lower glucocorticoid receptor expression in brain areas like the hippocampus, and went on to have much higher anxiety levels and startle responses. The rat pups that were given healthy amounts of attention had balanced receptor expression, were much calmer, and showed less fear (Weaver et al., 2004). Postmortem studies in humans corroborate these findings (Malavaez et al., 2009).

This knowledge of behavioral epigenetics certainly strengthens what we know about psychological work and CAM. It also inspires us to know that this work is not merely palliative or placebo but instead can actually change gene expression for the better in the current generation and for generations to come.

## NEUROTRANSMITTERS

A neurotransmitter is a chemical signal released from one end of a nerve fiber (usually called the presynaptic nerve terminal) into the synaptic cleft (space between neurons) that transfers an impulse to the next nerve fiber. The theory of brain neurotransmitter action has been the underpinning of psychiatric treatment for much the past 60 years.

The tricyclic antidepressant imipramine has been utilized since 1948 for the treatment of depression, although its mechanism of action was not understood. In 1965, the biogenic amine hypothesis suggested that reduced levels of the neurotransmitter norepinephrine were associated with depression (Schildkraut, 1965). This partly explained the reason why imipramine seemed to help some people with depression and motivated the continued interest in using drugs to manipulate neurotransmitters for depression.

Conventional care began utilizing tranquilizers for anxiety disorder in the 1950s as a means to calm anxious patients. In 1955, chlordiazepoxide (Librium) became the first benzodiazepine antianxiety drug. Benzodiazepines help calm the brain by binding to receptors for the neurotransmitter gamma-aminobutyric acid (GABA). GABA is the main inhibitory neurotransmitter in the brain and calms overall brain activity. Most of today's anxiety and sleeping medications still rely on this benzodiazepine effect.

Antianxiety and antidepressant medications rely on the neurotransmitter theory. However, I hope this book has already clued you in that your client's anxiety and depression are not as cut-and-dried as simply modulating levels of neurotransmitters.

When it comes to anxiety treatment, pharmaceutical therapy is clearly superior to placebo in all antianxiety drug categories. Benzodiazepines (e.g., alprazolam, lorazepam, and diazepam), which work on boosting the neurotransmitter GABA, and azapirones (e.g., buspirone), which upregulate serotonin and dopamine, were both shown equally effective (Mitte et al., 2005). When selective serotonin reuptake inhibitors (SSRIs) are used for anxiety, these also seem to have an effect greater than placebo, although they are not as effective at symptom management as the benzodiazepines. While antianxiety medications are effective and widely prescribed medications, they are best used in the short term. As discussed in the introduction of this book, long-term use of benzodiazepines for anxiety does not fix the underlying causes. Long-term use eventually leads to dependence, resistance, withdrawal syn-dromes, and increased rates for all-cause mortality. This is a reason that psychological therapy and holistic modalities are so important.

Both side effect profiles and efficacy are not good for antidepres-sants. They are linked to greater likelihood of headaches, insomnia, rashes, muscle aches, gastrointestinal symptoms, sexual problems, tera-togenic effects, and even depression and suicidal thoughts (Hyman, 1996). Even more, antidepressants may not actually work in most cases, for evidence suggests that depression is likely not solely a neurotransmit-ter issue. This would explain why antidepressant medications are not more effective than placebo (both have ~30 percent efficacy rate) in all but severe cases (Fournier et al., 2010).

## The Psychopharmacology–CAM Relationship

A holistic practitioner knows that even when the drugs are effective at relieving symptoms, the underlying cause of the mood problem has still not been addressed. From a psychology standpoint, it also seems to me that these drugs confer greater long-term vulnerability by giving the patient the sense that something out of a bottle is needed to feel healthy. This takes control away from the patient—lacking control over our lives is a central theme in anxiety and depression. I often tell my patients that "depression or anxiety is not a (insert name of drug du jour here) defi-ciency." Encouraging patients that they need something from a bottle, whether it is a drug or natural supplement, to stay balanced and healthy ultimately depletes the sense of control and reinforces anxiety and depression.

Even more, the use of a medication during the "hard times" does not allow a sufferer of anxiety or depression to healthily move through the difficult period to gain coping mechanisms and, ultimately, wisdom. I have worked with patient after patient who complain how weak they feel when there is a new traumatic life event (loss of a loved one or job, or moving a household), because they were put on drugs for the last event and never learned to cope on their own. I have also seen patient after patient who find, even after years of the initial event, that when they finally get off the medications, the original feelings of anxiety or depression come right back, necessitating the need for more medication.

This is why the CAM approach of addressing diet, lifestyle, and nutrients is so important. Medications do serve a purpose and can be miraculous in helping a patient move through a severely rough patch—in some instances, the drugs can be lifesaving. However, the CAM practitioner, along with the psychotherapist, will be invaluable in helping your client understand how to support the body to eventually heal, instead of simply focusing on neurotransmitters and symptoms.

In his book *Manufacturing Depression*, psychotherapist Gary Greenberg retells an old joke about an inebriated man dropped his car keys one night in a mostly dark parking lot. He was looking for them over and over in an area surrounding the only lighted lamppost that was lit. A police officer came up to him and said, "Hey friend, you could have lost your keys anywhere in this parking lot—why do you only looking over here?" The drunk man responded, "Because the light is better."

As you read this section, please remember that often in medicine we tend to keep myopically searching "where the light is better." The truth is, if neurotransmitters were the major issue in depression, medications that alter neurotransmitters would work most of the time. If anti-anxiety medications healed the underlying causes, people wouldn't relapse.

In this book, I refer to neurotransmitters probably too often. In my defense, I do this because the available research focuses on these—research that is driven mostly by pharmaceutical sales. Even research to study natural medicines is too often considered with regard to neurotransmitters and compares them to drugs in that light. Nevertheless, we can learn from this approach as long as we keep it in perspective as a smaller part of the whole picture.

Below is a summary of the major neurotransmitters considered when approaching anxiety and depression. Chapter 4 discusses natural ways to balance these.

## Dopamine

Dopamine is considered a monoamine and catecholamine and specifically is the precursor to epinephrine. It is implicated as a "feel good" neurotransmitter, where its release causes euphoria, focused attention to pursue a goal, and a sense of reward.

Evidence from clinical investigations supports the finding that depressed patients have reduced cerebrospinal levels of homovanillic acid, which is the main metabolite of dopamine (Robinson & Donald, 2007). Neuroimaging studies of medication-free depressed patients have found a functional deficiency of synaptic dopamine. Animals exhibiting "learned helplessness" behavior show dopamine depletion in the brain areas of the caudate nucleus and nucleus accumbens. This depletion can be prevented by pretreatment with a dopamine agonist. In the "forced swim test," another animal model of depression, the immobility of animals can be reversed by administration of the dopamine-norepinephine reuptake inhibitor nomifensine, as well as by tricyclic antidepressants. Dopamine antagonists have been shown to block the beneficial effects of antidepressants in animal models (Meyer et al., 2006). (*Agonists* are molecules that can dock to receptors and turn on an effect; *antagonists* bind to a receptor and block any effect from happening.)

Dopamine also plays an important role in fear and anxiety by modulating the medial prefrontal cortex activity on the output of the brain's amygdala. The amygdala's role is to help connect life situations with helpful emotional reactions. Dopamine has an important influence on the movement of impulses between the basolateral and central nuclei of amygdala (de la Mora et al., 2010). Adequate dopamine effects on the amygdala, and greater ability of the amygdala to store dopamine, seem to help it communicate best with a part of the prefrontal cortex called the anterior cingulate cortex, which keeps trait and baseline anxiety lower (Kienast et al., 2008).

**Some Basic Lifestyle and Herbal Methods to Support Dopamine:**
- *Creating a new goal*, and planning small steps to achieve that goal.

- *Meditation:* a study in 80 experienced meditation practitioners found meditating can raise dopamine 65 percent (Kjaer et al., 2002).
- *Regular daily exercise.*
- *Green tea:* a few cups a day.
- *Eating foods that contain tyrosine and phenylalanine,* which are dopamine precursors: chicken, turkey, eggs, beef, fish, yogurt, tofu, edamame, peanuts, sesame seeds, and pumpkin seeds.
- *Mucuna pruriens* (see Chapter 4 for more about this herb).

### Epinephrine and Norepinephrine

Epinephrine and norepinephrine are stress hormones made in the body's adrenal glands. The word *epinephrine* translates to "on the kidney" (*epi-* + *nephros*), in reference to the adrenal gland's anatomic location. Known as catecholamines, epinephrine and norepinephrine (called adrenaline and noradrenaline in the United Kingdom) are made in the outer cortex of the adrenal gland during stress and are responsible for feeling awake, alert, and motivated. Triggers of epinephrine include danger, surprises, light, temperature, and excitement. Epinephrine spurs the release of norepinephrine in the brain, which imparts psychological effects.

Epinephrine and norepinephrine were the first neurotransmitters to be considered in the mechanism of depression. According to the catecholamine theory of mood, the major symptoms of depression arise primarily from a deficiency in catecholamine neurotransmitters between nerve cells in the brain. Increasing catecholamine availability improves mood and has antidepressant effects (Millan et al., 2006). However, studies on middle-age adults found that higher levels of depression and anxiety symptoms are related to increased 24-hour urinary norepinephrine excretion, showing that depression and anxiety are associated with increased sympathetic nervous system activity (Hughes et al., 2004). In my experience with patients, those who exhibit depression over many years usually have low catecholamine levels, while those who have depression with anxiety, or recent-onset depression, usually have higher catecholamines.

Traditional antidepressants such as the tricyclic antidepressants and the seldom used monoamine oxidase (MAOI) inhibitors increase concentrations of catecholamine neurotransmitters in the brain by inhibiting either neurotransmitter reuptake or their breakdown. The catecholamine theory seems to have some validity, for it has been shown that these drugs have no effect in mice that cannot make any of their own norepinephrine.

**Suggestions for Lowering Epinephrine:**
- Regular healthy sleep schedule.
- Avoiding caffeine.
- Meditation.
- Ashwagandha and essential fatty acids (see Chapter 4 for these).

## Gamma-Aminobutyric Acid (GABA)

Like a gentle blanket for the brain, GABA is the primary calming and inhibitory transmitter in the central nervous system. Low GABA levels and GABA pathophysiology are associated anxiety, depression, irritability, and sleeplessness (Möhler, 2012). Interestingly, alcohol seems to stabilize GABA and increase GABA release, which may be why alcohol has a temporary calming effect.

**Some Methods to Naturally Raise GABA:**
- Tea—a specific type called oolong may enhance GABA response (Hossain et al., 2004).
- Meditation and relaxation work (see Chapter 5).
- Supplemental GABA (see Chapter 4) and valerian (see Chapter 2).

## Glutamate

While GABA is the main calming neurotransmitter, the neurotransmitter glutamate is one of the main excitatory neurotransmitters and also the most common neurotransmitter in the brain and a major mood player. Glutamate is also a player in the inflammatory process, where its buildup leads to toxicity and neuronal cell death, contributing to the pathophysiology of both anxiety and depression. The brains frontal cortex coordinates planning, decision making, and problem solving. Autopsy studies found elevated glutamate levels and more inflammation in the frontal cortex of depressed patients (Czyzewski, 2007) compared with those without depression. Stress will disrupt normal balance and clearance of glutamate. High-carbohydrate diets lead to impaired glutamate signaling and increased oxidative damage in the brain.

Glutamate binds to the N-methyl-D-aspartate (NMDA) receptor. Drugs that block NMDA receptors have a strong antidepressant effect. Ketamine is an anesthetic drug that has hallucinogenic properties. Known on the street as "special K," ketamine is an NMDA glutamate receptor antagonist, which effectively blocks NMDA receptors. Besides its recreational effects, ketamine has been shown to have an amazing antidepressant effect within 3 days of use (Berman et al., 2000)—the quickest-acting antidepressant known. Unfortunately, ketamine has a very high side effect profile and is limited by psychomimetic side effects (psychosis, delusions, and delirium) and high abuse potential.

### Natural Methods to Balance Glutamate:
- Avoid foods that contain monosodium glutamate.
- Stress reduction techniques: acupuncture, meditation, yoga, mindfulness-based stress reduction.
- Minimize intake of simple carbohydrates.
- Avoid environmental toxic metal exposure.

### Oxytocin

Oxytocin is the neurotransmitter best associated with feelings of love, meaningful touch, cuddling, and combating anxiety. Oxytocin helps reduce hyperactivity of the amygdala (a fear center of the brain) and helps block the perception of a threatening environment. High levels of oxytocin are consistent with bonding experiences, regular community interaction, and consistent social engagement. Oxytocin can even be released by petting a dog. Those who trust are able to release appropriate amounts of oxytocin, whereas humans who have social anxiety disorder have dysregulated oxytocin.

Oxytocin may play a dual role in the effect of social situations, reinforcing both positive and negative experiences. Adults who were abused in early life show lowered levels of oxytocin (Heim et al., 2009). Mice tested in stressful situations that did not have oxytocin receptors seemed not to show fear when the events were repeated, whereas those with working oxytocin receptors remembered interactions with aggressive mice and remained fearful (Guzmán et al., 2013).

Intranasal administration of oxytocin has shown to substantially increase trust among humans (Kosfeld et al., 2005). Oxytocin preparations are currently being tested as antianxiety drugs in several clinical trials (Hofman, 2013).

**Natural Methods to Increase Oxytocin:**
- Receiving a massage
- Hugging others and physical intimacy
- Cooking aromatic foods and then eating them
- Physical activity and exercise
- Community and social involvement
- Lithium supplementation (see Chapter 4)

### Serotonin

The focal point for many antidepressant and anxiety drugs, serotonin (5-hydroxytryptamine, 5-HT) has a widespread cellular distribution in the body and brain. It is considered to be calming and important for best sleep and appetite. Gaining confidence and feeling respect also trigger serotonin. High levels can promote agitation.

Interestingly, serotonin was originally discovered as the molecule that allowed the clam adductor muscle to remain chronically tight to keep its shell closed while expending minimal energy. Serotonin is found in many tissues, including blood platelets, intestinal mucosa, and the central nervous system. Some biologists called this molecule enteramine (*entera* refers to the gut) due to its high levels in squid and octopus digestive tracts; other researchers who found it in the blood named it serotonin. About 90 percent of our serotonin supply is found in the digestive tract—a likely connection between mood disorder and digestive dysfunction. With this pleiotropism (effects throughout the body), serotonin is implicated in many physiologic effects, including inhibition of gastric secretion (stopping enzymes needed for digestion), stimulation of smooth muscles (which can lead to diarrhea), vasoconstriction (tightening vessels for higher blood pressure), brain communication, and mood effect.

While there are numerous receptors for serotonin, this section focuses on 5-HT1A, the receptor for anxiety. Studies in mice showed that without the receptor they were much more prone to anxiety as adults (Donaldson et al., 2014). People may be predisposed to anxiety if serotonin levels are low. Serotonin is a likely factor in oxytocin levels, as there is evidence that oxytocin exerts anxiolytic (anxiety-relieving) effects via oxytocin receptors expressed in serotonergic neurons (Yoshida et al., 2009). SSRI (selective serotonin reuptake inhibitors) antidepressants preferentially increase serotonin levels by inhibiting its breakdown.

Serotonin was linked to depression in a landmark study by Coppen et al. (1965), who postulated serotonin's involvement in depressive illness. Serotonin's involvement may be due to low production, downregulation of its receptors, inability of serotonin to reach the receptor sites, or a shortage of tryptophan substrate (tryptophan is the amino acid the body uses to make serotonin). But serotonin is not the only actor on the depression stage. Some research suggests that synaptic depletion of serotonin may promote a fall in norepinephrine levels. Prange et al. (1974) wrote about the possibilities that alterations in mood were due to a deficit of serotonin plus either a deficit or excess of norepinephrine. This dual neurotransmitter approach lives on today in the debate as to whether single (SSRIs) or dual (*serotonin-norepinephrine reuptake inhibitors*) uptake blockers are actually more effective in treating depression.

Interestingly, the serotonin hypothesis of depression presumes that depression is caused by a serotonin deficiency. It is not well known that this has actually never been shown to be true. In fact, to confuse the situation, tianeptine, a medication that acts as a serotonin antagonist and decreases serotonin effects, is as effective as the SSRIs (Maas et al., 1984; Wagstaff et al., 2001). This tells us we still have a lot to learn about serotonin.

### How to Naturally Enhance Serotonin:
- Focusing on those who love and respect you, as well as working on increasing self-esteem
- Good sleep
- Morning bright light
- Supplemental tryptophan and 5-hydroxytryptophan (see Chapter 4)
- Supplemental melatonin at night (see Chapter 2)


## DETOXIFICATION AND MOOD DISORDER

The preceding section discussed the main neurotransmitters for brain chemistry and mood. This section shifts gears to look at a factor in neurodegenerative diseases like Parkinson's and cognitive decline and discusses how common environmental toxins such as heavy metals, bisphenol A from plastics, and pesticides can build up in the brain and nervous system and be a contributing factor to anxiety and depression. A controversial subject, there is relatively little information about the role toxins play in mood disorders. Hence, there is widespread disagreement as to the benefit of treatment. As we learn more, this subject will likely be at the vanguard of helping to balance mood.


### Heavy Metal Toxicity

Conventional medicine generally does not commonly consider neurologic problems with heavy metal toxicity, save for clear cause-and-effect situations. One example of such cause and effect is of lead paint exposure in children. Plentiful evidence shows that lead will cause insomnia, irritability, nervousness, aggressive behavior, and unwanted anxiety and depression-like symptoms.

CAM doctors and holistic clinicians are often criticized by mainstream care for treating "metal toxicity" because clear evidence does not warrant this approach except in clear-cut massive exposures. Nevertheless, this is a subject worth discussing. Emerging information reveals that toxic exposures can accumulate insidiously over time to cause slow degeneration of brain and nervous system tissue, resulting in more subtle mood dysregulation in predisposed individuals. Long-term heavy metal exposure may lead to apoptotic events (neuronal suicide) in susceptible brain and nervous system tissue. In an epidemiologic study, Stokes et al. (1998) compared 281 young adults who had environmental lead exposure as children with 287 nonexposed control subjects. Exposed subjects had significantly more neuropsychiatric symptoms 20 years after initial exposure.

The metals most commonly associated with depression are cadmium, lead (Shih et al., 2006), and mercury (Siblerud, 1989). These heavy metals are very common in our environment. Industry, dental amalgams, welding work, cigarettes, and galvanized water pipes are common sources. Natural medicines have even been implicated, as contamination of Ayurvedic (Saper et al., 2004) and Chinese herbs (Ko et al., 1998) has caused documented heavy metal exposures. Some preparations, such as rinchen rilbu ("Precious Pills") used in Tibetan medicine purposefully contain trace amounts of hundreds of ingredients, including mercury, gold, and iron.

Heavy metals create clear mechanistic changes in physiology. They deplete antioxidant reserves, which leads to inflammatory reactions and oxidative stress (Flora, Mehta, & Gupta., 2008). These metals have high affinity for thiol (sulfur) groups found within enzymes and proteins and impair cell function by inhibiting their normal metabolic workings. Metals that are lipophilic (able to go across fat membranes) are able to cross the blood-brain barrier easily and attach themselves to fatty myelin sheaths, as well as cell membranes (Nagamura et al., 2002). For example, if we eat oils or fish with heavy metals, these can easily get into the body and the brain. Once there, inflammatory levels in the brain skyrocket and contribute to mood disorder. In a cyclic fashion, inflammation further makes brain cells more vulnerable to a number of toxins.

The brain uses a very elaborate system to remove glutamate, a neurotransmitter that can be very toxic to brain cells. Mercury, aluminum, and other toxins can easily damage the reuptake proteins the brain uses to remove glutamate, thus rendering the brain cells more easily damaged (Aschner et al., 2007; Allen, 2002). Inflammation causes excess immune cytokine production, which can also affect these reuptake proteins, allowing smaller amounts of toxin to have a greater effect. This creates a cycle of toxicity, oxidation, and inflammation that becomes hard to break.

*Symptoms of anxiety and depression caused by heavy metals*
Exposure to mercury can give rise to the symptoms and traits often found in autistic individuals (Bernard et al., 2001). Heavy metals may contribute to anxiety as mercury is known to inhibit COMT, the enzyme discussed above that is needed to break down epinephrine. Evidence suggests that mercury will also inactivate the methionine/SAMe pathway needed to produce healthy neurotransmitter levels. (The SAMe pathway is discussed in Chapter 4.)

Self-registered symptoms of patients with mercury intolerance have revealed many commonalities with serotonin dysregulation (Mills, 1997), although test tube (*in vitro*) studies of mercury do not clearly show how mercury may regulate serotonin regulation to correlate to the psychosomatic symptoms (Marcusson, Cederbrant, & Gunnarsson, 2000). It may involve more inflammation and glutamate upregulation than serotonin—more needs to be learned.

Careful clinical history and presentation of specific symptoms may help the practitioner suspect toxicity. History of clinical exposure preceding symptoms would be a simple clue. Below is a short list of the most common symptoms. Certain compounds are specifically associated with other comorbidities, which may clues in the practitioner as to which metal may be playing a role (Bongiorno, 2010).

### Symptoms Associated with Heavy Metal Poisoning:
- Confusion
- Headaches
- Fatigue
- Numbness
- Tingling
- Tremors

### Adverse Health Effects Associated with Heavy Metals:
*Lead:* parkinsonism, cognitive decline, lower IQ, learning difficulties in children

*Mercury:* cognitive decline, mood problems, heart conditions, hypertension, infertility, immune dysfunction

*Cadmium:* osteoporosis, kidney damage, cancer

*Arsenic:* diabetes

*How to test for metal toxicity*

Clinicians can screen patients for heavy metal presence via hair, urine, or blood tests. Hair testing may be a valuable tool for evaluating methylmercury exposure but does not show the burden of elemental mercury in the body. Blood tests for heavy metals were initially developed by industry to document acute exposure. As a result, checking the blood for heavy metals is useful for current and acute high exposure but does not show past exposure, nor does it illustrate total body burden, meaning how much has settled out of the blood and into the tissues (Crinnion, 2009).

Urine tests can be done by simply checking the urine for the presence of metals, or by provocation, where the client first takes chelating agents (molecules that help pull metals out of the tissues and back into the blood, where it filters out into the urine). Urine tests without provocation will show current toxic exposure. Provocative tests using a heavy-metal chelating agent such as oral dimercaptosuccinic acid (DMSA) or intravenous 2,3-dimercapto-1-propanesulfonic acid (DMPS) will help assess if there is body burden of the metal. It is important to note that these tests are not controlled and do not suggest a reliable reference range. As such, it is unclear how accurate this is as a test for body burden. Unlike blood sugar tests, where there is a known standard and reference range, these chelation tests do not necessarily tell us whether a person's burden is supraphysiologic and pathologic to the level of causing disease (Hibbs, J., personal communication, 2013). Much more research and calibration are needed before these tests reliably assess metal body burden in a way that allows us to use this test as truly diagnostic. Nevertheless, for a patient with depression or anxiety that has not been helped by other dietary, lifestyle, and supplemental means, metal testing and detoxification may be a valuable next step.

If it decided to try to remove heavy metals from the body, chelation choices include foods and supplements with chelation properties, oral chelation, intravenous chelation, and rectal suppository chelation.

The characteristics of an ideal chelator include the following:

- Affinity for the toxic metal
- Low toxicity itself
- Ability to penetrate cell membranes
- Rapid elimination of metal
- High water solubility

It should be noted that some vitamins have a known protective role during metal chelation. In theory, when a person is being administrated chelation, release of the heavy metals may increase oxidant burden. Vitamin E (tocopherols and tocotrienols) is a fat-soluble vitamin known to be one of the most potent endogenous (made-in-the-body) antioxidants. Tocopherols and tocotrienols comprising vitamin E are potent, lipid-soluble, chain-breaking antioxidants that may prevent the propagation of free radical reactions. Vitamin C is a water-soluble antioxidant occurring in the body as an ascorbic anion that acts as a scavenger of free radicals and plays an important role in regeneration of the tocopherols. Supplementation with ascorbic acid and alpha-tocopherol has been known to alter the extent of DNA damage in arsenic-intoxicated animals (Ramanathan et al., 2005). Coadministration of antioxidants with another chelating agent has shown to improve removal of toxic metals from the system, as well as achieve better and faster clinical recoveries in animal models (Flora, Mittal, & Mehta, 2008).

There is unfortunately scant human clinical research studies supporting the use of chelation for any disease at this time. Anecdotal reports of patients (including a number I have seen myself) who have had chelation for mood care have noted less depression, more alertness, and better memory. As of this writing, there are no known published studies of chelation to treat any mood disorder. While a systemic review by Seely, Wu & Mills (2005) found that controlled scientific studies did not support chelation therapy for heart disease, the National Institutes of Health (NIH) Trial to Assess Chelation Therapy (TACT) begun in 2003 and completed six years later did find a very modest benefit for heart disease. This trial used a treatment originally used to remove lead from the body: office-based, intravenous disodium ethylenediaminetetraacetic acid ($Na_2EDTA$), a chelating substance that binds to lead and other heavy metals and removes them from the body through the urine. Post-heart-attack patients older than 50 who were administered 40 chelation infusions experienced 18 percent fewer cardiovascular events (a nonsignificant value) versus placebo in five years, and chelation was found to be safe (Lamas et al., 2013). This is interesting, for there are a number of underlying factors common to depression, anxiety, and cardiovascular disease—particularly regarding inflammation in the blood. Unfortunately, these studies did not track mood changes. Hopefully, future studies will look at possible mood benefits.

## Chemical Toxicity

Besides the ubiquity of metals, another environmental concern is the various chemical assaults that may also lead to depression. These often hail from the use plastics, insecticides, herbicides, and the thousands of other industrial and household chemicals. These chemicals are known contributors to diabetes, obesity, cancers, and hormonal challenges. These chemicals, found in the plastics that line our food packaging, receipts, water pipes, and medical tubing, are easily brought into the body and enter directly into the blood.

*Bisphenols*

Often referred to as endocrine disruptors, bisphenols occur in plastics and act as synthetic estrogens, increasing anxiety and depression, especially in kids. Females exposed prenatally to high levels of bisphenol A (BPA) are more likely to be anxious, depressed, and hyperactive by age 3 (Perera et al., 2012). Exposure in the womb or during early childhood in boys correlates with anxiety issues by age 7. Exposure by age 5 correlates with hyperactivity, internalizing challenges, anxiety, depression, inattention, and attention- deficit hyperactivity disorder in both girls and boys by age 7 (Harley et al., 2013). Boys were affected with greater levels of aggressive behavior. These effects are comparable to those found in other research on high exposure to toxins such as lead, mercury, and pesticides.

*Pesticides and solvents*

The primary toxic action of pesticides and solvents is disrupting healthy neurologic function. In addition to being neurotoxic, these compounds are particularly harmful to both the immune and endocrine (hormonal) systems (Crinnion, 2000). As discussed in Chapter 4, the production of the methyl group donor SAMe is integral for neurotransmitter production and mood regulation. SAMe pathway function is inhibited by both heavy metals and pesticides,. Vitamin B12 is a necessary component of the SAMe pathway and is itself reliant on the master body antioxidant glutathione for its own methylation. Excess oxidative stressors like pesticides and heavy metals deplete glutathione, which places B12 production in jeopardy (Watson, Munter, & Golding, 2004). Insufficient B12 production eventually leads to insufficient production of neurotransmitters. According to the World Health Organization, higher concentrations of a class of pesticides called organophosphates correlated with

Table 3.1 Sources of Toxins and How to Avoid Them

| Agent | Sources | How to avoid |
|-------|---------|--------------|
| Heavy metals | Shoes | • Take off shoes at entrance of home |
| | Pollution | • Use air filtration in home, or at least in the bedroom |
| | Fish | • Eat low-mercury fish |
| | Cigarettes | • Stop smoking and avoid second-hand smoke |
| | Dental fillings | • Avoid mercury or amalgam fillings |
| | Water pipers | • Change water pipes |
| | Drinking water | • Drink well-filtered water |
| | Rice | • Rinse rice; purchase California-grown rice |
| | Salt | • Check for contamination |
| | Vaccines | • Limit vaccines to only those absolutely necessary |
| | Antiperspirants | • Try natural deodorants |
| Pesticides | Foods | • Eat organic foods as much as possible |
| | Lawn | • Avoid pesticide use on lawn, in household, and on yard plants |
| Bisphenol A | Plastics | • Use glass and stainless steel containers |
| | Receipts | • Avoid and wash hands after touching receipts |
| | Packing | • Minimize foods in plastics and plastic-lined cans; especially avoid #7 plastic |

regions with higher rates of suicide and severe anxiety disorders (Zhang et al., 2009).

Intravenous glutathione may be a solution, albeit a temporary one, to naturally relieve mood disorder. Davies (2008) cites anecdotal evidence of over 100 depressed patients in a private naturopathic practice who have received intravenous glutathione. Glutathione supports the SAMe pathway by helping to create the intermediate complex glutathionylcobalamin, which is needed to keep B12 methylated. Davies (2008) reports these treatments have temporary results, which suggests that glutathione may not actually aid the removal of toxins but instead may reduce inflammation and help push the folate-methionine cycle for a limited time.

Table 3.1 summarizes sources and methods to avoid toxins in the environment that may factor into depression and anxiety.

# FOUR

# Effective Supplements for Anxiety and Depression

---

### *Case Study: Deanna*

*Deanna was a 35-year-old female who came to see me after spending eight years dealing with alternating bouts of anxiety and depression along with constant weight gain and, most recently, sleeplessness. She had seen a host of both conventional and natural medicine practitioners. When she came to see me she was taking Celexa, trazodone at night, SAMe, theanine, fish oils, valerian, B complex, vitamin C, and Bach Flower Remedies. She told me she thought the Celexa did help her stay less anxious during the day, and the trazodone knocked her out at night enough to get four or five hours of uninterrupted sleep.*

*For her first visit, we discussed diet, sleep rituals, lifestyle, exercise, and her supplements. Regarding her diet, Deanna and I rearranged her food intake, for generally she ate too many carbohydrates (even though they were healthier ones like bananas, yogurt, granola)—which may have played a part by creating a yo-yo effect with her blood sugar and mood. We added a good protein shake in the morning and made sure she ate some kind of protein in the afternoon (e.g., fish, beans, or poultry) to go with her daily lunchtime salad. She committed to get back to her exercise regimen, which she loved, but "got too busy for." We spent most of the time discussing all the supplements she was taking. When I asked her which ones were helping her the most, she stared at me with a blank look. So, I recommended she remove each of them (except for the fish oils), one every four days. At first she told me she was so surprised that "a naturopath would tell me not to take supplements" and then confided that she was a "bit scared to let them go." I told her it was clear to me that if any of them were getting the job done, she would not have made a visit to see me. So, she agreed to try my approach.*

*Deanna returned in a month feeling about "30 percent better," with much less anxiety, but still the low mood persisted. We discussed the need for meditation, added a multiple vitamin, increased her fish oil amount, and started a probiotic. She returned in two weeks and proclaimed her anxiety may have increased a bit, but the depression was lifting. In fact, at this visit, she was more worried about the weight gain she sustained over the last eight years simply from eating too much. While she blamed herself repeatedly, I reminded her that high levels of stress and cortisol, as well as the Celexa, are probably at fault for the weight issues. I also reminded her that blaming and beating herself up regularly will have to give way to talking nicely to herself—something her therapist had already started working on with her. At that point I took out a bottle of 50 mg 5-hydroxytryptophan (5-HTP). Because the moderately helpful Celexa artificially raises serotonin, I was thinking using some 5-HTP to help her body naturally produce more might do the trick. I told her I thought it may be the perfect choice for her for it is helpful as an appetite suppressant for weight loss, helps her stay asleep (two items not accomplished by Celexa), and works well for depression and anxiety—she fit the picture perfectly for this particular natural remedy. We started at 50 mg three times a day between meals for the first week and went up to 100 mg three times a day. By the third week, she was 90 percent better—and claimed it would be a 100 percent, but her job stress was high at the time. Within two months, her job stressed passed, she stayed at 100 percent, and began weaning off her medications over the course of two months. Within six months she no longer needed the 5-HTP and kept feeling well using diet, lifestyle, good sleep, and meditation.*

As Deanna already knew, there are a plethora of effective and promising supplements for the patient with anxiety and depression. There are more choices than the average patient could possibly try or tolerate. It is confusing to both practitioners and patients alike when deciding which may be the best. This chapter is designed to summarize both the available research-based evidence and the traditional use of these natural medicines. It will also, in naturopathic fashion, underscore particular clinical facets of each remedy to help best match the therapy for anxiety and depression.

When considering a supplement for the client with anxiety or depression, it is vital to keep in mind that supplementation should rarely be the focus of any holistic therapeutic regimen. This book has already outlined the overall determinants for health: sleep, diet, exercise, lifestyle, and toxin consideration. With Deanna, we had to reset her diet and lifestyle a bit. Even though the 5-HTP was the clincher, the setup of diet and lifestyle were a likely key to help the 5-HTP works its best. The determinants of health help balance and treat the myriad underlying causes of anxiety and depression. Like drugs, supplements by themselves will not likely get to the underlying cause. Having said this, choosing the right supplements for the right patient may prove to be mood balancing and create the desired health effect with much less chance of side effects than their pharmaceutical mates.

According to *Your Dictionary* (2013), *supplement* is defined as "something added, esp. to make up for a lack or deficiency." This is a succinct and effective definition, for it emphasizes the reasonable use of supplementation when deficiency is suspected. In comparison, the word *medication* is defined as "a substance for curing or healing, or for relieving pain." So, to compare the two, a supplement helps mitigate deficiency, whereas medications can be used to cure. Depending on the use of a supplement, it may satisfy either or both criteria. Supplements are typically used to correct a deficiency or for optimization of nutrient levels. However, certain supplements in proper doses may also act more like medication, often when prescribed in larger pharmacologic, rather than physiologic, doses.

Please note that most supplements described in this chapter also have food sources listed. If a patient is suspected to need a specific amount of a supplement, I encourage the holistic provider to also give that patient a list of healthy, whole foods, when available, that also focus on that nutritional element. As the patient learns to enjoy these foods, he or she will need to rely less and less on supplementation. It should always be noted that supplements, like drugs, should not be viewed as the "cure" but merely one step, of many healthful steps, to return the body and mind to balance.

The tables in appendix IV summarize the various supplements that can be considered for patients with anxiety or depression, which are described in further detail below. In particular, Table IV.1 lists general supplementation that should be considered for all patients with anxiety or depression.

## OILS AND FATS

The brain is made of mostly fats. Communities high in fish intake have low levels of anxiety and depressive illness. The word *essential* in nutrition means that the body needs to take something in for it cannot make its own. "Essential" fatty acid intake reduces stress hormones and perceived stress (Barbadoro et al., 2013). Very few of us take enough essential fats to combat our stressful world.

### Fish Oil

Fish oil is an important source of essential fatty acids and can be used to help form healthy brain and nervous tissue, and thus healthy mood. Numerous works have acknowledged likely benefit of using fish oil as first-line therapy or adjunctive care for anxiety and/or depression. Fish oil helps normalizes the membranes of brain tissues and simultaneously supports and calms the adrenal system during anxious and stressful times (Delarue et al., 2003), as well as encouraging a healthy cardiovascular system. Fish oil supports the nervous system by increasing nerve growth factor, a protein needed for the growth and repair of brain and nervous tissue (Thuret et al., 2007). Fish oils contain omega-3 fatty acids known as eicosapentatoic acid (EPA) and docohexanenoic acid (DHA). EPA and DHA have a long list of attributes that support mood and the nervous system (Song, Zhang, & Manku, 2009).

One of the most potent effects of fish oil is as global (throughout the body) anti-inflammatory. All cell membranes, including those of the immune system, are made of fats. Ingestion of too many saturated fats (the kind from grain-fed red meats and fried foods, sometimes referred to as omega-6 fats) make these membranes too rigid and inflexible. When they are too rigid, they can break off and cause greater inflammation in

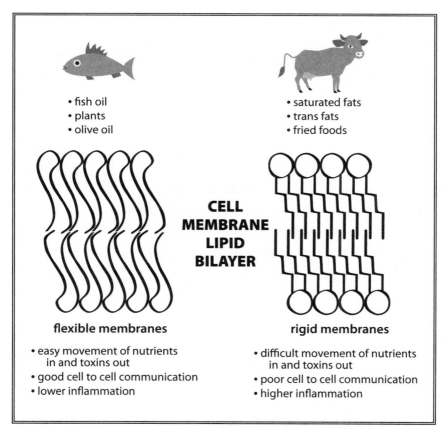

Figure 4.1. Dietary influence on cell membrane structure and function.

the body. Fish oils have unsaturated fats and create an immune system that is less able to get over inflamed.

## Some Benefits of Fish Oil

- Nerve growth factor enhancer
- Inflammation balance
- Adrenal gland support
- Cardiovascular support

Patients with both anxiety and depression report having mood-damaging imbalances in omega-3 fats, including significantly low EPA and DHA in cell tissues such as red blood cell membrane and plasma, as well as inadequate dietary intake. The lowest levels of EPA and DHA predict the presence and severity of anxiety symptoms in patients with depression (Liu et al., 2013).

Besides having low omega-3 fats, patients with depression have been shown to have an overabundance of arachidonic acid (an omega-6 fatty acid) compared with omega-3 fats (Adams, Lawson, & Sanigorski, 1996). Arachidonic acid comes from eating too many saturated fats. Lowering saturated fat intake while bringing in more fish oil helps create a more balanced ratio of omega-6 to omega-3. More balanced ratios will not only lower inflammation but also reduce the excessive clotting ability of platelets, which can potentially decrease the incidence of heart attacks and strokes. Given the relationship between depressive disorders and cardiovascular disease, it is possible omega-3 fatty acid deficiency and elevated homocysteine levels (discussed in Chapter 3), could be links between these two debilitating diseases (Severus, Littman, & Stoll, 2001).

Positron emission tomography (PET) in depressed subjects has shown low fatty acid content in specific brain regions that suffer from insuffi-cient glucose metabolism. In an uncontrolled study of 29 unmedicated depressed subjects, in which those subjects with lower levels of EPA and DHA had relatively poor glucose usage in the brain's temporoparietal lobe, Sublette et al. (2009) posited that low fatty acids discourage proper glucose metabolism in the temporoparietal area and may have an effect on depression-related cognitive problems, such as decision making and conflict resolution. The study also suggested that low levels of DHA promoted hyperfunction of the anterior cingulate and prefrontal cortex, areas known to be overactive in people with both depression and anxiety. DHA can calm these areas.

*Fish oil studies in humans*

People without diagnosed anxiety are shown to benefit from the anxiolytic (anxiety-breaking) properties of fish oil in times of stress—a reason we should probably all be taking some. Medical students are a well-known stressed-out group. Supplementation of 2.5 g/day of fish oil (2,000 mg EPA and about 350 mg DHA) or placebo given to 68 chronically stressed medical students in a placebo-controlled, double-blind, randomized controlled trial showed 14 percent lower levels of inflammatory cytokines, such as interleukin-6, and a 20 percent reduction in anxiety symptoms versus those who took a placebo over a 12-week period. It is not known if longer-term supplementation would increase the beneficial results. I give many talks at medical schools throughout the country, where I have presented this information and challenged the skeptical students to give it try. Numerous students have later reported how they really did feel the difference after taking fish oil.

A number of clinical studies support the use of fish oil for depression (Freeman, 2000). One 8-week, double-blind, placebo-controlled trial by Su et al. (2003) gave 28 depressed patients 6.6 g/day of fish oil or placebo, in addition to typical pharmaceutical and/or psychotherapy treatments. Patients taking the fish oil showed significantly improved ratings with the Hamilton Depression Inventory versus the placebo group. Su et al. suggested one reason for the benefit is fish oil's ability to install itself into neuronal membranes and support healthy electrical signal movement.

In a randomized double-blind controlled trial of 22 patients with major depressive disorder, Nemets et al. (2002) found highly significant benefits with the addition of the omega-3 fatty acid compared with placebo. These benefits were apparent by the third week of treatment. In a double-blind placebo-controlled pilot trial (da Silva et al., 2008), 31 Parkinson's patients with depression took omega-3 fatty acids for 3 months along with their antidepressant pharmaceutical therapy. Patients taking fish oil showed a clear increase of omega-3 fatty acids in red blood cell membranes, and these patients showed clear improvements in depressive symptoms. Tajalizadekhoob et al. (2011), in another double-blind, randomized, placebo-controlled study, gave low-dose fish oil therapy in 66 senior patients (1,000 mg total, breaking down to about 300 mg each of EPA and DHA), who showed clinical benefit and much greater effect over placebo, and clear differences in the Geriatric Depression scales after removing confounding factors such as body mass, thyroid dysfunction, and cholesterol. While omega-3 fatty acids have a clear albeit modest effect on anxiety, an 8-week trial using 1,050 mg/day EPA and 150 mg/day DHA suggested that those depressed patients without comorbid anxiety symptoms had a better positive response than patients who also exhibited anxiety (Lespérance et al., 2011). Double-blind placebo-controlled studies have also shown that omega-3 consumption is associated with a longer remission period in depressed patients (Parker et al., 2006).

For other mood-related disorders, Peet et al. (2002) found that 2 g/day of ethyl-EPA was the optimal dose for schizophrenia, another difficult-to-treat mood disorder. Fish oil also showed the ability to greatly reduce distress symptoms and basal cortisol secretion in abstinent alcoholics (Barbadoro et al., 2013), and 2,000 mg EPA lowered anxiety and anger scores in substance abusers (Buydens-Branchey et al., 2008). A 12-week study of bipolar depression showed that 1 or 2 g/day of ethyl-EPA significantly outperformed placebo based on the Hamilton Rating Scale for Depression and Clinical Global Impression Scale (Frangou, Lewis, & McCrone, 2006). Research is often completed on patentable forms of natural substances, such as ethyl-EPA, so that the compound can be treated as a drug and be called "FDA approved. " They thus can garner a higher price, as well as prescription status. As of this writing, it is not clear that ethyl-EPA has any greater benefit over high-quality, more natural fish oil versions.

There is also evidence that fish oil may benefit people who fail to respond to standard antidepressant medications (discussed in Chapter 6).

### Fish oil dosage

While dosages vary in different studies, a typical dosage of fish oil is 1,000 mg/day of EPA and about 800 mg/day of DHA. Read the fish oil label closely—if it does not break down the numbers, then purchase another one that does.

Also of note, you should encourage your clients to look for high-quality, pharmaceutical-grade fish oils only, for the lesser quality versions may have an increased chance of rancidity, as well as toxins and impurities. Because of our poor environmental stewardship of our seas, fish are at risk of high contaminant levels (mercury and other metals, dioxins, PCBs, etc.). Encouraging your client to purchase fish oil from a high-quality company is important. These companies use molecular distillation and assure their oil is certified contaminant-free. Molecular distillation to clear fish oil of contaminants is easily achieved by a company of integrity.

A small percentage of patients may experience reflux with fish oil, in which case they can try dosing with or away from a meal, either of which may resolve symptoms. Also, some patients report that capsules are better tolerated, while others think the liquid oil is best for them. Anecdotally, some patients report capsules kept in the refrigerator or freezer tend to minimize reflux or fishy breath. If none of the above ideas work to eliminate reflux effectively, try enteric-coated capsules. I recommend liquid fish oil taken from the a spoon if possible for three reasons: (1) capsules are significantly bigger to swallow and more expensive; (2) oil directly on the tongue sends a signal to the lower digestive tract to most adequately prepare for fat digestion; and (3) and most important, your grandmother probably recommended it this way.

*Safety of fish oil*

Fish oil is extremely safe to take (Kroes et al., 2003). Because of the concern of its anticlotting effect (commonly referred to as "blood thinning"), it is prudent to monitor clotting factors (using the blood tests thrombin time, prothrombin time, and INR) closely if considering fish oil supplementation along with anticlotting medication. I recommend discussing with the prescribing doctor about slowly adding the fish oil and checking clotting factors regularly until up to the full dose to give time for any medication adjustment, if needed. When using both together, it is important to stay consistent with the daily fish oil and medication intake. Actually, one recent study suggests fish oil does not have a negative effect on bleeding times during surgery (Kepler et al., 2012), so the concern may be exaggerated, but until we have more studies, it is important to be safe.

Many of my male patients contacted me due to one highly publicized report that fish oil increased rates of prostate cancer (Brasky et al., 2013). This was an extremely poorly designed study which surmised that higher levels of fish oils in the blood caused a 43 percent increase in low-grade prostate cancer, and an alarming 71 percent increase of high-grade cancer. The problem with this study is it was designed only to look at vitamin E and selenium intake, and never asked any of the volunteers about fish, and it based its conclusion on one sole time point of another 6 year study. Also, 80 percent of the men with prostate cancer were obese, a known factor for increasing risk of prostate cancer. Numerous studies previously have shown only safety. In fact, previous reports suggest decreases in prostate cancer risk (Terry et al., 2001; Augustsson et al., 2003). Another, *un*publicized meta-analysis of 21 studies, with almost 1 million participants, reported that consumption of fish oil and omega-3 fatty acids significantly reduces breast cancer occurrence (Zheng et al., 2013).

*Natural fish oil food sources*

Fish is by far the number one source for fish oil (big surprise). One small study supports the notion that portions of salmon or tuna twice weekly may be as effective as fish oil supplementation to raise fatty acid levels. Other studies show that intake through food may also allow for better omega-3 absorption (Harris et al., 2007; Elvevoll et al., 2006). Small fish such as anchovies, herring, and sardines are also potent omega-3 sources. Larger fish such as tuna, shark, swordfish, mackerel, and salmon may be contaminated with mercury and harmful pesticides, so caution regarding origination is important when choosing caught fish (please see list of low-mercury fishes in chapter 2). Chicken, eggs, and beef can also be sources of omega-3 fatty acids if the animals eat green plants and not just grains. Restraint-free grass-fed animals are recommended.

### Gamma-Linolenic Acid (GLA)

Related to fatty acids, another known factor in mood resides in some depressed people's genetic inability to manufacture enough prostaglandin E1 (PGE1), an immune system molecule that is important for best mood. Derived from EPA, PGE1 helps maintain neurotransmitter levels in the brain to support positive mood and calm. The first step to create this molecule is with an enzyme called delta-6-desaturase. It helps linoleic acid convert to the omega-6 fatty acid gamma-linolenic acid (GLA). If delta-6-desaturase is impaired for any reason, mood can decline—usually more toward depression.

Besides boosting mood, PGE1 also helps the cardiovascular system by decreasing clotting and lowering inflammation in the blood vessels. When PGE1 is low, it may also contribute to an increased risk of heart attacks and stroke, lead to high blood pressure, and contribute to nervous tissue degeneration.

The delta-6-desaturase enzyme can also be deficient or inhibited in people with diabetes or obesity, in older people, and when there is too much insulin in the blood or too much coffee, trans-fatty acids (hydrogenated oils), or alcohol is consumed. Experiments in rats suggest that prolonged stress also inhibits activity of this enzyme (Hibbeln & Salen, 1995). In these circumstances, taking supplemental GLA can be helpful

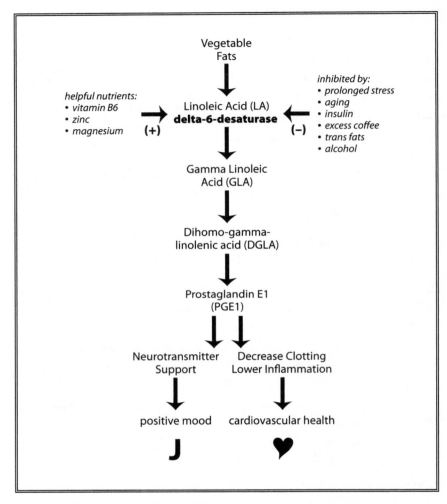

Figure 4.2. The gamma linolenic acid PGE1 pathway.

(Horrobin, 1993). The nutrients vitamin B6, zinc, and magnesium are cofactors in this reaction.

Delta-6-desaturase enzyme deficiency is especially common in people whose ancestry is 25 percent or higher Celtic Irish, Scottish, Welsh, Scandinavian, or Native Indian origin, and it is known these groups do have higher rates of alcoholism. Ever wonder why alcoholics like to drink? Well, it might be because it helps them feel better, temporarily— there's a link between alcoholism and this enzyme deficiency. In people predisposed, alcohol can temporarily stimulate production of PGE1 and help lift mood. But with cessation of alcohol, PGE1 levels fall again and depression returns. For some individuals, this will result in looking for alcohol as a way to get away momentarily from depression, thus contributing to an unhealthy cycle.

Even those individuals without delta-6-desaturase enzyme deficiency can deplete dihomo-gamma-linolenic acid with repeated drinking by preventing timely replenishment from linoleic acid. These individuals will also find the need for more and more alcohol to transiently increase PGE1 to lift mood (Greeley, 2000, chap. 11).

Supplemental GLA, in the form of evening primrose or borage oil, is easily converted to PGE1. For alcoholics, this can help support better mood and discourage the need to drink for relief. Premenstrual symptoms such as breast tenderness with feelings of depression, as well as irritability, swelling, and bloating from fluid retention, may also be indications for GLA supplementation (Horrobin, 1983).

*Dosage and toxicity of GLA*

The best indication for GLA would be for a depressed individual with alcoholic tendency, and for those who are Celtic Irish, Scottish, Welsh, Scandinavian, or Native American origin. Good sources of GLA include evening primrose oil, black currant seed oil, and borage oil. Dosage of GLA ranges from 1,000 mg to 2,500 mg once a day, whereas evening primrose oil is usually dosed between 4,000 mg and 8,000 mg/day. Doses of GLA >3,000 mg/day should be avoided due to possible exaggerated arachidonic acid levels, which may exacerbate inflammatory reactions (Yam, Eliraz, & Berry, 1996). GLA supplementation should not be used in patients with epileptic history, those with prostate cancer risk, or those who are pregnant (Hawkins & Ehrlich, 2011).

The only known food sources of GLA are black currants.

## Vegan Oils

The benefits of fish oils are multiple. The question then is, can practicing vegans get the same benefits by taking vegan oils? Vegan fatty acids have not been well studied in mood disorder. Plant foods are relatively low in alpha-linolenic acid (ALA) and higher in linoleic acid, an omega-6 fat. And these need to be converted to EPA and DHA in the body to have the mood benefits. Because fish oil already has EPA and DHA, it is likely that fish oil may be more beneficial than the plant oils. Also, some people do not do as good a job at making the conversion, which may predispose to mood problems.

For vegan oil dosage, an ALA intake of roughly 4 g/day is optimal. This level should provide enough to ensure that significant amounts of EPA and DHA are formed by the body. (Conversion rates are known to be around 5–10 percent for EPA and 2–5 percent for DHA.) However, it is also important for vegetarians to ensure that their intake of linoleic acid is not too high compared with ALA because a higher intake of linoleic acid interferes with the process in which the human body converts ALA into the even more beneficial EPA and DHA. An LA-to-ALA ratio of around 4–1 or slightly lower is considered to be the optimal (Vegetarian Society, 2009).

### Food sources of vegan oils

The best sources of vegan omega-3 fats are found in flaxseed, rape seed oil, walnuts, and tofu. Table IV.5 in Appendix IV reviews plant-derived oils that can be helpful for mood.

# PROBIOTICS

Chapter 3 established the importance of digestive function for mood balance. One aspect of optimal digestive health relies on its main resident: the gastrointestinal microbiome. The microbiome includes all the microorganisms that inhabitant our digestive tract—about 100 trillion bacteria. A healthy microbiome starts with vaginal birth: as the baby transcends the birth canal, the probiotics in the mother's vaginal fluid enter the baby's mouth and begin its healthful colonization of the digestive tract. It is possible that the high caesarian birth rate in the United States may be contributing to anxiety and depression due to lack of probiotic transference.

Gut bacteria, including both the healthy flora and pathogenic bacteria, can activate neural pathways and central nervous system signaling systems (Foster & McVey Neufield, 2013). The microbiome contributes to the bidirectional communication between the digestive tract and the brain. The autonomic nervous system, enteric (gut) nervous system, neuroendocrine system, and immune system all meet in the digestive tract and coordinate healthy physiologic and psychological responses. A healthy microbiome works to boost mood by generating healthy levels of brain-derived neurotrophic factor (Bercik et al., 2010) and gamma-aminobutyric acid (GABA) and enhancing brain receptors for GABA. Research has also shown that hypothalamic-pituitary-adrenal (HPA) axis dysregulation can be reversed by treatment with *Lactobacillus* and *Bifidobacterium* (Gareau et al., 2007; O'Mahony et al., 2005). This research verifies the two-way communication between the digestive tract and the brain and shows how the HPA axis is modulated by the enteric microbiota.

Animal studies to date clearly show probiotic supplementation benefits. In one mouse study, animals that received probiotics were, in general, more relaxed than the control mice. The probiotic mice had lower levels of corticosteroid release in response to stress, as well as lower anxiety and depression-related behaviors than those fed with just broth. In this study, they also performed a vagotomy (severing of the vagus nerve that communicates changes from the digestive tract to the brain) in some of the mice (Bravo et al., 2011). Other studies found that switching gut bacteria from a stressed mouse to a nonstressed one made the nonstressed one more stressed, and the reverse was also true when nonstressed animal gut bacteria was placed in an anxious animal (Ridaura et al., 2013; Bravo et al., 2011).

Probiotic supplementation has recently been referred to as 'psycho-biotic', for they can produce and deliver neurotransmitters such as gamma-aminobutyric acid and serotonin, with some experts going as far to suggest probiotics may become a useful alternative to pharmaceuticals due to their antidepressant and anxiolytic activity (Dinan, Stanton & Cryan, 2013). While still relatively few, emerging clinical research corroborates the animal studies showing supplementation can replenish a healthy microbiome in order to gain psychological benefit. In healthy people not diagnosed with a mental disorder, strains of the probiotic *Lactobacillus* and *Bifidobacterium* given for just 30 days lowered psychological distress and depression, decreased anger and hostility, lessened anxiety, and improved problem solving, compared with the placebo group (Messaoudi et al., 2011). In another double-blind, placebo-controlled trial, Benton et al. (2007) fed healthy subjects either a probiotic-containing milk drink or placebo for 3 weeks, with mood and cognition assessed before treatment and after 10 and 20 days of consumption. Subjects who initially scored in the lowest third for depressed mood showed significant improvement in symptoms after probiotic treatment. In one pilot study, Rao et al. (2009) gave patients with chronic fatigue *Lactobacillus casei* every day for 60 days. Based on the Beck Depression and Anxiety Inventories, these patients showed far less anxiety symptoms than placebo group.

*Probiotics dosage and best application*

Identified in the 1800s with Ilya Ilyich Mechnikov's groundbreaking work, probiotics were virtually ignored until recently and thus represent a relatively new field of research. Human studies have used various probiotic dosing and strains, so study comparisons are not possible until dosing procedures become standardized. Studies utilized a range of 6.5–24 billion colonies of *Lactobacillus casei* per day, while another supplemented with only 3 billion colonies of both *Lactobacillus helveticus* and *Bifidobacterium longum* per day. In our clinic we use a *Lactobacillus acidophilus* and *Bifidobacterium lactis* at a dose of 4 to 8 billion one to three times a day. Given that antibiotics are known to disrupt the microbiome and create feelings of anxiety and depression (Denou et al., 2011), it is recommended to dose probiotics during any antibiotic treatment. Probiotics are possibly contraindicated in digestive tract issues when there is active bleeding (e.g., active ulcerative colitis or active Crohn's disease) due to concern of bacteria moving into the bloodstream at a high volume.

### Probiotic toxicity

While probiotic studies have not demonstrated toxicity, oversight for using live bacteria in foods or food supplements is also relatively new and evolving. There have been many controlled clinical trials on the use of probiotics that demonstrate safe use (Snydman, 2008). I recommend these are purchased from high-quality companies that provide evidence for absence of any pathogenic germs, for these have been detected in inferior-quality products (Wassenaar & Klein, 2008).

### Food sources of probiotics

Yogurt is the most familiar source of probiotics, although for people who are lactose intolerant or have a dairy sensitivity or allergy there are other choices: natto (a traditional Japanese fermented soy food), kimchi (traditional Korean fermented vegetables), miso, and sauerkraut.

## VITAMIN AND MINERAL CHOICES

Vitamins and minerals can be supportive to patients both on and off medications. This section first reviews multivitamins, and then a few specific vitamins and minerals that are most pertinent for anxiety and depression. Keep in mind that some vitamins and minerals may already be dosed in a multiple vitamin in adequate levels, while others may need to be increased for optimal dosing. Also, while most vitamins can be ingested safely in doses higher than the recommend daily allowance, it is best to be careful to not overdose certain vitamins, especially the fat-soluble ones (vitamins A, D, E, and K), which can become toxic when the levels are too high.

Table IV.2 in Appendix IV reviews the reviews the most commonly used vitamins for anxiety and depression, which are described in detail below.

## Multiple Vitamins

There is good reason to consider the shotgun approach of a high-quality multiple vitamin. There is a demonstrated association between poor mood and deficiency in several micronutrients. The standard American diet (with the appropriate acronym SAD) is low in vegetables and whole foods and woefully deficient in many nutrients (e.g., folic acid, B vitamins) necessary for metabolic processes, antioxidant protection (e.g., vitamin E and C) needed to protect cells, and levels of protein and amino acid precursors (e.g., tryptophan) needed to make chemical neurotransmitters.

Dietary studies also show us that even people who are trying to eat healthy are in trouble. Misner (2006) reviewed 70 dietary analyses of 20 different diets from a cross section of people, ranging from elite athletes (who had pristine dietary intakes) to sedentary people who did not exercise or take good care of themselves. All diets fell short of 100 percent of the recommended RDA micronutrient levels. Even more, the more athletic and active the person, the greater the tendency toward deficiency.

In one randomized, double-blind, placebo-controlled trial in Australia, Harris et al. (2011) gave a multivitamin and mineral formulation or a placebo to 50 healthy men ranging in age from 50–69 years. Compared with the placebo, the multiple vitamin led to significant reduction in depression and stress scales, as well as better wakefulness and higher daily function. A meta-analysis of eight studies on the effect of a multivitamin on mild psychiatric symptoms found that the multiple vitamin reduced the levels of mild psychiatric symptoms, perceived stress and anxiety, and fatigue and confusion but had no benefit for depression (Long & Benton, 2013).

### Multivitamin dosing

The better-quality vitamins are usually made out of capsules that have powder in them (as opposed to hard tablets), and higher-quality vitamins are usually dosed around four to six capsules a day. Once patients are doing well and have been replete for a few months at full dose, I often will recommend a half dose of a high-potency multiple as maintenance. Because vitamins vary in potency, it is recommended that the dosage on the bottle be followed and taken with food unless otherwise indicated.

### Multiple vitamin safety

A study by the U.S. Preventive Services Task Force (Fortmann et al., 2013) suggests multiple vitamins have no reportable toxicity. The study did find two large trials of over 27,000 men that reported lower cancer incidence when taking a multivitamin for more than 10 years, but there was no benefit for cardiovascular disease and no extra benefit for either condition in women. Multiple vitamins have a good safety record, although it is controversial whether there is clear benefit by itself for any specific disease.

### Foods source of multiple vitamins

Generally, the best source for a wide array of healthy vitamins is in green vegetables and fruits.

## B Vitamins, Folate, and Inositol

As discussed in Chapter 3 in the section on blood testing, B vitamins play an important role in neurotransmitter production, prostaglandin formation, and homocysteine regulation, all of which correlate with mood. An association between low blood levels of B vitamins (especially folate and vitamins B6 and B12) and higher prevalence of anxiety and depressive symptoms has been reported in several epidemiologic studies (Sanchez-Villegas et al., 2009b). This section discusses the benefits of a few vitamins from the vitamin B family that are most relevant to anxiety and depression: vitamins B3, B6, and B12 and inositol and folate.

### Vitamin B3 (niacinamide)

Known for its effectiveness as a treatment in anxiety conditions, vitamin B3 helps mood in two ways. One is its ability to inhibit the liver enzyme tryptophan pyrrolase (Badawy & Evans, 1976). This enzyme breaks down tryptophan, making it less available to produce serotonin. Vitamin B3 is also responsible for activating the enzyme that converts tryptophan to 5-hydroxytryptophan. Vitamin B3 supplementation in the form of nicotinamide was found to prevent development of anxiety in baby animals that were exposed to low oxygen around the time of birth compared with a placebo group (Morales et al., 2010).

### Vitamin B6 (pyridoxine)

Vitamin B6 is a main cofactor for enzymes that convert L-tryptophan to serotonin, a likely reason vitamin B6 deficiency contributes to low mood. In females with known evidence of serum vitamin B6 deficiency due to oral contraceptive use, supplementation with 40 mg/day of vitamin B6 improved both anxiety and depression (Bermond, 1982). Studies supplementing vitamin B6 found modest anxiety benefit in anxious females with premenstrual disorder when given 200 mg magnesium along with 50 mg vitamin B6, over either alone or placebo. Another study found little improvement using solely supplementation with vitamin B6 versus placebo in depressed patients (Villegas-Salas et al., 1997). This suggests that B6 deficiency alone is not a likely cause and that using it in conjunction with other nutrients, especially magnesium (see below), is probably best due to synergistic effects (De Souza et al., 2000).

### Vitamin B12 (methylcobalamin)

Vitamin B12 is a key player in the synthesis of serotonin. There is some evidence that people with depression respond better to treatment if they have higher levels of vitamin B12. Anecdotal reports suggest weekly intramuscular administration of vitamin B12 (in the form of hydroxocobalamin) may improve unexplained anxiety patients with normal serum vitamin B12 (Gaby, 2011). One study showed a full response to antidepressant medications when B12 levels were higher (discussed further in Chapter 6 in the section on vitamin B12).

### Folic acid (folate)

Folic acid has been studied in the literature for its mood benefit over the last 30 years. The word *folate* comes from the Latin word *folium*, which means "leaf," emblematic of the high levels of this vitamin in leafy greens. Populations whose diets that are rich in folate have high serum folate concentrations and tend to have very low lifetime rates of major depression (Coppen & Bolander-Gouaille, 2005). Depletion can be encouraged by eating poorly, intestinal malabsorption, certain drugs (e.g., antiepileptic medications or birth control pills), and chronic alcohol intake.

Low folate status seems to be more associated with low mood and depression and less associated with anxiety (Bjelland et al., 2003). Folic acid status is also important for bipolar patients who are looking to gain benefit from lithium (Coppen, Chaudhry, & Swade, 1986). In his study of the interaction between folic acid and the opioid system, Brocardo et al. (2009) reviews for us how folic acid has been well implicated in depressive disorders, and folic acid deficiency has been noted among people with depression, with some estimates suggesting up to 33 percent of depressed individuals are folate deficient. He notes several studies that regard its role in the pathophysiology of depression, showing that patients with depression often have a functional folate deficiency, and the severity of such deficiency correlates with depression severity. Low folate status makes it much less likely a drug treatment will work, for folate is required for the synthesis of serotonin.

Besides being an important factor in serotonin synthesis, folic acid is also needed to support dopamine, norepinephrine, and epinephrine (Stahl, 2008). Folate also helps to reduce homocysteine levels (Slot,

2001), a cardiovascular risk factor that tends to be elevated in depression. Homocysteine is discussed in chapter 3.

### Inositol

Inositol is an abundant carbohydrate molecule with half the sweetness of sucrose. It is derived from component of plant seeds known for benefit in cancer care (Vucenik & Shamsuddin, 2003). While it is not actually related to the B vitamin family, it is often combined with B vitamins when treating mood challenges. Early animal studies on inositol have reported efficacy in relieving symptoms of depression (Einat et al., 1999) via serotonin receptor modulation (Brink et al., 2004) and neurotransmitter reuptake (Einat et al., 2001).

While two studies looked at 6–12 g/day of supplemental inositol for depression resulted in positive therapeutic improvements similar to common antidepressant drugs (Levine et al., 1993, 1995), a Cochrane review of four trials with a total of 141 participants did showed mixed evidence of therapeutic benefit (Taylor et al., 2004).

Inositol may be best for patients with anxieties, especially those who exhibit traits of obsessive-compulsivity and panic. Dosages of 18 g/day were found effective in small patient groups with obsessive-compulsive disorder (Fux et al., 1996). A follow-up double-blind, controlled, randomized crossover study looked at 20 patients taking 18 g/day followed by 1 month of fluvoxamine (150 mg/day). In the first month, inositol reduced panic attacks per week by 4.0 compared with a reduction of 2.4 with fluvoxamine.

### B complex studies

One workplace study of 60 nonanxious, nondepressed participants given a B complex who completed the 3-month, double-blind, randomized, placebo-controlled trial found the B complex group reported significantly lower personal strain and a reduction in confusion and depressed/dejected mood (Stough et al., 2011), suggesting that work productivity may increase with the administration of B complex to combat the stressors many workers experience.

A large study by Skarupski et al. (2010) looking at over 3,500 adults showed that higher intakes of B6, folate, and B12, whether through foods or supplementation, was associated with a decreased likelihood of incident depression for up to 12 years of follow-up. For each additional 10 mg vitamin B6 and additional 10 µg vitamin B12, there was a 2 percent decreased risk of depressive symptoms per year. In a randomized, double-blind, placebo-controlled trial, Lewis et al. (2013) evaluated the efficacy of a B complex nutritional supplement that included vitamins B1 (1.7 mg), B2 (as riboflavin-5-phosphate; 1.6 mg), B5 (3.3 mg), B6 (as pyridoxal 5-phosphate; 3 mg), B12 (263 µg), and folate (as folinic acid; 1,000 µg) and inositol hexanicotinate (30 mg) for improving anxiety and depression symptoms in 60 depressed adults for 60 days. The Beck Depression and Anxiety Inventories showed significant, moderate improvements in both depressive and anxiety symptoms compared with placebo. Interestingly, the B complex group showed greater improvement on the anxiety scale, while the placebo group demonstrated greater improvement on the depression scale (25 percent vs. 22 percent, and 34 percent vs. 39 percent, respectively), suggesting that B vitamins may be more effective for symptom relief in anxiety cases than in depression cases. The vitamin group achieved a more continuous decrease throughout the protocol, while the placebo group had less or no improvement from 30–60 days, suggesting a subtle but longer-lasting effect. Also, there was significant improvement on the mental health scale of the Medical Outcomes Study Short Form 36 compared with placebo. It should be noted that this study was supported by the company that made the vitamins, and a main contributing author received rumuneration from this company as well.

### Dosages of B vitamins, folate, and inositol

For anxiety and depression support, generally I recommend using a B complex, which includes vitamins B2, B3, B5, B6, and B12. It typically will also include folate (400–1,000 µg). Depending on the individual case, I often dose extra vitamin B12 (up to 5,000 µg/day) and folate (up to total 15 mg/day), and I may also consider adding a powdered inositol (up to 18 g/day) if there is a strong anxiety, obsessive, or panic aspect.

Certain forms of the vitamins are best utilized by the body. For vitamin B6, the activated form of the vitamin, pyridoxine 6-phosphate, is recommended. For vitamin B12, methylcobalamin is best, and for folate, the methyltetrahydrofolate form is best and is most like the form that appears in natural vegetables. In fact, some studies are now suggesting that using the common form of the supplement folic acid, which is employed in most vitamins, pregnancy formulas, and enriched foods, may actually make the more bioavailable L-methylfolate form less available for the body to use to protect against cancers. Those with the a MTHFR gene mutation (see the section on the *MTHFR* gene test in chapter 3) will benefit even further from using the methtyltetrahydrate form of the this vitamin.

In treatment-resistant cases of depression, oral doses of both folic acid (800 µg/day) and vitamin B12 (1 mg/day) should be tried (Coppen & Bailey, 2000). Folic acid intake for treatment-resistant depression may be dosed as high at 15 mg/day (see Chapter 6). Taking 100 mg vitamin B3 several times daily with meals may also enhance the effectiveness of supplemental tryptophan doses, which is useful in both anxiety and depression.

*Toxicity of B vitamins, folic acid, and inositol*

Prolonged high doses of vitamin B6 of 200 mg/day or more may cause a reversible tingling or neuropathy in the hands and feet, along with fatigue (Beers & Berkow, 1999, 1526). Do not use more than 100 mg/day of B6 (or pyridoxine 6-phosphate) to be safe.

Because the drug methotrexate's anticancer effect works via interference with folate metabolism, it is best not to take any folate when treating cancer (Fugh-Berman & Cott, 1999) with methotrexate. However, folate can be used supportively for patients using methotrexate to treat rheumatoid arthritis (RA) without blocking its general effect, because methotrexate works by another non-folate-mediated mechanism to treat RA. A 48-week, randomized, double-blind, placebo-controlled trial where patients supplemented with 1 mg/day folate did need slightly higher levels of the drug to be fully effective in RA, but these patients enjoyed lower liver enzymes than the group given only the drug (van Ede et al., 2001). Folate has also been reported to reduce the effectiveness of several anticonvulsants, potentially leading to seizures, so clients should not take folate if they are taking any epilepsy medications (Fugh-Berman & Cott, 1999). A 2004 Cochrane review (Taylor, et. al, 2004) of 18 g/day of inositol showed good tolerability. In my office, I have had two clients with obsessive-compulsive disorder complain of apparent minor gastric distress with gram doses of inositol, with full resolution once the supplement was discontinued.

*Food sources of B vitamins, folic acid, and inositol*

Sources of vitamin B3 include chicken, turkey, beef, liver, peanuts, sunflower seeds, mushrooms, avocado, and green peas. Best vitamin B6 sources include bell peppers, spinach, and turnip greens. Great sources of B12 are snapper and calf's liver, and very good sources of vitamin B12 include venison, shrimp, scallops, salmon, and beef. Vegetarian food sources have significantly lower available B12. The best vegetarian sources are sea plants (e.g., kelp), algae (e.g., blue-green algae), brewer's yeast, tempeh, miso, and tofu. High levels of methylfolate are in spinach, asparagus, romaine lettuce, turnip greens, mustard greens, calf's liver, collard greens, kale, cauliflower, broccoli, parsley, lentils, and beets. Inositol sources include most vegetables, nuts, wheat germ, brewers yeast, bananas, liver, brown rice, oat flakes, unrefined molasses, and raisins.

## Vitamin D and Iron

Please refer to Chapter 3, which discusses testing and supplementation of these important nutrients.

## Minerals

Like the B vitamins, minerals are quite supportive for healthiest mood. Minerals like zinc, magnesium, and selenium are important for neurotransmitter production, blood sugar balance, oxygen-carrying capacity, hormonal balance, and antioxidant status. Minerals such as calcium, magnesium, zinc, selenium, and manganese may competitively inhibit the absorption and utilization of toxic metals like lead, mercury, and aluminum (Baumel, 2003, p.50). Thus, it is possible that dietary deficiency of minerals may increase one's ability to absorb unwanted toxic metals.

Table IV.5 in Appendix IV reviews the minerals most commonly used to support anxiety and depression, which are described in detail below.

### Magnesium

Magnesium is one of my all-time favorite nutrients. Beneficial to the heart and cardiovascular system, relaxing to the muscles, and calming to the mind, it may not always be the first nutrient thought about for anxiety and depression. Nevertheless, I have relied on magnesium for my own optimal mood and consider it a strong ally for many of my patients.

Magnesium is an essential trace mineral that is often quite low in most American diets, as many nutrients get stripped away with processing. For example, only 16 percent of the magnesium found in whole wheat remains in refined flour, and magnesium has been filtered from most drinking water supplies, setting the stage for human magnesium deficiency (Eby & Eby, 2006). As explained in the "Foods to Avoid" section of Chapter 3, low magnesium can also be caused by high carbohydrate consumption because minerals literally flush out our system with carbohydrates (Pennington, 2000). This makes simple carbohydrates like breads, cakes, and cookies doubly problematic, because not only do they not provide any good-quality nutrients, but they also dysregulate blood sugar and deplete minerals from the body. Lowered magnesium intake will also contribute to another mood factor: inflammation. With magnesium deficiency, nervous tissue becomes damaged easier, thus increasing inflammation throughout the body. This can increase levels of the inflammatory marker C-reactive protein (Pakfetrat et al., 2008), another factor in mood disorder. (See chapter 4 for more about C-reactive protein.)

People with mood issues are even more prone to deficiency. Magnesium deficiency is found in 80 percent of depressed individuals (Shealy et al., 1992) and may play a strong role in anxiety by causing dysregulation of the HPA axis (Sartori et al., 2012). Suicidal patients show low levels of magnesium in their cerebral spinal fluid (Banki et al., 1985). One study that included 23 elderly patients with type 2 diabetes and hypomagnesemia (low magnesium in the blood) showed that magnesium chloride treatment was as effective to improve depressive symptoms as imipramine (Barragán-Rodríguez, Rodríguez-Morán, & Guerrero-Romero 2008). It seems the less magnesium in the body, the more anxiety and depression. One Norwegian study of community-dwelling men and women consisted of 5,708 individuals 46–74 years of age where magnesium intake was recorded (Jacka et al., 2009). A clear inverse correlation was found between magnesium intake with anxiety and depression symptoms. This study adjusted for age, gender, body type, blood pressure, level of income, and lifestyle variables. Another four case histories showed rapid recovery (<7 days) from major depression using 125–300 mg magnesium (in the forms of glycinate or taurinate) with each meal and at bedtime (Eby & Eby, 2006). That's pretty fast action—but not unusual, for the body responds when given what it needs to heal.

***Magnesium dosage and best application.*** Typical dosages of magnesium range from 300 to 800 mg/day (Jee et al., 2002; Magnesium, 2002). For patients with mood issues, I typically recommend the magnesium glycinate or magnesium taurate form over other types. (Glycine and taurine are discussed under "Amino Acids," below.) Magnesium in the form of Epsom salts can be used in a relaxing bath, with one to two cups in a standard size bathtub.

***Magnesium toxicity.*** Toxicity from magnesium is exceedingly rare, even at higher than normal doses. Supplementation is not recommended for patients who have compromised renal function or are undergoing dialysis. Supplementation can sometimes cause a looser stool, especially in higher doses. Nonchelated forms such as magnesium sulfate (as found in

Epsom salts), oxide, hydroxide, or chloride will typically encourage diarrhea sooner than the malate, citrate, glycinate, and taurate forms.

*Magnesium food sources.* Magnesium is found in mineralized hard water. In fact, many experts believe it is the mineral water that keeps French hearts healthy, despite the tendency to eat richer foods. Also, Swiss chard, summer squash, blackstrap molasses, spinach, mustard greens, halibut, turnip greens, and seeds (pumpkin, sunflower, and flax) are higher in magnesium content.

### Chromium

As discussed in chapter 3, poor blood sugar control (low blood sugar, fluctuating blood sugar, or high blood sugar and diabetes) will contribute to mood problems. The essential trace element chromium is a component of glucose tolerance factor, a complex molecule in the body used balance insulin levels and blood sugar. Chromium's modus operandi may also be its activation of brain serotonin (Attenburrow et al., 2002), as well as ability to increase insulin sensitivity (Anderson, 1998). Like other minerals, increased carbohydrate intake increases chromium loss.

Atypical types of major depressive disorder constitute more than 20 percent of all cases of depression. The atypically depressed patient can experience extreme reaction to events as well as a greatly increased sensitivity to rejection, resulting in depressed overreaction. Atypically depressed patients can also have greater physical feelings, such as extreme sense of physical heaviness (lead legs), weight gain or increased appetite, and these patients can sleep too much. These symptoms are summarized as follows.

### Atypical Depression Symptoms

Adults: Somatic (bodily) symptoms: lead legs, headache, fatigue, digestive disorders

Seniors: Confusion, lowered cognitive ability, overall low function

Children: irritability, decline in school, lowered social interest

A placebo-controlled, double-blinded, pilot study of chromium piccolinate was conducted in 15 patients with atypical types of major depressive disorder. Ten patients with atypical depression were started on a low dose of 400 µg/day of chromium, which was increased to 600 µg/day for a total of 8 weeks. The other five patients took a placebo. An impressive 70 percent of the patients (7 of 10) on the chromium responded positively to the treatment; none of the placebo patients had a positive response. The chromium piccolinate was well tolerated, with no noticeable side effects (Davidson et al., 2003). Although this was a small study given the safety and potential benefit of chromium, it is certainly worth trying as part of an overall naturopathic protocol, especially if imbalanced blood sugar is part of the picture.

***Chromium dosage and best application.*** With no known side effects at the standard dosage of 200 µg/day, chromium is a reasonable choice for any anxious or depressed patient showing atypical depression symptoms or challenges with blood sugar, either reactive hypoglycemia or diabetes. Chromium can be given up to 600 µg/day, or even higher under the supervision of a health care practitioner. I have personally seen excellent results with both anxiety and depression symptoms in my patients when chromium was taken to help support blood sugar regulation.

***Chromium food sources.*** Onions, romaine lettuce, and tomatoes are top sources for chromium. Brewer's yeast, eggs, liver, bran cereal, and oysters are also good sources. For those brave enough to try it liver should be obtained from naturally raised animals so there is a lower burden of toxins.

### Selenium

Selenium is mineral known for the ability to replenish glutathione, a master antioxidant in the body, by acting as a cofactor for the enzyme glutathione peroxidase, the enzyme that helps make glutathione. Selenium supports neurologic function, helps the body produce mood-lifting neurotransmitters, and is especially important in the conversion of the thyroid hormone thyroxine (T4) to its more active form tri-iodothyronine (T3). One review looked at five studies, all of which indicated that low selenium intake is associated with poor mood (Benton, 2002). Studies giving selenium revealed that selenium improved mood and diminished anxiety (Shor-Posner et al., 2003; Duntas, Mantzou, & Koutras, 2003).

**Selenium dosage and best application.** Typical dosage of selenium is 100–200 μg/day. Selenium is best used for the anxious and depressed patient who also has low thyroid function and/or low T3 levels.

**Toxicity of selenium.** Large doses of selenium can be toxic. Doses larger than 400 μg may cause symptoms of dermatitis, hair loss, and brittle nails.

**Food sources of selenium.** Best sources of selenium include meat, fish, nuts (especially Brazil nuts), and garlic.

*Lithium orotate*

Lithium is a mood stabilizer with both antidepressant and antimanic properties. However, its mechanism of action is unclear. In the carbonate form, it is prescribed for patients with bipolar disorder, although now newer drugs are available. Geographical areas with higher natural lithium concentrations in the drinking water are associated with lower mortality rates from suicide (Kapusta et al., 1987). Bipolar disorder patients who take lithium carbonate have lower rates of Alzheimer's disease, as well as less cognitive impairment, suggesting lithium may have a neuroprotective quality as well (Lowry, 2011).

The supplemental form of lithium is lithium orotate, which is a salt of lithium and orotic acid. Lithium orotate may be the preferred form, for the orotate ion is known to more easily traverse the blood-brain barrier than the drug version, which uses the carbonate ion of lithium. As a result, the orotate form can be used in much lower doses with reasonable results and no side effects (Lakhan & Vieira, 2008). Typical lithium orotate dosages can be as low as 5 mg/day, versus up to the 180 mg needed for the lithium carbonate form.

While considered more natural, lithium orotate has been minimally studied. In one evaluation, alcoholic patients prescribed 150 mg lithium orotate (approximately 5–7 mg/day of elemental lithium) four to five times a week along with a diet low in simple carbohydrates that assured moderate amounts of protein and fat were studied by Sartori et al. (1986). Of 42 patients, 10 had no alcoholic relapse for over 3 and up to 10 years, and 13 patients remained without relapse for 1–3 years. The remaining 12 had relapses between 6 and 12 months.

It is suggested that lithium's beneficial effects on mood may be due to its oxytocin-raising properties. In one small study by Winstock et al., 20 long-term marijuana smokers took 500 mg lithium carbonate twice daily for seven days. Three months later, most were getting high less, and some had quit entirely. Winstock et al. also noted that those that stopped completely had greater levels of happiness than those who smoked less. This corroborates previous studies on rats that showed higher levels of oxytocin with lithium supplementation (Cui et al., 2001).

*Lithium orotate dosage and best usage.* Lithium orotate is commonly dosed at 5–20 mg/day of elemental lithium. Lithium might be best used with someone who is anxious or depressed and has demonstrated doing well with oxytocin-building activity like receiving a massage. More study is clearly needed to understand who will best benefit from lithium supplementation.

*Lithium orotate toxicity.* While common supplemental doses show no toxicity, high doses can cause muscle weakness, loss of appetite, mild apathy, tremors, nausea, and vomiting. In high doses, lithium may also cause dulled personality, reduced emotions, memory loss, tremors, or weight gain (Waring, 2006), as well as impair kidney function (Smith & Schou, 1979). One case of an 18-year-old who ingested 18 tablets (2,160 mg total) of a lithium-containing over-the-counter relaxation supplement had normal vital signs but complained of nausea and vomiting and presented with tremor, which resolved after 3 hours of intravenous fluids and observation (Pauzé & Brooks., 2007).

*Food sources of lithium.* Primary food sources are grains and vegetables.

### Zinc

Known as a mineral cofactor, zinc is responsible for many aspects of health, including wound healing, as well as immune and nervous system balance. Deficiency will contribute to emotional instability and depression. Low zinc status may cause lower levels of GABA, increasing anxiety symptoms. Zinc deficiency has been found to be associated with GABA receptor impairment (Takeda et al., 2006). It has been reasoned that zinc may protect the brain by blocking the toxic effect of glutamate (Nowak et al, 2003).

Patients with anxiety have been shown to have low zinc levels, especially in relationship to copper levels. In these patients, zinc piccolinate daily for 8 weeks restored that balance and improved symptoms (Russo, 2011). For depression, lower zinc correlates with increased severity. As is the case with folic acid, low serum zinc increases the likelihood antidepressants will not work (Maes et al., 1997a). (This is discussed further in Chapter 6.)

*Zinc dosage and toxicity.* Optimal zinc dosage is 15–30 mg/day. It should be taken with food due to the possibility of gastric upset. It may be most indicated for patients with mood problems along with acne or low immune status. If taking zinc for more than 2 months, and high copper is not a concern, it is best to take 1–2 mg/day copper, for extra zinc supplementation can cause the body to lose copper.

*Zinc food sources.* Known to accompany animal protein, zinc is found in highest levels in beef, lamb, turkey, chicken, pork, crabmeat, lobster, clams, and salmon. The best vegetable source is pumpkin seed.

162

## Amino Acids

Amino acids are the precursors to neurotransmitters. Adding supplemental amino acids can create happy mood and help avoid the need for medications. While most vitamins and minerals act as cofactors in the production of neurotransmitters, the amino acids are the building blocks of the neurotransmitters and can play a central role in changing mood for the better.

Table IV.6 in Appendix IV reviews the top supplemental amino acids used for anxiety and depression, which are described in detail below.

### Gamma-aminobutyric acid and phenibut

Gamma-aminobutyric acid (GABA) is a natural calming brain neurotransmitter that may act like a natural benzodiazepine. People who suffer with anxiety, insomnia, epilepsy, and other brain disorders often do not manufacture sufficient levels of GABA. Supplemental GABA helps open chloride channels in neurons, which hyperpolarizes them so that the positive charges remain on one side of the membrane, which inactivates the nerve cell. This slows firing and calms the brain.

While supplemental GABA is widely accepted in the CAM community, relatively few studies have been conducted with this amino acid, but they do suggest benefit. One randomized, single-blind, placebo-controlled, crossover study over 2 days looked at 63 healthy adults taking 100 mg GABA or placebo. Electroencephalogram activities showed more balance in alpha waves (alpha waves are generated in states of peacefulness, e.g., during meditation and before sleep) and beta wave activity (used in wakefulness) with GABA compared with placebo when mental stressors were given (Yoto et al., 2012b). Abdou et al., (2006) conducted two separate trials using supplemental GABA. The first showed GABA-enhancing alpha wave activity over beta waves in 13 normal volunteers. The second looked at eight acrophobic subjects (those afraid of heights) given the task of crossing a high suspension

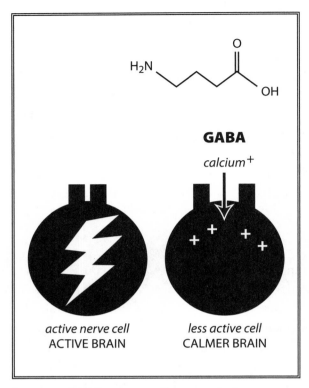

Figure 4.3. GABA's calming influence on the brain.

bridge and found GABA was able to keep secretory and immune function normal, whereas the placebo group was not able to keep normal physiologic function.

Phenibut is a supplement you may find some of your clients using, as it is used in the holistic community and is sold by a number of nutraceutical companies as a calming agent. Phenibut is a form of GABA known as beta-phenyl-gamma-aminobutyric acid, which is a GABA receptor agonist (binds and stimulates the GABA receptor to cause a calming reaction). Used as a prescription drug in Russia, it is available as a supplement in Western countries. Like its GABA counterpart, this supplement has little evidenced-based research.

**GABA dosage, best application, and toxicity.** The typical dosage for GABA is 100–200 mg up to three times daily away from food, although some practitioners dose higher for better effect. Though no side effects have been reported, as a general guideline it is recommended to take no more than 1,000 mg within a 4-hour period and no more than 3,000 mg within a 24-hour period. The best application for GABA is either as a "natural Xanax" where a patient would like something relatively quick as a calmative, or for enhancing the process of falling asleep in times when he or she cannot wind down and move into the alpha state.

**GABA toxicity.** No known toxicity is associated with GABA when used in recommended dosages. Phenibut has limited research, with one case report suggesting dependence, tolerance, and withdrawal symptoms (Samokhvalov et al., 2013).

**Food sources of GABA.** The highest levels of GABA are found in green, black, and oolong teas, which is probably why sipping these can be relaxing. Fermented foods (e.g., yogurt, kimchi, and sauerkraut), as well as oats, whole grains, and brown rice, also include GABA.

### Glycine

The simplest of the amino acids, glycine is a calming amino acid known to reduce neuronal excitement, optimize GABA, and bind to the locus coeruleus to decrease the release of norepinephrine. Glycine, like GABA, is also known to help open chloride channels, which calms electrical activity.

Two double-blind, placebo-controlled studies in 14 and 16 healthy patients exposed to loud sounds found that high doses of glycine (0.8 g/kg body weight—about 44 grams for a 120 pound person) calmed the brain's cortex and decreased reaction to the sound by lessening auditory evoked potentials (O'Neill et al., 2007; Leung et al., 2008). Several double-blind trials in patients with schizophrenia using 0.4–0.8 g/kg body weight/day for 6–12 weeks along with antipsychotic medication improved negative symptoms by 15–30 percent, over using medication by itself. Heresco-Levy et al., 1999). One trial of 0.8 g/kg saw no benefit in cognitive in already healthy young people (Palmer et al., 2008), suggesting it's best use may be in people could use calming.

***Dosage and best application.*** Glycine usually comes in a powder that can be taken in a little water. The studies described above used very high doses (0.8 mg/kg is equivalent to a whopping 44 g/day of powder) to achieve benefit. In my experience, prescribing lower doses (two or three teaspoons a day—about 10–15 g total), along with other lifestyle and dietary changes and supplements, can help keep anxiety at bay. Patients experiencing or anticipating panic attacks can take 5–10 g in one dose before anxiety-provoking situations. Glycine tends to work within 30 minutes of ingestion. Often, I will have patients mix one teaspoon of glycine powder with passionflower tincture to take three times a day for anxiety.

***Glycine toxicity.*** While glycine has no known toxicity, no long-term studies at very high doses (0.8 g/kg) have been conducted. Patients with kidney or liver disease should talk to their doctor before using high doses of amino acids.

### Lysine and arginine

Lysine deficiency is implicated in anxiety, because lysine helps lower amygdala activation. L-Lysine has also been shown to act as a partial serotonin receptor-4 (5-HT4) antagonist, decreasing the brain-gut response to stress (Smriga & Torii, 2003). Arginine helps balance corticotropin-releasing hormone release from the hypothalamus, as well as lower cortisol levels. Arginine also helps lower blood pressure.

Two human studies have looked at supplementation of both of these amino acids. Jezova et al. (2005) performed a randomized, double-blind, placebo-controlled trial performed in 29 high-trait-anxiety males. High-trait anxiety is defined as a preset level of anxiety or a tendency to be anxious. These individuals typically have long-term chronic stress that segues into HPA dysregulation, resulting in low cortisol, an effect that is seen in some long-term depression. Given 3 g of each amino acid a day for 10 days, participants improved in their ability to handle induced stress (public speaking) by enhancing cortisol, adrenaline, and nor-adrenaline levels, while the placebo had no benefit.

In the second trial, Smriga et al. (2007) worked with 108 healthy non-trait-anxiety volunteers. After 1 week of treatment with 2.64 g of an L-lysine and L-arginine supplement, basal levels of salivary cortisol decreased in males but not in females. Supplementation also resulted in significant reductions in state anxiety (which is a condition-specific acute experience of apprehension, tension, and fear) and trait anxiety in both males and females Taken together, these two clinical trials suggest that arginine and lysine may have an adaptogenic quality, meaning they can help raise cortisol if too low, and lower it when it is too high.

**Lysine and arginine dosage and best application.** Typical dosage for both of these is 2–3 g twice a day, away from food. These amino acids are considered in anxiety, but no information exists regarding benefit for depression.

**Lysine and arginine toxicity.** Lysine and arginine are safe long term. Some research suggests arginine may increase likelihood of herpes type 1 break outs and may need to be avoided if these increase in frequency. When treating herpetic sores, natural medicine protocol usually recommends avoiding arginine sources (e.g., nuts and chocolate) and taking supplemental lysine to suppress virality.

### L-Theanine

L-Theanine is a unique amino acid found in the tea plant (*Camellia sinensis*). This amino acid possesses neuroprotective, mood-balancing, and relaxation properties. Theanine is known to increase brain-derived neurotrophic factor and create a more beneficial ratio of cortisol to dehydroepiandrosterone by lowering cortisol (Miodownik et al., 2011).

Paradoxically, theanine has been shown to have both stimulant and relaxant effects, with animal studies suggesting that low doses have more of a stimulatory effect and higher doses are more relaxing. This would explain the effect of "relaxed alertness" often mentioned with theanine. Theanine can help support dopamine, GABA, and serotonin activity and is known to generate alpha wave activity at bedtime (although not as robustly as supplemental GABA can).

Theanine (400 mg/day) with concomitant antipsychotic medications in 40 patients with schizophrenia and schizoaffective disorder was helpful in curbing positive signs, activation, and anxiety symptoms, without negative interactions with medication (Ritsner et al., 2011).

**L-Theanine dosage and best application.** At 200–400 mg/day, L-theanine may be best for someone with consistently anxiety and a tendency for obsessive/running thoughts, where the person cannot stop thinking about them. Because theanine has been shown to lower blood pressure in anxious adults, it may be best used in an anxious person who also exhibits higher blood pressures when anxious, such as "white coat syndrome" (Yoto et al., 2012a). Because studies show it works best for chronic versus anticipatory anxiety (Lu et al., 2004), it should be dosed daily to achieve desired relaxation effect.

Studies using 200 mg twice a day for six weeks have also been performed in 98 boys aged 8 to 12 years with ADHD, and found clear benefit to help the boys fall and stay asleep (Lyon, Kapur & Luneja., 2011).

### L-Tryptophan and 5-hydroxytryptophan

Tryptophan is an amino acid precursor to serotonin and may be one of the most popular amino acids for mood and sleep. It has also been established that circulating plasma tryptophan is also a potent antioxidant (Maes et al., 1994b). Research shows that tryptophan is significantly lower in major depression subjects than in normal controls. Low levels may increase the risk of a suicide attempt in patients who are depressed (Maes et al., 1997c) and will increase panic response (Miller, Deakin, & Anderson, 2000).

The desired therapeutic effect of antidepressant drugs known as serotonin reuptake inhibitors (SSRIs) is to increase levels of serotonin in the

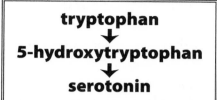

Figure 4.4. The conversion of tryptophan to serotonin.

brain by slowing the brain from breaking down this neurotransmitter. The idea of supplementing with tryptophan or 5-hydroxytryptophan (5-HTP) is to give the body more building blocks to make more serotonin. Many natural medicine practitioners like myself believe tryptophan or 5-HTP might be a better method of a achieving the same goal because it allows the body more control over this process and may mitigate side effects associated with SSRIs.

As an aside, when considering serotonin abnormalities in an anxious or depressed patient, from a naturopathic standpoint it is important to consider the role and health of the digestive tract. The naturopathic notion of "treating the gut" may be important in treating primary mechanisms of anxiety and depression by increasing overall serotonin levels. As discussed in Chapter 2, evidence linking digestive dysfunction, abnormal serotonin levels, and psychiatric illness is emerging. Effectively treating digestive dysfunction and combining of foods to optimize tryptophan uptake may rebalance tryptophan and serotonin levels, thus working to alleviate mood challenges.

Despite the widespread use and anecdotal reports, there are relatively very few studies using tryptophan and 5-HTP for mood disorder. Research on using these is scarce because the advent of the SSRI drugs precluded more study. In a small double-blind, placebo-controlled, crossover pilot study, Hudson et al. (2009) gave seven social phobia subjects a 2-week protocol of eating a type of seed called a deoiled gourd seed, which is a rich source of tryptophan. This was prescribed with or without a high-glycemic-index carbohydrate to raise insulin levels, which helps increase absorption of tryptophan into the brain. The tryptophan given with the carbohydrate had significant anxiety improvements.

In a double-blind placebo-controlled study of 5-HTP and the tricyclic antidepressant clomipramine (Anafranil) with 45 anxiety patients (Khan et al., 1987), clomipramine showed superior improvement on all rating scales versus placebo, but the 5-HTP held its own, with moderate reduction of the symptomatology and its best effect on agoraphobia and panic. However, the 5-HTP did not help the depressive symptomatology. One study by Schruers et al. (2002) used a carbon dioxide inhalation challenge to induce panic in 24 panic disorder patients and 24 controls. 5-HTP at 200 mg 90 minutes before the challenge significantly reduced the reaction to the panic challenge in panic disorder patients, affecting subjective anxiety, panic symptom score, and number of panic attacks, whereas the placebo had no effect.

A meta-analysis by Shaw, Turner, and Del Mar (2002) looked at all the depression studies of tryptophan and 5-HTP, but few were well done: of 108 studies, only two with a combined total of 64 patients met sufficient quality criteria to be included. However, these studies did suggest 5-HTP and L-tryptophan are better than placebo at alleviating depression. While this is promising, more quality research on a larger number of individuals would be welcome.

*Tryptophan and 5-HTP dosing and best application.* When considering either tryptophan or 5-HTP supplementation for overall mood, I recommend starting with 5-HTP, which is more effective at crossing the blood-brain barrier. The conversion to serotonin is also better with 5-HTP than with tryptophan (70 percent 5-HTP vs. ~3 percent of tryptophan gets absorbed), so it takes significantly less to obtain the same mood effect.

For anxiety states and panic disorder, as well as depression with a social anxiety or panic component, I highly recommend considering a high-quality tryptophan or 5-HTP. Because more research is needed to optimize dosing schedule and amounts, a good place to start would be 500 mg/day of tryptophan taken with a simple carbohydrate (slice or apple or a cracker) on an empty stomach and work up to 2 g/day if needed. Dosages of 5-HTP can start at 100 mg three times a day and work up to 200 mg three times a day, also taken on an empty stomach. If patients have trouble staying asleep at night, I often recommend 500 or 1,000 mg tryptophan taken with some simple carbohydrate, about 30 minutes before bed. Because conversion of 5-HTP to serotonin can increase gut motility, it is not recommended in patients with anxiety or depression who are already experiencing diarrhea, for supplementation may exacerbate this.

*Tryptophan and 5-HTP safety.* When dosed accordingly, tryptophan appears to be quite safe and effective. The most common and reversible adverse effects are gastrointestinal: nausea, vomiting, and diarrhea. Much less common, patients have complained of headache, insomnia, and palpitations.

About 20 years ago, there was a lot of misinformation about the safety of tryptophan. In 1989 more than 1,000 people fell ill after consuming the supplement, causing concern for eosinophilia-myalgia syndrome (EMS) in the United States. This syndrome consisted of severe muscle and joint pain, high fever, swelling of the arms and legs, weakness, and shortness of breath. Sadly, more than 30 deaths were attributed to EMS caused by tryptophan supplements (Belongia et al., 1990). Although the supplement itself was originally blamed and then banned in the United States, it was actually poor quality control that was at fault due to contaminants in the supplement—it had nothing to do with tryptophan itself. No new cases of EMS have been reported since (Das et al., 2004).

More salient to our conversation would be discussion of "serotonin syndrome." This is a theoretical situation where combined SSRIs drugs or an SSRI drug and serotonin-promoting natural therapy (e.g., tryptophan, 5-HTP, or St. John's wort) might increase serotonin levels. This syndrome is characterized by severe agitation and confusion and may include symptoms of hallucinations, fast heart beat, blood pressure changes, feeling hot, coordination issues, hyperreflexes, and gastrointestinal tract symptoms such as nausea, vomiting, and diarrhea. Severe cases can cause rapid fluctuation of temperature and blood pressure, mental status changes, and even coma.

Although polypharmacy (taking several drugs at the same time) has caused this syndrome (Gnanadesigan et al., 2005), no reports of natural substances being the cause have been reported to date. This chapter, along with Chapter 6 presents a number of studies showing the benefit of using tryptophan or 5-HTP together with SSRIs and tricyclic antidepressants. For example, in 870 patients taking medications with 5-HTP, there has not been one case of serotonin syndrome (Turner, Loftis, & Blackwell, 2006). Nevertheless, to be safe, any integrative care practitioner should watch for signs of serotonin syndrome until more study is done. With careful dosing of SSRI drugs along with tryptophan or 5-HTP, supplementation may prove a side-effect-free integrative approach. 5-HTP has also been used clinically in combination with tryptophan, with no signs of serotonin syndrome (Quadbeck, Lehmann, & Tegeler, 1984).

***Tryptophan and 5-HTP food sources.*** Tryptophan can be found in all protein foods in small amounts. Relatively high amounts are present in pumpkin seeds, bananas, turkey (which some believe contributes to the post-Thanksgiving meal sleepiness—but research suggests this is really the effect of excess food intake), red meat, dairy, nuts, seeds, soy, tuna, and shellfish. There are no food sources of 5-HTP.

*Phenylalanine and tyrosine*

Because tryptophan and 5-hydroxytryptophan are the building blocks for serotonin, L-phenylalanine and tyrosine are the precursors that convert to the two neurotransmitters dopamine and norepinephrine (Gelenberg & Gibson, 1984). As such, people experiencing mild to moderate depression who have low dopamine or norepinephrine may find it helpful to "preload" with these precursors.

Phenylalanine is a precursor of brain phenylethylamine, an amino acid derivative that promotes overall energy and elevation of mood

(Sabelli et al., 1986). Phenylethylamine converts to tyrosine, which is in turn converted to dopamine and subsequently norepinephrine and epinephrine. Given orally, phenylalanine will mildly stimulate the nervous system.

Tyrosine has a mild antioxidant effect, binding free radicals that can cause damage to the cells and tissues. Tyrosine may lessen tobacco withdrawal symptoms with the addition of glucose tolerance factor (McCarty & Mark, 1982) by enhancing tyrosine and catecholamine levels in the brain (more about chromium and glucose tolerance factor earlier in this chapter).

Tyrosine can help the body deal with stress and difficult challenges. In a double-blind, placebo-controlled crossover study, Banderet and Lieberman (1989) looked at the possibility of using tyrosine to decrease the adverse consequences of a 4.5-hour exposure to cold and lack of oxygen in volunteer subjects. At a dose of 100 mg per 2.2 pounds of body weight, tyrosine significantly helped the symptoms, adverse moods, and performance problems in subjects exposed to these harsh conditions. Tyrosine has also been shown to significantly improve mental performance in those with sleep deprivation (Neri et al., 1995).

Studies of people who were both phenylalanine and tyrosine depleted paint a picture of those who are less content and more apa-

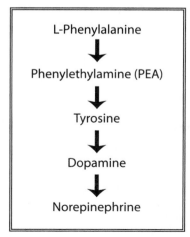

Figure 4.5. The phenylalanine–norepinephrine pathway.

thetic (McLean et al., 2003). Unfortunately, few clinical studies have examined the effects of these two amino acids for depression. The rationale behind supplementation has been further fueled by a study in which injections of tyrosine hydroxylase, an enzyme in the brain that helps make more tyrosine, resulted in significant improvement in behavioral despair in animal depression models (Fu et al., 2006).

Fischer et al. (1975) conducted a small study of 23 subjects with depression after a previous unsuccessful treatment with common antidepressive drugs. D-Phenylalanine was given in daily in oral doses of 50 or 100 mg/day for 15 days. Normal mood was seen in 17 subjects between 1 and 13 days of treatment. No important adverse reaction was observed. A second study showed that L-phenylalanine supplementation elevated mood in 31 of 40 depressives with doses of 14 g/day (Sabelli et al., 1986).

Gelenberg et al. (1990) performed a randomized, prospective, double-blind comparison of 65 outpatients with major depression given oral L-tyrosine or imipramine. Although both treatments trended toward some improvement, imipramine showed greater improvement, with little difference between placebo and tyrosine. The only effect noted to achieve statistical significance was greater dry mouth with imipramine. Gelenberg et al. concluded that "the idea that a natural product with negligible side effects would turn out to be an effective treatment for depression appeared too good to be true—and our data suggest that it was." Thus, although there is certainly promise with phenylalanine and tyrosine, more studies are clearly needed. I still find both tyrosine + penylalanine useful as adjunctive to the other supports for clients, especially in the cases of low motivation and pain.

*Phenylalanine and tyrosine dosages and best application.* The L form of phenylalanine may be dosed of up to 14 g/day in divided doses. The D form of phenylalanine has been studied in doses of 350 mg/day. As an antidepressant strategy, L-tyrosine may be used in doses of 500–1,000 mg two or three times a day, with some studies dosing up to 6,000 mg/day in total. Because tyrosine can be stimulating and possibly affect sleep, a reasonable clinical strategy would be to prescribe tyrosine during the daytime and supplementing at night with 1000–1500 mg L-tryptophan or 50–100 mg 5-HTP in patients with mild to moderate depression. No known studies have used phenylalanine and tyrosine at the same time.

These amino acids would be useful for a depressed person but would not be recommended for anxiety. The best choice would be an overweight client with a strong appetite who experiences regular pain (maybe suffering migraines or arthritis) and has many physical stressors and/or low motivation and apathy. Using tyrosine and glucose tolerance factor (a nutrient found in brewer's yeast) or chromium may lessen tobacco withdrawal symptoms and may increase the chance of success in a smoking cessation program if your client smokes.

*Phenylalanine and tyrosine toxicity.* Taking too much of these amino acids may result in increased blood pressure and emotional jitters, trouble sleeping, or headaches. Phenylketonuria (PKU) is a disorder in which the body fails to turn phenylalanine into tyrosine properly. Those with PKU should not supplement with phenylalanine. Tyrosine seems to be generally safe, though reports of nausea, diarrhea, headache, vomiting, or excessive nervousness have occurred with doses >9 g. Insomnia can be prevented by avoiding evening supplementation. Tyrosine should not be taken by anyone who is taking monoamine oxidase inhibitors for depression, or by patients with hypertension. The Parkinson's drug levodopa may interfere with the absorption of tyrosine and could reduce tyrosine levels in the blood. Tyrosine may also be contraindicated in multiple myeloma, a cancer of bone marrow cells. Patients with Grave's disease and an overactive thyroid should use caution when supplementing with tyrosine because it can boost thyroid hormone levels (L-Tyrosine, 2007).

*Dietary sources of phenylalanine and tyrosine.* Some of the most concentrated sources of phenylalanine are torula yeast, soybean protein isolate and concentrate, peanut flour, dried spirulina, seaweed, defatted and low-fat soybean flour, dried and salted cod, tofu, Parmesan cheese, almond meal, dry roasted soybean nuts, dried watermelon seeds, and fenugreek seeds. Tyrosine is found in fish, soy products, chicken, almonds, avocados, bananas, dairy products, lima beans, and sesame seeds.

*Phosphatidylserine*

Along with fatty acids, phosphatidylserine is a major component of nerve cell membranes. It plays a crucial role in many activities: activation of enzymes, communication between cells, transport in and out of the cell, maintenance of the cell's internal environment, cell-to-cell communication, and regulation of cell growth.

Known mostly for memory enhancement, supplementation of phosphatidylserine may also have a potent effect on the modulation of the stress hormone cortisol, which can destroy areas of the brain when it is sustained at high levels. Phosphatidylserine can help reduce cortisol and protect the brain.

In two clinical trials by the same researchers, healthy men were given 800 mg/day of phosphatidylserine followed by exercise. Both trials resulted in a blunting (lowering) of cortisol and adrenocorticotropic hormone (Monteleone, Maj, & Beinat, 1992; Monteleon et al., 1990). Another study of 30 subjects (10 elderly women with major depressive disorders, 10 age- and gender-matched healthy controls, and 10 young healthy controls) found 200 mg daily of phosphatidylserine supported a significant improvement in depressive symptoms and memory (Hellhammer et al., 2012). Researchers interested combining the anxiety-supporting power of phosphatidylserine with omega-3 fats gave 60 healthy men under high stress either an omega-3 fatty acid supplement with 300mg of phosphatidylserine per day or placebo for 3 months. Phosphatidylserine with the omega fats had stress-reducing effects in those who have chronically high stress and helped restore balanced cortisol response in this group, but not in the other subjects, suggesting the treatment worked in an adaptogenic fashion. (Adaptogens raise levels when too low, and lowers levels when too high.) This was impressive, given this was quite a low dose of phosphatidylserine and omega fats.

*Phosphatidylserine dosage.* Phosphatidylserine is dosed anywhere between 200 and 800 mg/day in divided doses on an empty stomach, and it may be especially useful before the onset of an acute stressor. I will typically recommend phosphatidylserine for the highly stressed or depressed person who is under great physical stress and who has high cortisol and poor memory. Also, phosphatidylserine may work best when taken in conjunction with essential fatty acids.

*Phosphatidylserine toxicity.* In a tolerability and toxicity study of 130 elderly patients given 300 mg or 600 mg daily in divided doses for 12 weeks. Hematologic safety parameters, blood pressure, heart rate, and adverse events were assessed, and no significant changes were noted in blood tests, except for a favorable change in liver enzymes (Jorissen et al., 2002; Phosphatidylserine, 2008). While more studies are welcome, there is no evidence of toxicity for phosphatidylserine.

*Food sources of phosphatidylserine.* The sources with the greatest amounts of phosphatidylserine are mackerel, herring, chicken liver, tuna, soft-shell clams, and white beans.

### N-Acetyl-cysteine

Known for years in conventional care as an emergency intravenous treatment to thwart the effects of acute liver toxicity (e.g., eating a poison mushroom), N-acetyl-cysteine (NAC) has found a strong place in the natural medicine armamentarium due to its glutathione-regenerating capability as well as its ability to balance levels of glutamate in the brain. Glutathione is the body's master antioxidant and is produced in the liver.

NAC's effect on anxiety has been shown to be helpful in cases of obsessive-compulsive disorder, gambling issues, and trichotillomania (hair pulling) (Grant, Odlaug, & Kim, 2009). NAC has also been given to children and adolescents with autism by helping resperidone more effectively treat irritability symptoms (Ghanizadeh, & Moghimi Sarani. 2013).

NAC has also been studied for use of depressive symptoms. One study of 17 patients with bipolar disorder found that 8 of the 10 patients taking NAC over 24 weeks achieved a very beneficial effect on mood (Magalhães et al., 2011). However, a larger open-label trial of 149 patients did not confirm these results (Berk et al., 2012).

**N-Acetyl-cysteine dosage and best application.** Typical dosages of NAC are 500–600 mg two or three times a day.

**N-Acetyl-cysteine toxicity.** Occasional headaches or stomach discomfort might occur, but it is known to be quite nontoxic. One study did report considerable headaches, agitation, social withdrawal, and severe aggression in a few young patients being studied for pathologic nail-biting habits (Ghanizadeh, Derakhshan, & Berk, 2013). NAC may interfere with certain cancer treatments and could be avoided with chemotherapy.

**N-Acetyl-cysteine food sources.** While there are no direct food sources of NAC, cysteine is a precursor of NAC and is found any high-protein food (meats, tofu, eggs, dairy products, etc.).

### Taurine

Made from cysteine with the cofactor vitamin B6, taurine it is thought to act by supporting levels of glycine and GABA to help relax the brain and nervous system while keeping levels of toxic glutamate low (Mori, Gähwiler, & Gerber, 2002). It is also known as a cardiovascular support and prevents aggregation of platelets to help decrease excess clotting. While animal studies do suggest an anxiolytic effect (El Idrissi et al., 2009), no clinical studies to date have evaluated the direct use of taurine in anxiety or depression. Overall, studies are lacking to fully support the use of this nutrient.

**Taurine dosage and best application.** Taurine is usually dosed about 500 mg up to three times daily and may be good for a person with anxiety, low energy, and cardiovascular concerns who would do best to relax.

Taurine can also be obtained by using the magnesium taurate form of magnesium.

**Taurine toxicity.** One study using doses of 1,500 mg/day did not find significant toxicity in patients with epilepsy. Four of 25 patients did report headaches, nausea, nosebleeding, or temporary balance disturbance (Takahashi & Nakane, 1978). Because taurine may lower blood pressure or cause slight drowsiness, bedtime may be a good time to take it, and persons taking antihypertension medications should monitor their blood pressure.

**Food sources of taurine.** Taurine is present only in animal foods, so meats and eggs would be top sources.

### S-Adenosyl-L-methionine

S-Adenosyl-L-methionine (SAMe) is a naturally occurring molecule derived from the amino acid methionine and adenine triphosphate (ATP—the main energy molecule in the body). SAMe is involved in the synthesis of various neurotransmitters in the brain and is not a newly identified substance—its chemical structure was described as early as 1952. It has been in use for decades in Europe. While it is a prescription medication in most other countries, it is found over-the-counter in the United States. Even the American Psychiatric Association (2010) has acknowledged it "might be considered" as an alternative to pharmaceutical medications—that's a rave from them as far as natural substances are concerned.

Known best as an antidepressant, SAMe serves in many biological reactions by transferring molecules called methyl groups to DNA, proteins, fats, and amino acid compounds. Methylation (carbon-molecule-donating) reactions supported by SAMe have been shown to form monoamine neurotransmitters such as dopamine, serotonin, and norepinephrine (Miller, 2008; Bottiglieri, 2002)—all of which are needed for good mood.

This chapter has already discussed the importance of B vitamins and folic acid. In depression, folate, vitamins B6 and B12, and unsaturated omega-3 fatty acid deficiencies all affect the biochemical processes in the central nervous system, as folic acid and vitamin B12 participate in the metabolism of SAMe. The deficiency of these vitamins results in high homocysteine levels. Research shows that approximately 45–55 percent of patients with depression develop significantly elevated serum homocysteine. This homocysteinemia causes a decrease in SAMe. This stops the needed methylation, which is a process needed to make neurotransmitters and fatty myelin sheaths for nerve cells. Electrical conduction along the nerve cells does not work well when the myelin sheaths are not well made or if they are damaged. Hyperhomocysteinemia also leads to increased glutamate, a brain toxin linked to mood disorder. It also affects the cardiovascular system by causing breakdown in the linings of the vessel walls, which contributes to inflammation and heart disease. All this promotes the development of various disorders, including depression (Karakula et al., 2009).

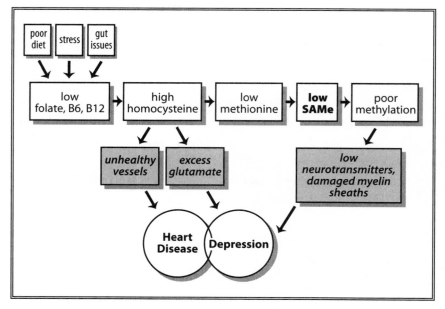

Figure 4.6. The SAMe pathway.

Folate and B12 help get things back on track by methylating the homocysteine to create methionine. SAMe is the downstream metabolite of methionine, which needs folic acid and vitamin B12 to stay at high enough levels to make neurotransmitters and to keep the nervous system in good working condition.

SAMe has been found to be safe and effective in the treatment of mild and moderate depression and, according to some accounts, has a faster onset of action than conventional antidepressants (Mischoulon & Fava, 2002; Nguyen & Gregan, 2002). In a meta-analysis of 47 studies of people with mild to moderate depression, SAMe produced significant improvements in mood. SAMe tested significantly better than placebo and worked at least as well as conventional drug therapy (U.S. Department of Health and Human Services, 2002).

One uncontrolled trial administered in doses of 800–3,600 mg/day for 10 weeks in 13 depressed patients with Parkinson's disease. Eleven patients completed the study, and 10 had at least a 50 percent improvement per depression mood questionnaires. Only one patient did not improve. In terms of possible side effects, 2 of the 13 patients did prematurely terminate participation in the study because of increased anxiety, 1 patient experienced mild nausea, and another 2 patients developed mild diarrhea, which resolved spontaneously.

SAMe has also been tested in patients who have the genetic variants in the catechol-O-methyltransferase (COMT) enzyme gene called 22q11.2DS deletion syndrome. Because these patients have only one copy of the gene responsible for the enzyme COMT (see Chapter 3 for more information), these patients have much higher likelihood of psychiatric morbidity and cognitive deficits. Patients given 800 mg SAMe twice a day for 6 weeks in a randomized double-blind cross-over placebo-controlled trial enjoyed a larger numerical improvement on relevant clinical scales compared with those given placebo, and they exhibited no manic or psychotic symptoms during the SAMe treatment (Green et al., 2012).

No research has been done using SAMe to treat severe depression, so it is unknown whether SAMe would have the same benefits as seen in mild to moderate depression. SAMe is considered expensive and may be a good second-line choice if other natural treatments are not effective or a first-line choice in older patients with other health challenges such as cardiovascular disease, Parkinson's disease, or dementia.

A number of studies directly compared SAMe to tricyclic antidepressants, with about eight studies showing equal benefits and lower side effect profiles. Pancheri, Scapicchio, and Chiaie (2002) ran a multi-center study where patients with depression received 400 mg/day via an intramuscular injection, or 150 mg/day by mouth. A total of 146 patients received SAMe, and 147 received 150mg per day of imipramine, for a period of 4 weeks. The drug or SAMe worked equally as well in both groups, but SAMe was significantly better tolerated. Another study by the same group compared 1,600 mg/day of SAMe by mouth, or 400 mg/day via intramuscular injection, with the tricyclic antidepressant Tofranil (imipramine; 150 mg/day) and found the same positive results (Delle Chiaie et al., 2002). The conclusion drawn from these studies is that the antidepressant effect of SAMe at 1,600 mg/day orally or 400 mg/day intramuscularly is comparable with that of 150 mg imipramine/day orally, with much better toleration of SAMe over its pharmaceutical counterpart.

**SAMe dosage, toxicity, and best application.** Because oral SAMe may cause nausea in some people, it is suggested to start a dosage of 200 mg twice daily, then increase to 400 mg twice daily on day 3, then to 400 mg three times daily on day 10, and finally to the full dose of 400 mg four times daily on day 14. Of course, if there are any noticeable side effects, then SAMe may need to be ramped up slower. SAMe has been used safely in children as well and has been studied doses of 200 mg up to 1,400 mg over a 2-month period in young teens (average age of 14 years) to help with functional abdominal pain, with no side effects or change in liver function (Choi & Huang, 2013). For maximal absorption, SAMe is best taken away from food.

The best application for SAMe is in a depressed patient who has low energy and little motivation. SAMe may increase anxiety in patients who are already anxious, and is contraindicated in bipolar disorder.

**SAMe food sources.** The body makes SAMe, but there are no known food sources.

## BOTANICAL MEDICINES

From time immemorial, plants have been a source of nutrition and medicine for humans. Botanical medicines (also known as herbs) may be used as a supplement in the sense of using plant material as a source of certain vitamins or minerals. Botanicals can also be used to create more physiologic or biological effects in the body, similar to how a drug may work.

Herbs are typically safe because herbal medications, as natural plants, contain many ingredients that will communicate with the body and create warning messages before toxicity can occur. For example, we can look at the herbal plant *Digitalis* (foxglove) and the medication digoxin (Digox). The Native Americans used foxglove for apparent cardiovascular distress, as they noticed a positive effect on energy and circulation upon consumption of the plant. From foxglove, modern medicine extracted the component digoxin, which works as a positive inotrope (strengthens heart muscle contractions). The problem with digoxin is it has a narrow therapeutic window—you take too little and it doesn't work, but take too much and it can cause bradycardia and quickly kill a person. The whole plant foxglove, on the other hand, tends to make a person vomit and creates great digestive distress well before levels of digoxin become too high. While both the drug and the plant can be toxic, the multiple molecules in the plant will usually create nonfatal signs of toxicity first, whereas processing has removed the drug's ability to do this. This example underscores the reason that, in general, natural herbal substances tend to be safer, and also that it may be best to use whole herbs, instead of extracting and studying certain molecules and "active ingredients" only.

Table IV.7 in Appendix IV reviews the top botanical medicines for anxiety and depression, which are described in detail below.

## Turmeric (*Curcuma longa*)

Turmeric enjoys a long and rich history stemming from both Chinese and Ayurvedic Sanmukhani studied for its anticancer properties, neurologic support, and anti-inflammatory benefits. It is known as a powerful ally to reduce relapse rates in ulcerative colitis, heal proctitis, and reduce polyp formation (Hanai et al., 2006). Posited benefits for the brain and nervous system include its anti-inflammatory and neural regenerative capacity, with ability to create new neurons in emotional centers of the brain (Kulkarni et al. 2009).

Curcumin comprises up to 5 percent of turmeric and is considered the most likely active component in this spice. Studies show curcumin's significant antianxiety abilities in stressed mice (Gilhotra & Dhingra, 2010), possibly through changes of serotonin expression in the brain (Benammi et al., 2014). Curcumin has been shown to normalize the depressive-like behaviors of neuropathic mice (mice modeling pain syndromes) (Zhao et al., 2014). Animal studies using a highly absorbable form of turmeric called BCM-95 with fluoxetine (Prozac) or imipramine (Tofranil) found benefits when added on as a medication (Sanmukhani et al., 2011). The combined research suggests that curcumin's positive effect may be due to its anti-inflammatory abilities, as well as direct support of neurotransmitters, specifically increasing norepinephrine, dopamine, and serotonin.

A clinical study by Sanmukhani et al. (2014) of 45 depressed patients taking fluoxetine, curcumin as BCM-95, or both, found greatest number of responders in the group taking both interventions (about 78 percent), with the single-therapy groups having practically identical results (65 percent and 63 percent, respectively). Even more, all three groups found similar benefit levels among those that positively responded, showing that curcumin may be used to treat major depressive disorder.

### Dosage and safety

The study by Sanmukhani et al. (2013)used 1,000 mg/day of the BCM-95 form of curcumin, which is known to have bioavailability up to seven times greater than regular curcumin (Antony et al., 2008). While side effects are uncommon, curcumin supplementation may cause mild gastritis and mild nausea, and for effectiveness is best taken away from meals.

### Passionflower (*Passiflora incarnata*)

Passionflower has a long and rich history of use as calmative agent in folklore for its anxiolytic properties and is considered an official plant medicine in many countries. Although there are many possible active ingredients in passionflower, they are likely alkaloids and bioflavonoids (Mitchell, 2003, p. 126).

Like the pharmaceutical Xanax, passionflower reduces anxiety in part by binding to benzodiazepine receptors in the brain. It has chrysin and other flavonoid-like compounds with confirmed antianxiety, anti-inflammatory activities (Zhou Tan & Deng, 2008).

A 2007 Cochrane meta-analysis looked at two studies with a total of 198 participants and showed that passionflower had the same effect as the benzodiazepine medications (Miyasaka, Atallah, & Soares, 2007). One double-blind, placebo-controlled study of 36 patients compared passionflower to the benzodiazepine oxazepam, in patients with generalized anxiety disorder. While the drug had a faster onset, the passionflower and medication worked at the same efficacy and while the herbal remedy showed fewer side effects than the drug, such as job impairment performance (Akhondzadeh et al., 2001). Another study looked at 60 patients given passionflower or placebo for anxiety 90 minutes before surgery and found much lower anxiety using the botanical, without inducing sedation or negative postoperative effects (Movafegh et al.,

2008). Other positive effects were noted in a multicenter, double-blind, placebo-controlled general practice study where 182 patients with anxiety and adjustment disorder were given passionflower along with a few other herbs, including hawthorn (*Crataegus oxyacantha*) and valerian (*Valeriana officinalis*).

### *Passionflower dosage and best application*

Like many herbs, passionflower can be dosed in capsules or tablets, as a tea, or as a liquid tincture. I typically prescribe passionflower in tincture form at 1 or 2 dropperful (about 30–60 drops) three times a day. It may be placed in a little water or taken in tea.

Passionflower is known by herbalists as helpful with overthinking and swirling thoughts that exaggerate anxiety in the mind. Patients who mention how their mind is "spinning" and "reeling out of control" often do well with passionflower. Passionflower's Latin name is *Passiflora incarnata*, or "passion incarnate," and can be suggested for people who are unsure of where there life is going.

### *Passionflower toxicity*

Passionflower has no known toxicity when taken in typical doses. One study above (Akhondzadeh et al., 2001) found minor dizziness, drowsiness, and confusion in one patient. Because it has a sedative effect, it should not be combined with alcoholic beverages or prescription sedatives without working with an experienced practitioner. There is a theoretical concern when used with monoamine oxidase inhibitors due to interaction with passionflower's alkaloids. Passionflower should not be used by pregnant or lactating women or given to children under 6 months old (Fisher, Purcell, & Le Couteur, 2004).

### Kava Kava (*Piper methysticum*)

Translated as "intoxicating pepper," kava hails from the Western Pacific for its ability to calm and relax without acting as a sedative. Animal studies suggest its likely mechanisms are through GABA receptors, as well as dopamine reuptake inhibition by its kava lactone constituents. Kava may also inhibit both norepinephrine uptake and sodium and potassium channels (Weeks, 2009). Its effect is anxiolytic, producing a reduction in skeletal muscle tension.

Since the late 1990s, a number of controlled trials have been conducted to look at the effectiveness of kava in anxiety. A meta-analysis of six trials of patients with nonpsychotic anxiety disorders showed excellent overall results, with particular benefit in women and younger patients (Witte, Loew, & Gaus, 2005). A separate earlier Cochrane meta-analysis (Pittler & Ernst, 2003) looked at 11 trials with a total of 645 participants and also found it to be effective versus placebo. Most of the research concluded that when kava is used as an anxiolytic alternative to benzodiazepines or tricyclic antidepressants, individuals typically suffer from fewer side effects. While in the minority, a few studies did not find benefit in reducing anxiety symptoms. Two of these studies showed no significant difference between kava treatment and placebo (Sarris et al., 2009; Jacobs et al., 2005) with one very small pilot suggesting placebo was actually more effective for symptoms in patients with higher baseline anxiety scores (Connor & Davidson, 2002). Overall, though, the majority of studies show substantial benefit.

Malsch and Kieser (2001) utilized a kava kava extract in a 5-week randomized, placebo-controlled, double-blind study for 49 patients looking to wean off their anxiety medications. The kava was increased from 50 mg to 300 mg/day during the first treatment week, and the patient's benzodiazepine medication was tapered off over 2 weeks. This was followed by 3 weeks solely with kava or placebo. This study used the Hamilton Anxiety Scale and a subjective well-being scale, along with monitoring for benzodiazepine withdrawal symptoms. Treatment safety was checked by regular patient interviews. The kava was clearly better than placebo based on scale measures, as well as secondary measures. Also, kava was as well tolerated as the placebo over the weeks of the study.

*Kava kava dosage and best application*

In my clinic, I often use 30 drops of tincture two or three times a day as a mental relaxant, which can be placed in a little water, or into hot water as a calming tea. The above trials suggest that an extract dosage of 400 mg/day in capsule form is useful and should not cause any side effects. It may best serve younger patients and women. I have used it clinically in female patients who suffer from interstitial cystitis. Effectiveness in men was also found in the above trials. Kava is especially useful in anxiety that manifests with muscle tension. Kava can also be used to help wean off benzodiazepines by starting with 50 mg and moving up to 300 mg/day while tapering the benzodiazepine medication tapers off over 2 weeks, with a subsequent 3 weeks of 300 mg/day of kava.

*Kava kava toxicity*

While the trials above describe no toxicity with kava, the FDA published a consumer advisory warning in 2002 about the potential for severe liver damage from kava-containing supplements due to some reports that suggested hepatotoxicity (U.S. Food & Drug Administration, 2002). It has since been shown that the vast majority of studies and traditional use do not identify toxicity with kava and that it is possible these case reports may be secondary to polypharmacy, overdose, or poor quality and adulteration of the herbs. From 1992 to 2002, over 450 million daily doses of kava extract, equating to 15 million of monthly doses, were sold in Germany and Switzerland alone, without major incident (Teschke, Schwarzenboeck, & Akinci, 2008). A few anecdotal reports suggest a paradoxical increase in anxiety.

## Lavender (*Lavendula angustifolium*)

For centuries, different species of lavender flowers have been relied on in times of anxiety. Today, various preparations are well known for benefit in anxiety, as well as being a support for depression.

Studies are starting to pile up in favor of lavender for mood. A multicenter study of 221 patients with anxiety showed clear benefits of an immediate-release capsule preparation of lavender over placebo (Kasper et al., 2010b). A double-blind study by Woelk and Schläfke (2010) compared a commercial lavender oil preparation (Silexan) and lorazepam (Ativan) for general anxiety disorder and found 40 percent of the patients that received lavender achieved remission, versus 27 percent using the drug. The herb achieved this without any sedative side effects. While the study design was quite strong, it should be noted the authors of the study were employees of the study's sponsor.

### Lavender dosage and toxicity

Lavender can be taken in the immediate-release capsule mentioned above, using one capsule a day, which contains 80 mg lavender oil. If a client has significant anxiety then I recommend placing a few drops of lavender essential oil in a warm bath with some Epsom salts. A randomized controlled trial of 80 women who took daily baths with lavender oil experienced improved mood, reduced aggression, and a more positive outlook (Morris, 2002). I may also recommend a separate lavender tincture at 30 drops three times a day. Lavender may also be taken as a tea by using 1 or 2 teaspoons of herb per cup or two of water, and it is especially good for an upset stomach resulting from nervousness. Remember, essential oils are used externally, either for the bath or for aromatherapy. Essential oils are not supposed to be taken orally. There are no problems with toxicity when lavender is used in the proper form.

### Ashwagandha (Withania somnifera)

Of all the supplements discussed in this book, ashwagandha may have the richest history, dating back three millennia to the time Ayurvedic practitioners began to enjoy its benefits. The word ashwagandha translates to "smell of horse" for two reasons: the herb itself does have that interesting smell, and traditional belief is that consumption can help its user gain horse-like strength and vitality (Shastry, 2001).

While ancient medicines view it as a overall tonic for the body, modern research has keyed in on its advantage for inflammatory conditions, Parkinson's disease, neurologic disorders and as an adjunct in cancer care to support drops in white blood cell counts (Mishra, Singh, & Dagenais, 2000). While this herb possesses numerous compounds that help balance physiology, this plant's alkaloids and lactones (known as withanolides), acting as hormonal precursors, have been the center of much research on ashwagandha (Withania somnifera, 2004).

In holistic care, ashwagandha is seen as adaptogenic and can bind to receptors to increase effect when available ligands (receptor stimulators) are low but block excess stimulation when ligand availability is high (Bhattacharya et al., 2000). While most understanding of ashwagandha is based on its long history and animal studies, a few studies do show benefit for anxiety.

A study by Chandrasekhar, Kapoor, and Anishetty (2012) randomized 64 people to either placebo or 300 mg of high-concentration extract from the ashwagandha root, as one capsule twice a day, for 60 days. During the treatment period (on days 15, 30, 45, and 60), follow-up telephone calls were made to all subjects to check for treatment compliance and to note any adverse reactions. The treatment group exhibited a significant reduction in scores on all the stress-assessment scales on day 60 relative to the placebo group. Serum cortisol levels were substantially reduced compared with the placebo group. The adverse effects were mild and comparable in both groups. A case study (Kalani, Bahtiyar, & Sacerdote, 2012) showed benefit in women with adrenal hyperplasia (a situation where the adrenal glands have swollen due to chronic stress). The women found improvements in levels of cortisol, progesterone, and pregnenolone, as well as noticeable improvement in alopecia (hair loss). In another case study, men with stress-related fertility issues showed higher antioxidant status and healthier sperm (Mahdi et al., 2009).

### Ashwagandha dosage and best usage

Typical dosage is 300 mg once or twice a day of ashwagandha with standardized withanolide content (considered an active component of ashwagandha) of at least 1–5 percent. Ashwagandha's best use is for someone with anxiety and a stressful life accompanied by nervous depletion and sleeplessness. I have taken ashwagandha myself and can attest to its value to help support stressful situations by making the body less reactive.

### Ashwagandha toxicity

No toxicity was noted in any studies with this botanical medicine, save one case report that documented a woman who presented with hirsutism (body hair growth) who appeared to have increased levels of dehydro-epiandrosterone sulfate along with lowered testosterone levels while taking ashwagandha. While not clear if the ashwagandha was the cause, this resolved once she stopped the herb (Nguyen et al., 2013). One senior patient of mine reported vomiting with this herb.

### Rhodiola (Rhodiola rosea)

Rhodiola was originally observed in the Russian literature as a plant medicine useful to combat physical, biological, and chemical stressors (Kelly, 2001). Like ashwagandha, rhodiola is adaptogenic in that it can increase lower levels of hormones and neurotransmitters and bring down levels that are too high. As an adaptogenic herb, studies show it acts as a neuroprotective, cardioprotective, antifatigue, antidepressive, anxiolytic, and nootropic (cognitive enhancing), with effects that increase life span and stimulate the central nervous system (Panossian et al., 2010).

Looking at a unique molecule in rhodiola called rosavin, mouse studies have shown both antidepressant and anxiety-reducing effects (Perfumi & Mattioli, 2007). Animal studies have suggested that rhodiola's ability to effect GABA is minimal, suggesting that other mechanisms throughout the nervous system and body (other than acting like a benzodiazepine) are involved in its calming and protective effects (Cayer et al., 2013).

One small pilot study looked at 10 patients with a diagnosis of generalized anxiety disorder. They received a total daily dose of 340 mg rhodiola extract for 10 weeks and showed significant decreases in the Hamilton Anxiety Rating Scale (Bystritsky, Kerwin, & Feusner, 2008).

A clinical trial assessed the efficacy of a standardized extract rhodiola in the treatment of patients with mild to moderate depression comparing it to placebo (Darbinyan et al., 2007). Over a 6-week period, one group A (31 patients) was given 340 mg/day of standardized rhodiola extract, Group B (29 patients) was given 680 mg/day, and Group C (29 patients) was given a placebo. Groups A and B showed a statistically significant reduction in overall depression; group C did not improve. Of all the mood parameters tested, the only one not affected for the better at the lower dose was "self-esteem" (which is an important one). However, at 680 mg/day, self-esteem also improved significantly with no side effects noted.

### Rhodiola dosage and best application

Dosages in studies have ranged from 340 mg/day up to 680 mg/day. Rhodiola may be standardized for 1 percent of the molecule rosavin. Longer-term studies of this adaptogen are needed, but what we know so far seems to make rhodiola a great choice if a patient is depressed and/or anxious and feeling burnt out in the process.

### Rhodiola toxicity

Within given dosages, no toxicities have been reported. Other studies have used rhodiola for up to 4 months without reported side effects. One study (Bystritsky et al., 2008) found mild to moderate side effects of dizziness and dry mouth, which might have been attributable to the subjects' anxiety.

### St. John's wort (Hypericum perforatum)

While ashwagandha may have the longest history of use of all the supplements discussed in this book, St. John's wort (SJW) is the most studied herb of all time. The Latin name Hypericum perforatum means "above a ghost," and this botanical was gathered as a way to ward off evil spirits. SJW is a plant with five-petal yellow flowers and is notable for its effectiveness in both anxiety and mild to moderate depression. As a result,

SJW is now becoming one of world's standard treatment consideration for low mood. Like SAMe, even the American Psychiatric Association (2010) has acknowledged it "might be considered" as an alternative to pharmaceutical medications—again, that's pretty much another rave from them as far as natural substances are concerned.

SJW is best known as an antidepressant, and most conventional circles consider it, at a cursory glance, as simply another antidepressant drug with some SSRI capability. While SJW may exhibit some SSRI mechanisms, it has numerous other effects in both the brain and the central nervous system. In truth, despite all the study, the exact antidepressant mechanism of action of SJW is still not fully understood—likely because it, likely other botanical medicines, has numerous chemical components that cause multiple gentle effects throughout the body. Initially it was believed to work like the first drugs used for depression, the monoamine oxidase inhibitors, which act by slowing the breakdown of neurotransmitters (Müller et al., 1997). Other studies then suggested it stops the breakdown of acetylcholine (Re et al., 2003) and has a serotonin-like activity (Helgason, 2007), where it can act like a weak SSRI with fewer side effects (Morelli & Zoorob, 2000). It also gently balances other neurotransmitter levels, including norepinephrine and dopamine, as well supporting GABA (Nierenberg Lund & Mischoulon, 2008; Hammerness, 2003). Other studies show this wonderful herb to have anti-inflammatory and nerve protective properties (Wong et al., 2004). What we can take from all this is that SJW has pleiotropic effects—all around the body and brain—and in total they seem to lower both depression and anxiety symptoms.

With hundreds of studies reviewing SJW for depression, the most recent meta-analysis as of this writing is a 2008 study from Munich (Linde, Berner, & Kriston, 2008) that reviewed only randomized and double-blind studies of patients with depression. Compared with previous reviews, this meta-analysis included newer well-designed studies published between 1995 and 2006. SJW for 4–12 weeks was compared with placebo and, in 17 studies published between 1997 and 2006, with standard antidepressants, including fluoxetine, sertraline (Zoloft), imipramine, citalopram (Celexa), paroxetine (Paxil), and amitriptyline (Elavil). In all, it included 29 studies with 5,489 patients. The studies came from many of countries, tested several different SJW extracts, and mostly included patients suffering from mild to moderately severe symptoms. Overall, the SJW extracts tested in these trials were superior to placebo and were at least as effective as standard antidepressants. Furthermore, patients given SJW extracts dropped out of trials less frequently due to adverse effects than those given older antidepressants. Further research goes on to suggest that antidepressant side effects are between 10- and 38-fold higher than those of SJW (Kasper et al., 2010a). Given the same benefits as the drugs, and fewer side effects, there is no reason not try it first for mild to moderate depression.

While SJW is well studied for depression, newer studies are starting to unearth its antianxiety power. Animal studies in diabetic rats given SJW showed clear benefits toward lowering glucose levels, as well as minimizing anxiety and depression behaviors (Husain et al., 2011). Another study found benefit for mood and anxiety in postmenopausal women (Geller & Studee, 2007). However, study of 60 subjects did not see benefit for obsessive-compulsive disorder (Kobak et al., 2005).

*St. John's wort dosage and best application*

SJW dosage is usually given between 900 and 1,800 mg of standardized extract/day, usually divided into three doses throughout the day, although some literature reports one or two larger doses a day can be as effective (which makes compliance easier). Common tincture dose ranges from 20 to 60 drops three times a day. Extracts from fresh herb are typically dosed 5 mL two to three times a day. It is best to check the label for the type of medicine and concentration. With my patients, I typically use a capsule or tablet form standardized for 0.3 percent of the compound hypericin.

Overall, the literature supports the use of SJW for mild to moderate depression. I would add that there's likely benefit for anxiety associated with diabetes and for postmenopausal depression with anxiety. At this point, results are not clear that there is any benefit for anxiety by itself, and it should not be used as a monotherapy in severe depression, especially if used in place of pharmaceutical medications known to have quicker and more effective response.

For patients with preexisting conductive heart dysfunction or elderly patients, high-dose *Hypericum* extract has found to be safer with regard to cardiac function over tricyclic antidepressants (Czekalla et al., 1997) and may be indicated as a better choice for cardiac patients with depression. Also, two studies show that SJW (300 mg one to three times a day) can actually improve the effectiveness of the platelet inhibitor clopidogrel (Plavix) up to 36 percent in patients who are poor responders to this medication (Lau et al., 2011).

*St. John's wort toxicity and interactions*

The side effect profile of SJW extract is minor, especially compared with the well-known side effects of antidepressant medications (Henry, Alexander & Sener, 1995). Symptoms of agitation and others matching possible excessive levels of serotonin should also be considered and monitored when using SJW with antidepressant medication, tryptophan, or 5-HTP (see the discussion of serotonin syndrome in the tryptophan section above).

Although SJW has been demonstrated to induce photosensitivity in some patients (less than 1 percent of people taking it), this not likely with standard dosages and has occurred mainly in HIV patients using larger than normal quantities for an antiviral effect (Gulick et al., 1992). It has been suggested that using a tincture may avoid photosensitivity while still achieving the mood benefits (Barendsen, 1996).

It has been shown that SJW can either enhance or reduce circulating levels of many drugs (Izzo, 2004; Tannergren et al., 2004; Hall et al., 2003; Peebles et al., 2001). SJW is known to increase the effect of enzymes of the liver (the cytochrome P450 system), as well as compounds in the intestinal wall (P-glycoprotein) that are used to detoxify drugs. As a result, it is important for patients to check with a doctor or pharmacist if they are taking medications, before they start SJW.

## Saffron (*Crocus sativus*)

Hailing from the Persian traditional medicine pharmacopoeia (Akhondzadeh et al., 2004), saffron is known for its vibrant color and flavor and also for being the world's most expensive spice. With a high amount of antioxidative carotenoids (which give it its burnt orange color) and B vitamins, saffron has been traditionally used as a calmative, antidepressant, and anti-inflammatory, with a digestive specialty of relaxing the muscles of the digestive tract to reduce spasms and help digest food, as well being an appetite enhancer (Yarnell, 2008).

A number of recent preclinical and clinical studies indicate that the stigma of the plant (the top of the plant where the pollen is, which is technically called the "saffron") and petal of the *Crocus sativus* plant both have antidepressant effects. Animal studies show that the compounds safranal and crocin may exert antidepressant effects by keeping balanced levels of dopamine, norepinephrine, and serotonin (Hosseinzadeh, Karimi, & Niapoor, 2004).

In an 8-week double-blind randomized trial, Akhondzadeh et al. (2007) randomly assigned 40 depressed adult outpatients to receive either a 15-mg capsule of petals of the crocus plant in the morning and evening or 10 mg Prozac, in the morning and in the evening. At the end of trial, the crocus petal capsules were as effective as the drug, with no significant differences in percentages of responders: fluoxetine had an 85 percent responder rate (17 of 20 patients, an unusually high rate for this drug) and crocus petal capsules showed a similar 75 percent responder rate. A 6-week comparison with imipramine found significantly better Hamilton Depression Scale outcomes with the herb (Akhondzadeh et al., 2005).

### Crocus dosage and toxicity

For the above clinical studies, 15 mg of the petal or stigma (saffron) was given twice a day. Crocus petal is reported to have the same antidepressant effect as the stigma in at least three clinical trials (Noorbala et al.,

2005; Akhondzadeh et al., 2004, 2005)—the petal costs significantly less than saffron but with the same benefit.

No toxicity has been reported at these dosages or when ingested in culinary amounts. One study on rats with exceedingly high levels of the herb injected directly into their abdomen showed reductions in red blood cells, as well as changed liver and kidney function. However, these are much higher doses than used clinically, and intraperitoneal (abdominal) injection doses are not processed through the digestive tract as oral doses would be (Mohajeri et al., 2007). As a precaution, patients with liver and kidney problems may not want to use this herb if other treatment choices are available. Interestingly, in rats given the chemotherapy drug cisplatin, crocus, along with the amino acid cysteine and vitamin E, actually protected the kidneys from toxicity (el Daly, 1998).

### Mucuna (*Mucuna puriens*)

Known as the velvet bean, this herb hails from traditional use in Ayurvedic medicine. Used as medicine since 1500 BC, mucuna has not been studied for use in depression, although some animal studies suggest possible benefit.

This plant contains more L-dopamine than any other known source. Chapter 2 discussed how this neurotransmitter is known to boost mood and raise motivation. Mucuna has been studied for its effectiveness in helping patients with Parkinson's disease, a condition where the area of the brain that makes dopamine does not function. Three open label studies where patients took an average of 45 g/day of mucuna seed powder extract (which is equivalent to about 1,500 mg L-dopamine) reported significant symptom improvement (HP-200 in Parkinson's Disease Study Group, 1995; Vaidya et al., 1978; Nagashayana et al., 2000). Another study suggested the mucuna might have fewer side effects than the standard Parkinson's medication (Katzenschlager et al., 2004).

I mention this herb for depressed patients who may be benefiting from dopamine-boosting medications like bupropion or aripiprazole.

Patients who have found these to help with motivation, self-esteem, and a general good mood may be able to use low doses of this herb to help them wean off the medication while maintaining their better mood. Some patients may be able to use this as an alternative to the medications—please note, though, that this idea has not been studied clinically, although my personal experience with patients suggests it works.

### Mucuna dosage

For support with medication, I recommend starting with 200 mg of the extract and moving up to 200 mg twice a day after 2 weeks (which supplies ~120–240 mg L-dopamine). This is a relatively low dose. Higher doses may be appropriate if patients are not on dopamine-boosting medications.

### Mucuna toxicity

Mucuna may cause some bloating and nausea in some people and can interfere with anticoagulant (blood-thinning) drugs. It may boost testosterone and could aggravate polycystic ovarian syndrome in women. There have been reported cases of severe vomiting, palpitations, difficulty in falling asleep, delusions, or confusion. To be safe, I recommend that a patient work with a knowledgeable practitioner when using this herb.

## HOMEOPATHY

The term *homeopathy* is derived from the two Greek words *homeo*, which means "similar," and *pathos*, which refers to suffering. Homeopathy is one of the most interesting and controversial modalities in the holistic armamentarium. Homeopathy can be a staple treatment or point of contention for the integrative medicine practitioner, as well as a focus of vitriol for those looking to discredit natural medicine.

Homeopathy is also one of the more difficult natural medicine approaches to explain from a Western science standpoint. Despite this, it has prescribed as a part of successful care in Europe and India for over a 100 years. The theory of homeopathy suggests that a given remedy may play a role in changing the energetics of a person's condition to allow the body to heal from the inside.

Developed by physician Samuel Hahnemann in the late eighteenth and early nineteenth centuries, homeopathy is a system of therapy based on the concept that each naturally occurring element, plant, and mineral compound will, when ingested or applied, result in certain symptoms and physiologic change. Using this knowledge, a given disease may be treated with minute homeopathic doses of the substance thought capable of producing in healthy people the same symptoms of that disease. This is known as the concept "like cures like" (Medicine.net, 2009).

Using this principle, Hahnemann's work found clinical value and gained acceptance. The first homeopathic medical college was established in Allentown, Pennsylvania, in 1835 (which is today's Medical College of Pennsylvania). The American Medical Association (AMA) was founded in 1847 and from its inception pursued policies to discredit natural medicines and specifically homeopathy. Despite the AMA's influence, by the latter half of the nineteenth century homeopathy continued to grow and gain acceptance. With a reputation for efficacy, it spread throughout Europe, as well as in Asia and North America. Today, it is well accepted in India and Germany for use along with conventional care.

## Homeopathic Studies in Anxiety and Depression

Studies using homeopathic medicines for psychiatric illness are scant. Probably one of the strongest studies to date for homeopathic treatment of anxiety and depression is a 1997 study out of Duke University that examined selected remedies given on an outpatient basis to treat 12 adults who had major depression, social phobia, or panic disorder (Davidson et al., 1997). The patients either requested homeopathic treatment or received it on a physician's recommendation after partial or poor response to conventional therapies. Patients were prescribed individual homeopathic prescriptions based on their presentations. Duration of treatment was 7–8 weeks. Response rates were 58 percent for overall improvement, as scored using clinical global improvement scales, and 50 percent according to the Symptom Checklist-90-R or the Brief Social Phobia Scale. Type and potency of the remedies, duration of treatment, and cointerventions varied across patients, as did the initial diagnoses, which makes it difficult to truly understand the efficacy of the intervention. The authors concluded that homeopathy "may be useful in the treatment of affective and anxiety disorders in patients with mildly to severely symptomatic conditions" (Davidson et al., 1997). Unfortunately, this trial also did not have a control. However, this study was considered relevant, and valuable as a preliminary report, by an independent study review (Pilkington et al., 2005).

One well-designed uncontrolled clinical trial of the use of individualized homeopathy was conducted to assess symptom relief in 100 patients with cancer (Thompson & Reilly, 2002), 39 of whom had metastatic disease—a pretty tough group in which to gain symptom relief. There was significant improvement in mean depression score for the whole study group. Overall, 52 percent of patients had some improvement in depression scores after four to six consultations. Seventeen patients suffered an aggravation of symptoms during this study. Symptom scores for fatigue and hot flushes, but not pain scores, improved significantly over the study period. No side effects were noted. Of the 52 patients who completed the study, patient satisfaction measured by self-completion questionnaire was high; 73 percent (38 of 52) regarded homeopathic treatment as having been "helpful" or better.

A meta-analysis conducted at Duke University by Wayne Jonas MD (former head of the former Office of Alternative Medicine at the National Institutes of Health—now called the National Center of Complementary Medicine) and his colleagues (Davidson et al., 2011) found 25 eligible studies from an initial pool of 1,431 subjects. Efficacy was found for the functional somatic syndromes group (fibromyalgia and chronic fatigue syndrome), but not for anxiety or stress. For other psychiatric disorders, homeopathy produced mixed effects. As mentioned above, there have been no placebo-controlled studies for depression. Meaningful safety data were lacking in the reports, but the superficial findings suggested good tolerability of homeopathy for treatment of psychiatric illness.

One recent randomized, double-blind, placebo-controlled study looked at a combination homeopathic remedy in stressed women (Hellhammer & Schubert, 2013). For 14 days, 40 female subjects took three tables of a homeopathic comprising respinum, gelsemium, passionflower, coffea, and veratrum. On the 15th study day, participants took three pills in the morning and upon arrival at the study site. Subjects were assessed for salivary cortisol, plasma cortisol, adrenocorticotrophic hormone, epinephrine, norepinephrine, and heart rates; well-being, anxiety, stress, and insecurity during the stress test; and sleep and quality of life. While cortisol levels did not differ between groups, homeopathically treated participants had better sleep quality and lower norepinephrine levels. The authors concluded that the homeopathic helped regulate the neuroendocrine stress response during acute stress and impaired sleep.

Combined, these studies show that when studying homeopathy using conventional parameters, results are mixed, with some suggestion of efficacy. It is highly possible, however, that studying homeopathy from a more systems-based paradigm (food, sleep, work, stress reduction, nutrients, etc.), and more specific prescribing for the individual, may show better results in the future.

Appendix V lists homeopathics commonly used for depression and anxiety. The tables suggest mental and emotional patterns, as well as physical appearance and/or peculiar or idiosyncratic aspects, that may be found in your client. It is likely that not all clients will display all of these, but ideally you will see an overall pattern that may fit. Please note that a few remedies may be appropriate for either anxiety or depression. If you are more interested in homeopathy, you may want to purchase a homeopathic material medica, which describes the remedies in greater detail.

## Dosage of homeopathics

As is true for many forms of natural medicines, different sources recommend various methods of dosing. One simple low-potency method is to take one dose of 30X potency every 6–12 hours and look for change in about a week. Clients should stop taking the remedy once symptoms are better. If there is no change, or if symptoms worsen after dosing, then consider another remedy.

# FIVE

# Mind-Body Medicine

---

### Clinical Case Study: Anxious Alice

*Alice is a 43-year-old mother of three girls, ages three, seven, and nine. About five years ago she started having her first panic attacks while driving over a bridge. While she drove (albeit with great discomfort), her anxiety slowly moved into the realm many anxious moms report: "Dying and leaving my children motherless." To make it worse, last year her husband's sister died at the age of 34, leaving two children behind.*

*She continually worried that something would happen to her, either an accident or, she felt more likely, an illness. Her focus centered on breast cancer. Given that she is from Long Island, an area of New York known for its record-high breast cancer rates, she found much fuel for this thought. She started seeing her current therapist about four years ago. This helped her function better and get out and drive, but the daily stress did not let up. Mammogram after mammogram was negative, which gave her a few days of relief until she learned that mammograms themselves might cause breast cancer! In her mind now, she didn't know what to do: keep checking and increase her risk more, or let a cancer go undetected.*

*One year ago, she decided to visit another naturopathic doctor who put her on a solid regimen of health food and vitamins for anxiety and cancer prevention support. This helped as well. When she came to see me, she had her "good days" when she could distract herself enough with being busy, and "bad days" when nothing could stop her from thinking about death. Either way, she still went to bed thinking in detail about the various scenarios her death would take and picturing the milestone events in her daughters' lives coming up without her.*

*I asked Alice if she ever had anxiety before five years ago, she first told me no. But, as we talked, she told me she could never stay still. "My mind is never quiet. Even as a kid, I was always worried about the next thing. I thought that was normal." I asked her if she every meditated. Her face tightened, and almost paled as she said, "That is the worst thing—it makes me crazy. I won't do it." I explained to her how the mind is like a puppy, and if we let the puppy run around undisciplined, it will grow up very unhappy, and in a sense, her mind is a puppy that needs some gentle but firm discipline.*

*Starting very, very slowly (30 seconds twice a day), she began to deeply breathe and meditate—learning to deal with the thoughts that flooded in. In two months, she was up to 10 minutes twice a day. She also added yoga once a week to her regimen. Today, she still has fleeting thoughts of death but uses them as a moment to appreciate her life and to enjoy her family. In fact, after doing more therapy work, she now states how death is "a natural part of life" and "I can't teach my kids to fear death." There's an old adage that says sometimes "the thing you hate the most is what you need the most." In Alice's case, this was true.*

Once relegated to the world of "placebo," it is quite clear that mind-body modalities are not simply "feel-good" distractions but instead can be an effective part of healing anxiety and depression. In fact, given the research, it may be argued that these therapies are the most elegant method to create change in the hypothalamic-pituitary-adrenal (HPA) axis, thus altering the neuroendocrine, digestive, and inflammatory pathways of the body for the benefit of the patient. This chapter touches on some of the top mind-body methods, but this is by no means an exhaustive list.

## YOGA

At least 5,000 years old, the practice of yoga predates Hinduism. The Sanskrit word *yuj* means "yoke" or "to unite" and points to creating an awareness that unites our physical, spirit, and emotional worlds. While today's Western practices focus on movement of the body, yoga inspires us to bring synergy to all aspects of life, mental, physical, and emotional, by using breath and movement and changing thoughts. In our modern society, these aspects of life are often missing and can predispose us to anxiety and depression. Yogic controlled breathing helps to focus the mind and achieve relaxation (in contrast to meditation, which aims to calm the mind). Like exercise, yoga is an excellent method to deepen the breath and keep the blood flowing.

From a spiritual standpoint, yoga is a strong practice that can help modify emotional processing. *Sukha* is the Sanskrit word for happiness, which literally translates to "unobstructed peace." Yoga practice is thought to clear blockages within the body, which leads to greater sense of calm and contentment with reality as it is, often with greater sense of happiness and connectedness with others (Weintraub, 2005).

Numerous studies point to yoga's ability to modulate HPA function. Yoga's ability to lower cortisol, modulate hormones, and regulate the activity of both the parasympathetic and sympathetic nervous systems may underlie some of the benefits it offers for both anxiety and stress (Kerstan et al., 2007). Yoga also helps mood by balancing the neurotransmitter serotonin and stabilizing blood sugar. Physiologically, yoga has been shown to lower cortisol and decrease inflammatory markers such as C-reactive protein, and may be effective at lowering blood pressure. For example, a significant decrease in salivary cortisol was seen following a 90-minute session of Iyengar yoga, an important physiologic finding that may help to explain yoga's beneficial effects for stress and anxiety (Michalsen et al., 2005). Yoga practitioners experienced a significant increase in GABA levels following a 60-minute yoga session compared with a control group who read magazines and fiction (Streeter, 2010).

A systematic review by Kirkwood et al. (2005) that included only controlled clinical trials of patients with anxiety disorders found positive results with the use of yoga for anxiety. Shannahoff-Khalsa et al. (1999) conducted a hospital-based randomized controlled trial in the United States with a group of participants diagnosed with obsessive-compulsive disorder. After 3 months, an experimental group practicing Kundalini yoga along with a number of other yoga techniques, including mantra meditation, experienced significantly greater improvements on the Yale Brown Obsessive Compulsive Scale, as well as other scales, than a control group that practiced a meditative control regimen.

Five randomized controlled trials have also reported positive results for patients with reactive depression (depression due to a specific event) (Broota & Dhir, 1990), melancholic depression (depression with strong aspects of not enjoying activities and guilt) (Janakiramaiah et al., 2000)' major depression (Rohini et al., 2000) and even severe depression (Khumar, Kaur, & Kaur, 1993), with no side effects noted. Woolery et al., (2004) looked at the Iyengar style of yoga, which focuses on body alignment. The asanas (postures) recommended are those that involve opening and lifting of the chest, inversions, and vigorous standing poses. Patients were randomly assigned to two 1-hour yoga classes each week for 5 weeks or control group. A total of 5 patients withdrew (3 out of 13 in the yoga group, 2 out of 15 in the control group), without reported reasons. Of the subjects who remained, significant reductions in depression and anxiety scales were observed in the yoga but not in the control group who had received no intervention. The effects emerged about 2.5 weeks into the study and were maintained at week 5.

*Yoga contraindications*

While yoga presents very few contraindications and practically no interaction with Western medications, certain poses may need modification to work with pregnancy, and there is special caution for those with glaucoma, high blood pressure, and sciatica (National Center for Complementary and Alternative Medicine, 2013b).

## MEDITATION AND MINDFULNESS-BASED THERAPY (MBT)

### Meditation/Qigong

Meditation hails from yoga and Buddhist traditions going back 7,000 years. There are a number of types of meditation practices, including yogic meditation, Buddhist style, Zen Buddhism, and transcendental meditation. While different styles have developed, there is a central theme of meditation encouraging deeper awareness in the present moment.

Anxiety and depression are associated with the destruction of cells in the brain's hippocampus, an area needed for both memory and mood (Sapolsky, 2001). While medicine had considered damaged nervous tissue an irreversible event, research has shown that it can regenerate (Erickson et al., 1998). Chapter 2 discusses how exercise can accomplish this, and meditation can accomplish this feat as well.

Compelling evidence has revealed that meditation helps to increase the birth and growth of nerves. In one study (Cromie, 2006), volunteers meditated an average of about 40 minutes a day. Depth of the meditation was measured by the slowing of breathing rates. Those most deeply involved in the meditation showed the greatest healthful changes in brain structure. The meditators literally had altered brain structure compared with people who did not meditate: MRI scans revealed that meditation can boost the thickness of brain areas dealing with attention, sensory input, and memory functions. The thickening was found to be more noticeable in adults than in younger individuals—in the same sections of our brain cortex that atrophy with increased age. It is plausible, then, that meditation can slow or stop the effect of aging on the brain. Eight week pilot studies using 12 minutes a day of meditation for Alzheimer's and cognitive impairment have shown clear promise (Innes et al., 2012; .Moss et al., 2012).

Meditation is also known to boost brain activity, organize brain wave activity, strengthen neural connections, and thicken gray matter (Cromie, 2006). Admittedly, medical science doesn't fully understand how or why meditation benefits and rebuilds nerve tissue. Mediation also enhances vagal nerve tone: when stimulated, the vagus nerve can turn off inflammation and help turn on digestive function (Das, 2007). It is possible that helping digestion might be another key of how meditation to balances the mind. More studies are needed to learn if specific meditative techniques may be most beneficial.

Regarding anxiety and depression, studies dating back to the early 1900s have shown that meditation training programs can effectively reduce symptoms of anxiety and panic and will help maintain these reductions in patients with generalized anxiety disorder, panic disorder, or panic disorder with agoraphobia (Kabat-Zinn et al., 1992). A meta-analysis by Chiesa and Serretti (2009). found that mindfulness meditation can reduce stress in healthy people. It has also been shown to reduce ruminative thinking and trait anxiety, both factors contributing to stress. Compared with other relaxation techniques, mindfulness meditation may offer a greater ability to significantly reduce cortisol levels (Tang et al., 2007). Meditation has been shown to alleviate depressed symptoms significantly in 51 treated versus 41 control subjects (Sephton et al., 2007).

While likely great for just about everyone, meditation may be best for those depressed patients who have a strong anxieties. In cases of sole depressed mood without any anxiousness, sometimes I prefer the patient get up and do some movement, in which case qigong (which involves breathing practice with gentle movement) might be more balancing than stationary meditative work. One study by Gaik (2003) of 39 subjects suffering from major depression, dysthymia, or bipolar disorder were taught a qigong technique in a one-day training session with two follow-up sessions 1 and 2 months later. Supportive audio and videotapes were also given to the volunteers. The subjects were directed to practice for at least 40 minutes each day and to keep a log of their practice sessions. Gaik found that "all subjects improved over the treatment period" and observed "a very significant level of improvement in the majority of the subjects who were measured at serious levels of depression."

## Mindfulness-Based Therapy (MBT)

Hailing from Buddhist and yoga practices, MBT includes mindfulness-based cognitive therapy and mindfulness-based stress reduction. This modern mindful movement was made popular with the work of John Kabat Zinn (see, e.g., Kabat-Zinn, 2003) and has gained popularity for parallel use with psychotherapy.

In order to calm anxiety, depression, and feelings of being overwhelmed, the client is taught to process thoughts in a nonjudgmental way that allows for feelings (both emotional and physical) to be experienced and resolved while allowing for a nonjudgmental experience of the present moment. Remaining in the present moment is incompatible with anxious and depressed feelings.

While wonderful in theory, until recently it was unclear if this type of approach was actually clinically effective. In an effort to provide a quantitative, meta-analytic review of the efficacy of MBT, Hofmann et al. (2010) analyzed the most well-constructed 39 studies of a possible 723 studies, totaling 1,140 participants who worked with mind-body therapies. They found anxiety and depression responded quite well and the effect size was "robust" in favor of symptom improvement.

### Contraindications to meditation and MBT

According to the National Center for Complementary and Alternative Medicine of the National Institutes of Health (2014), meditation is considered quite safe, with virtually no side effects reported. There have been some isolated and rare reports of worsening of symptoms in persons with psychiatric illness, but this has not been well researched (Arias et al., 2006). Patients with physical limitations (e.g., inability to sit in a certain position) should also seek the assistance of a knowledgeable health care provider or an experienced meditation practitioner in choosing a style that is right for them.

## MASSAGE THERAPY

Massage therapy is one of the most ancient of health care practices. First recorded in Chinese medical texts more than 4,000 years old, massage has been advocated outside of Asia at least since the time of Hippocrates, who said "The physician must be acquainted with many things and assuredly with rubbing [massage]."

Mechanistically speaking, massage therapy is shown to reduce pain perception (Ferrell-Torry, 1993), to significantly balance electroencephalogram currents in the brain (Jones & Field., 1999), to decrease cortisol an average of 31 percent (Field et al., 1996), and to increase dopamine and serotonin 31 percent and 28 percent, respectively (Field et al., 2005).

Massage helps circulation of blood, the flow of blood and lymph and can reduce muscle tension, improve weakness, balance the nervous system, and enhance tissue healing. Although more studies are needed, some have shown massage to be effective in reducing both state and trait anxiety, blood pressure and heart rate, pain, and depression (Kutner, et al., 2008).

The ability of massage to alter HPA axis dysregulation and help balance neurotransmitters helps to explain the findings of an extensive review that showed benefits of massage to rival even psychotherapy in depression and state anxiety (a temporary anxious change spurred on by an outside situation). A review by Moyer, Rounds & Hannum. (2004). looked at 37 randomized, controlled trials on massage and included 17 studies on trait anxiety and depression from 1998 through 2002. On average, the massage therapy participants experienced a reduction in state anxiety of at least 77 percent compared with controls, with 73 percent decreases in depressive symptomology compared with nonmassage therapy controls. Comparatively, psychotherapy for these conditions has been shown to have a 79 percent benefit rate over untreated patients. It is possible that using both in tandem may give even more substantial results.

## ACUPUNCTURE

Practiced for the last three to four millennia, traditional Chinese medicine (TCM) is a medical system based on the concept of comparing the state of the human body to the natural world and then attempting to balance the human body to be in harmony with the laws of nature. Acupuncture is a central modality in TCM, which involves inserting fine needles into the body in order to balance the energy of the body to create a healing effect.

TCM uses the basic concept of yin and yang, as depicted in figure 2.1. The white areas represent yang, which is full of light, energy, daytime, and movement. Yang represents the male energy, going outward, and heat. The darker area is the yin part, representing quiet, female, nourishment, dark, nighttime, stillness, cool, and energy in reserve. In the body, yang and yin work together to create harmony and move in and out of each other all the time. When the body is experiencing disease of balance, TCM would say that yin and yang are out of harmony, and one is taking over the other, either because one is too strong or the other is too weak.

In the paradigm of TCM, anxiety is often an issue of excess yang, or deficient yin, whereas depression is more typically a deficient yang or excess yin problem. When these are out of balance, people become very anxious and agitated, depressed and withdrawn, or both. In TCM, emotional illness is often due to accumulated anger, sorrow, and other unprocessed emotions that lead to dysfunction and imbalances in yin and yang. Chronic outside stress, poor food choices, lack of sleep, and inadequate movement can also unbalance the life energy force known as "qi." As a result, "knotted qi" accumulates, and a disruption of the body and mind results (Jilin & Peck, 1995). As a result, anxious people may act too "yang" while depressed people act much more "yin."

In TCM, emotional problems often center on a particular organ. The emotional issue can decide which organ in the body has the most problems. For example, some patients tend toward excess fear, which can cause a kidney imbalance. Please note, this does not suggest there is a problem with the physical organ in the Western biomedical sense—it is the Chinese sense of the kidney, which stores our life energy to keep our physical and emotional well-being maintained. Other people will have a lot of anger, hostility, or lack of motivation, which is a liver-centered issue. Excess amounts of sorrow or even too much happiness will attack the heart. Grief and loss will affect the lungs.

### Clinical Case Study: Mel the Firefighter

*Practicing here in New York City, I have had the honor to work with many people who experienced extreme loss during the 9/11 crisis. As is well documented, many of these people have lung and respiratory problems, such as asthma, breathing difficulty, and sarcoidosis. While conventional medicine suggests that there must have been unknown particulates in the air causing these lung problems that no one could figure out, the Chinese medicine practitioner would suggest it was the incredible amount of loss around them that "attacked the lungs" to cause their breathing symptoms, asthma, and other respiratory problems. I have found that besides using Western herbal approaches to support breathing and the lungs, using acupuncture and Chinese herbs to address these while looking closer at the sense of loss has been invaluable to help move people through this grief.*

*A first responder named Mel who arrived at the scene of 911 was diagnosed with "chronic bronchitis" and "possible sarcoidosis" about three years after this traumatic event. I noticed, as I would ask Mel about his symptoms, that his discussion ultimately returned to the death he saw around him, with special memory of watching people jump out of smoked-filled windows and falling to their deaths. Once we discussed the Chinese view of the lungs and the grief, he lightened, suggesting that, for the first time, he believed his illness made sense. We used herbs specific for the lungs and acupuncture twice a week—in two months he was better. I have, numerous times, seen this varied approach centering on the TCM aspect work amazingly well when other approaches failed. Sometimes, TCM sees patterns and formulates a plan in a way other medicines do not.*

The exact mechanism of acupuncture action is unknown. Present Western medical interpretation of the treatment effect is that acupuncture stimulates nerves called afferent group III nerve fibers. These fibers are like electrical wires that transmit impulses to various parts of the central nervous system and induce the release of serotonin, norepinephrine, dopamine, beta-endorphin, and other emotional supportive molecules called enkephalins and dynorphins (Wang et al., 2008; Samuels, Cornelius, & Shepherd, 2008). Many of these are secreted and modulate the hypothalamus, suggesting a direct mode of influence on mood disorder (Wang et al., 2007). Other possible modes of action may include acupuncture's ability to influence changes of the autonomic nervous system (the part of the immune system that governs the ability to get stressed or stay calm), the immune system, inflammation, and hormones, as well as its ability modulate the recognition of serotonin, norepinephrine, and acetylcholine in brain and body (Gurguis et al., 1999).

A literature review by Pilkington et al. (2007) looked at the benefits of acupuncture for anxiety in 12 controlled trials, of which 10 were the more stringent randomized controlled kind. The authors found positive results for generalized anxiety disorder or anxiety neurosis (a diffuse type of anxiety) but concluded more research is needed for clear conclusions to be drawn. They were also not able to find studies on obsessive-compulsive disorder or panic attacks. Interestingly, the study found a good deal of benefit using auricular acupuncture (acupuncture using small needles on the outer ear) for anxiety before operations. In my experience, patients with mild to moderate anxiety do well with calming acupuncture treatments, but sometimes those with very high anxiety may overthink the administration of needles and find the treatments unpleasant. For some, this can be an opportunity to work with anxiety, and messaging using mindfulness therapies may help the patient move through these moments while in a secure setting. I personally was introduced to acupuncture during my early twenties when I experienced great stress, anxiety, and insomnia. When conventional medicine offered me drugs, which I didn't want to take, I decided to try acupuncture, although I didn't believe in it. I was very impressed how, from the first treatment, I started sleep better and how it clearly lowered my anxiety.

Research studies are somewhat conflicting regarding the benefits of acupuncture for depression. While one randomized controlled study of 151 depressed patients showed that 12 sessions of acupuncture failed to prove more effective than sham acupuncture (Allen et al., 2006), another positive study compared electroacupuncture and Prozac. In this evaluation, Luo et al. (2003) gave patients a type of acupuncture with gentle electrical stimulation placed on the needles 45 minutes in the morning for 6 weeks. In 90 subjects divided into drug only, acupuncture only, or controls, acupuncture was found as effective as using Prozac. Another positive study used electroacupuncture with patients already taking Paxil. This treatment showed superior efficacy to using only the drug—and those who used both had an even quicker response rate (Zhang et al., 2007). A thorough meta-analysis by Wang et al. (2008) of eight small randomized trials with sham (fake) acupuncture as control comparisons, with a total of 477 patients, concluded that acupuncture could significantly reduce the severity of disease in the patients with depression. This is an important study, for sham acupuncture uses real needling on body points not considered real acupuncture points. This helps us realize the specific points used make a difference, and that it is not merely a placebo effect making people feel better.

In my own clinic, I find clear benefits using acupuncture as therapy instead of and adjunctively to conventional medicine and other natural remedies for anxiety and depression. Acupuncture allows the pharmaceutical medications to work quicker and typically allow for a lower effective dose. It is also very effective to support the patient while weaning off conventional medications when they are ready to do so.

### Acupuncture safety and contraindications

One of the benefits of acupuncture is that, when used properly, there are virtually no contraindications to treatment, and it does not adversely interact with other treatments, such as conventional pharmaceutical therapy. It is safe with pregnancy and does not interfere with lactation for breast-feeding women. Large-scale studies have reviewed millions of treatments.

One systematic review of nine studies of nearly a quarter of a million acupuncture treatments found adverse events to be exceedingly rare when acupuncture is performed by a competent acupuncturist (Ernst & Adrian, 2001). In a large survey by Witt et al. (2009) with 2.2 million consecutive acupuncture treatments provided for 229,230 patients, two patients were found to have had a pneumothorax (non-life-threatening for either patient) and one had a lower limb nerve injury that persisted for 180 days. While there are some reports of hepatitis spread due to improper and illegal acupuncture techniques (U.S. Food & Drug Administration, 1996), when preformed properly it is exceedingly safe.

## EMOTIONAL FREEDOM TECHNIQUE

Emotional freedom technique (EFT) is a therapy that employs acupressure palpation (a form of acupuncture, but without needles) combined with a type of talk therapy in order to reprogram negative thinking patterns. Developed in the early 1990s by Gary Craig, a Stanford engineering graduate, it can help accelerate the process of reaching underlying issues for a patient.

While it is new, some studies are showing it can be beneficial. Successful application has been observed in treatment of phobias (Wells et al., 2003), and one study looking at 30 moderately to severely depressed college students 3 weeks after having four 90-minute EFT sessions (Church, De Asis, & Brooks, 2012).

My personal experience working with this simple technique has generally yielded mild to significant results in approximately 70 percent of patients, using it for such conditions as grief, pain, guilt, anxiety, posttraumatic stress disorder, stuck emotion, and functional digestive illness. This represents a very loose and informal review of my cases—certainly not a scientific study. Nevertheless, I believe it is especially valuable for it is something clients can try for their own self-care and does not have any known contraindications. Please visit www.emofree.com for more information.

Table 5.1 lists several effective mind-body therapies.

## Table 5.2 Most commonly Effective Mind-Body Therapies for Anxiety and Depression

| Method | |
|---|---|
| Yoga (30 to 90 minutes twice a week or more) | • Anxiety<br>• Depression<br>*Caution with pregnancy, glaucoma, high blood pressure, and sciatica |
| Meditation | • Anxiety<br>• Depression<br>*May be best for depressed patients with strong anxiety |
| Qigong | • Depression without anxiety |
| Mindfulness-based therapy | • Depression<br>• Anxiety |
| Massage | • anxiety<br>• depression<br>• when anxiety and depression are associated with high blood pressure |
| Acupuncture | • Anxiety<br>• Depression<br>*Excellent as adjunctive care to medications and helping to wean from medication |
| Emotional freedom technique | • Depression<br>• Anxiety<br>• Posttraumatic stress disorder<br>• Pain issues<br>• Digestive issues |

# SIX

# Working Integratively with Medications

I'm not confused. I'm just well mixed.　　　—Robert Frost

Mixing one's wines may be a mistake, but old and new wisdom mix admirably.　　　　　　　—Bertolt Brecht

### Clinical Case: Jim on Celexa

*Like many patients, Jim came to me after three years on antidepressant medication. Jim had had a minor form of fibromyalgia since his mid-twenties. Following the death of both his parents in an accident, Jim's depression came on during his mid-thirties. Interestingly, Jim was a grief counselor and, with his background, was very familiar with psychology, medications, and loss. Unfortunately, his own loss left him with a very low mood that threatened his job security and his ability to live his life.*

*When Jim came in, I could tell he was in great physical shape. He exercised every day and slept pretty well for the most part. His protein intake was a little low for his exercise level, and blood testing revealed low normal vitamin D and low total and free testosterone. Jim had been just about every medication and did not find benefit. He was currently on Celexa at 40 mg/day.*

*After adjusting his protein intake and starting some acupuncture for two months, Jim's mood was no better. We finally ran his MTHFR test*

*and found mutations in this gene. I explained the role of the methylenetetrahydrofolate reductase enzyme function (see Chapter 3), and we talked about how a special form of folic acid might benefit him. He was skeptical, since every drug he tried with his Celexa did not help. We started with 5 mg L-methylfolate and within two weeks moved up to 10 mg/day. Within two weeks of increasing to the 10 mg dose, he claimed the fog lifted. Within the next year, Jim met a woman, got married, and was able to discontinue first the Celexa and then the folate without any recurrence. The fibromyalgia that plagued him for years also dissipated and returned only when he was especially tired. He was grateful the folic acid helped get his brain back on track so he could move his life forward.*

Most of the patients who visit me for the first time are already on medication. Likely you see the same with your clients. There are three scenarios a patient will present with:

1. *The medications are helping.* In this case, I tell my patients we can consider the medication a blessing, for they can then help us work on what's needed to eventually not need the drugs in the long term. This is where working on sleep, diet, lifestyle, supplements, and mind-body therapies can help us get to the point where they will no longer be needed.

2. *The medications are not helping.* In this situation, patients often find themselves switching drugs, seemingly randomly, or medications are just piled on top of each other. Generally, this approach is hard on the body. It can also be psychologically traumatic as different medications bounce neurotransmitters around.

3. *The medications are helping but are causing unwanted sexual side effects.* This is a main complaint, especially from SSRI users. Patients are placed in a tough spot, for they are glad to feel better but their sexuality and relationships suffer.

This chapter addresses the second and third scenarios. It reviews the emerging literature about using natural medicines alongside conventional drugs to help foster better outcomes and efficacy and to lessen their sexual side effects. It then broaches the often psychiatrically taboo subject of using natural medicines with drugs to help the patient safely get off the medications.

The conventional media and the medical establishment often warn us about the dangers of mixing vitamins and herbs with medications, which unfortunately has persuaded many psychiatrists and patients to think about conventional and natural medicines as a "can't have both" scenario in which the very natural things that can help the body heal the most are considered secondary, or mistaken as dangerous. My hope is this chapter will start to debunk some of the unsubstantiated concerns, while noting safety concerns when merited.

## HELPING ANXIETY AND DEPRESSION MEDICATIONS WORK THEIR BEST

In my practice, whether a patient is utilizing medications or not, I have seen again and again how the naturopathic model of balancing sleep, exercise, healthful diet, counseling work, and the right supplementation can help a person with mood disorder optimally rebalance. Just to reiterate what is discussed in chapter 4, focusing only on supplementation will not serve the best results in the long term. But sometimes starting with a focus on one lifestyle or supplement—especially if that is all the patient can realistically handle in the beginning—will help kick-start a better mood. A better mood will help clients to do even more helpful lifestyle work later on when they are ready.

The suggestions below may be considered first for patients coming to the holistic practitioner's office who are already taking mood medications. Please remember that this is a fairly new field of research, so unfortunately information is limited. Nevertheless, my experience is this work can create an important bridge to getting clients better quicker. Also important is that a patient should never simply stop taking antianxiety or antidepressant medication without good reason and careful monitoring.

## Exercise

Can a good walk help a medication work? Can it be better than adding another drug to a current drug that is not working all that well? One study seems to suggest it can. Trivedi et al. (2011) looked at 126 patients whose selective serotonin reuptake inhibitors (SSRIs) were not working for them. Their next treatment choice is usually an add-on drug that has a 20–30 percent success rate (also known as a 70–80 percent failure rate), typically with a higher risk of side effects.

These patients had never exercised before and were allowed to choose exercise instead of an add-on medication. One group chose a daily easy, light exercise, like strolling at two to three miles an hour, or gentle exercise biking. A second choice was following the American College of Sports Medicine recommendations of exercising a bit more vigorously by walking in a brisk manner, at the rate of 4 miles an hour, every day.

For both groups, overall about 30 percent of patients felt better in 4 months—a little better than one would expect from a second medication. Interestingly, more people stopped their exercise if they were in the more vigorous group; thus, more people were able to stick to the lighter exercising. This tells us that a patient should start at his or her own comfort level, beginning with lighter exercise (especially if new to exercise) and then gradually increasing intensity. In truth, the exercise did not do much better than the medication—but my clinical experience tells me that the benefits of exercise help the underlying causes of mood issues, and are more substantial and long lasting. (For more about exercise, see Chapter 2.)

## Thyroid Hormone

Chapter 2 discussed the multiple important actions of thyroid hormone to help the mind and body of a person with depression. Thyroid hormone can also be an important ally to a medication that is otherwise not working.

As early as 1969, astute researchers had shown that when patients on tricyclic antidepressants were given tri-iodothyronine (T3), the result was an "enhanced and accelerated recovery" (Prange & Loosen, 1982). About 55–60 percent of patients who previously failed to respond to tricyclic antidepressants will respond when they have enough thyroid hormone (Barowsky & Schwartz, 2006). In one study of almost 300 patients, those treated with T3, or a more natural glandular thyroid support, were twice as likely to respond than to placebo and almost three times more likely to respond than to thyroxine (T4) (Joffe & Singer, 1990).

Joffe's (1992) review of the literature supports the successful utilization of T3 in patients taking SSRIs. Lack of energy was especially common in patients given Prozac, but when the T3 was added the low energy went away, with no side effects noted.

If a patient is using a medication that is not working well, checking thyroid levels may be in order. If these are normal but on the low-normal side, a small dose of T3 (Cytomel) or natural glandular supplements like Armour Thyroid or Nature-Throid could be tried to see if there is benefit, while monitoring blood tests and looking for signs of excess thyroid hormone (fast heart rate, palpitations, sweating, greasy skin and hair, and anxiety). Since excess levels of thyroid may contribute to anxiety feelings, it may be best to avoid in anxious patients.

## Estrogen

As mentioned in Chapter 3, estrogen levels play a role in mood. Estrogen will affect the level of serotonin and also modify the reactivity of serotonin receptors. As some women with imbalanced menstrual cycle may attest, estrogen fluctuations can also bounce mood around. If a woman is predisposed to anxiety or depression, especially around the time of menopause and postmenopause, these estrogen changes will allow the mood issues to fully manifest. In postmenopausal women being treated for depression, estrogen replacement therapy has improved the effects of conventional antidepressants (Schneider, Small, & Clary,

2001). In a number of cases in my practice, administration of a little extra estrogen in the form of a skin cream made all the difference in allowing both anxiety and antidepressant medications work their best. (Please refer to Chapter 3 for more about estrogen.) While I prefer women first work with sleep, lifestyle, diet, and other natural ways to balance the body before considering hormones, natural estrogen replacement may be a good second-line option.

## Progesterone

As discussed in Chapter 3, optimal levels of progesterone are known to help calm the brain, improve sleep, and strengthen libido. Both animal and human clinical research suggests that progesterone and its metabolites may have a calming effect by enhancing GABA in the brain, an action similar to that of the common benzodiazepine medications. Balbalonis et. al (2011) looked at whether progesterone can potentiate the effects of the benzodiazepine triazolam (Halcion). The natural bioidentical form of progesterone called oral micronized progesterone (at 0, 100, and 200 mg doses) along with oral triazolam (0.00, 0.12, and 0.25 mg/70 kg) was given to 11 healthy premenopausal women who had documented low levels of sex hormones. Triazolam alone produced expected sedative-like effect and the progesterone alone also had some, albeit weaker, sedative effects that were shorter in duration. Most notably, progesterone increased and extended the duration of triazolam effects, suggesting that progesterone may alter how a benzodiazepine will work in the body. This concerned the researchers, who raised the question about whether progesterone could increase the risk of addiction.

I have two thoughts about this study: one, it used an oral progesterone, which has a first pass through the liver before going into the general circulation. This may increase the effects of altering the liver metabolism of the benzodiazepine medication. Any hormone taken orally will have to first pass through the liver, before going out to the general circulation. This first pass will have a stronger effect on the processing of other drugs and hormones. A better method might have been using a transdermal cream, that would go through the skin and diffuse into the general blood circulation, creating less of a progesterone "hit" in the liver. Also, we may consider the possibility that use of progesterone might supplant the need for benzodiazepines in women who are low in progesterone, or may lower the required dosage of the drug. More research is needed, and progesterone might be considered for an anxious woman alongside a benzodiazepine as long as she is well monitored for any signs of addiction to the drug.

## Testosterone

Chapter 3 discussed the importance of this hormone when discussing blood tests. While some testosterone may helpful for anyone who suffers from anxiety and depression and has low testosterone levels, it may be even more beneficial in patients already taking medications but not getting good results. In a randomized controlled trial of 56 men with treatment-resistant depression, Pope et al. (2003) found that 24 of these men had morning serum total testosterone levels of ≤350 ng/dl (normal range, 270–1,070 ng/dl). Of these 24 men with low testosterone, 23 entered the study. One man responded quickly to a 1-week single-blind placebo period, while the 22 others were subsequently randomly assigned to either 10 g/day of a 1 percent testosterone gel or a placebo, while continuing their antidepressant drugs. Ten subjects receiving testosterone and nine receiving placebo completed the 8-week trial. Subjects receiving testosterone gel had significantly greater improvement in scores on the Hamilton Depression Rating Scale than subjects receiving placebo. A significant difference was also found on the Clinical Global Impression severity scale but not the Beck Depression Inventory. One subject assigned to testosterone reported increased difficulty with urination, suggesting an unconfirmed exacerbation of benign prostatic hyperplasia; no other subject reported adverse events attributable to testosterone. This study also showed that it is possible to use pharmaceutical medications with transdermal testosterone concurrently.

In a second, smaller randomized controlled trial by Barowsky and

Schwartz (2006), 19 men with difficult-to-treat depression who also had low or even normal testosterone levels completed an 8-week, randomized, placebo-controlled study. Participants were given either 10 g/day of transdermal testosterone gel or an equivalent amount of placebo cream. Each subject continued his existing antidepressant regimen. The testosterone-treated patients had a significantly greater decrease in depression questionnaire scores than the placebo-treated patients.

I have seen many cases of healthy mood adjustments using a little testosterone in both men and women. I have also witnessed cases of patients with low testosterone not able to successfully wean off medication until their testosterone was adjusted.

## Fish Oil

As discussed in Chapter 3, fish oil is immensely supportive of the nervous tissue and the adrenal system and as gentle but consistent anti-inflammatory support. Of all the supplements, this is my first choice for anyone with mood issues, whether they are taking medication or not (unless, of course, they have a fish allergy).

One study of 20 patients taking anti-depressant medications found the addition of fish oil in a 4-week, parallel-group, double-blind evaluation found highly significant benefits with the addition of the omega-3 fatty acid compared with placebo by the third week over those that did not take fish oil. (Nemets et al., 2002). In a study of 70 patients with persistent depression, despite ongoing treatment with an adequate dose of a standard antidepressant, Peet and Horrobin (2003) found benefit from 1 g/day of ethyl-eicosapentaenoate (ethyl-EPA) versus placebo. Interestingly, this 1g/day dose may have had greater benefit over the 2 and 4 g doses. Ethyl-EPA is a pure, prescription form of EPA that is devoid of other essential fatty acids (and is discussed in Chapter 4). Strong beneficial effects were seen while patients were monitored for depression, anxiety, sleep, fatigue, low sex drive, and thoughts of suicide.

## Tryptophan and 5-HTP

SSRIs are standard therapy for most of your clients prescribed drugs for anxiety and/or depression. As discussed in Chapter 3, tryptophan and 5-HTP are amino acid precursors helpful in supporting the body to make its own serotonin. While most conventional psychiatrists are uncomfortable or cite "serotonin syndrome" as a concern when combining these with medication, research discussed in chapter 3, as well some specific studies reviewed here, suggests this is a missed opportunity.

One 8-week randomized controlled trial of 30 patients with major depression found that combining 20 mg Prozac with 2 g tryptophan daily at the outset of treatment for major depressive disorder appeared to be a safe protocol that had both rapid antidepressant effects and a protective effect on slow wave sleep, with no need for monitoring of drug levels (Levitan et al., 2000). I know of only one relevant study of the combination of 5-HTP with SSRIs, in which Meltzer et al. (1997) administered single doses of 200 mg 5-HTP to 16 patients taking fluoxetine (Prozac) and to 14 patients taking tricyclic antidepressants (which inhibit serotonin reuptake to varying degrees). None of these patients showed evidence of serotonin syndrome.

In a study of 26 patients, Nardini et al. (1983) used 5-HTP to augment clomipramine (Anafranil), a potent inhibitor of serotonin reuptake. There were no signs of serotonin syndrome or other serious adverse events, and the group who received clomipramine (50 mg/day) combined with 5-HTP (300 mg/day) enjoyed better mood, less anxiety, and fewer uncomfortable physical symptoms. In addition, a trial with fibromyalgia patients taking 5-HTP together with monoamine oxidase inhibitors, a class of antidepressants notorious for its many drug interactions, did not indicate any side effects attributable to serotonin syndrome (Nicolodi & Sicuteri, 1996). Instead, this combination of significantly improved fibromyalgia symptoms, whereas the other treatments yielded poorer benefits.

Typically, if patients are taking medications, I would recommend they start with a small dose of either L-tryptophan (500 mg/day) or 5-HTP (50 mg/day) and continue dosing up to 2,000 mg/day of tryptophan or 300 mg/day of 5-HTP in divided doses until benefit is achieved. Of course, monitor closely, and if symptoms worsen, then boosting the serotonin pathway may not be appropriate for that particular patient.

## Folic Acid

Folic acid in the form of methyltetrahydrofolate is becoming well known in the conventional psychiatric community as a support for antidepressants. Fava et al. (1997) were among the first to study this, when they examined the relationships among levels of folate, vitamin B12, and homocysteine with response to fluoxetine (Prozac) treatment in 213 outpatients with major depressive disorder. For a baseline assessment, a blood sample was collected from each patient. Subjects with low folate levels were more likely to have melancholic depression and were significantly less likely to respond to the Prozac. Fava et al. concluded that there was a link between low folate levels and poorer response to antidepressant treatment. They suggested that folate levels be considered in the evaluation of depressed patients who do not respond to antidepressant treatment. It makes sense to me to look at folate levels before starting any kind of treatment.

A more recent second research study by the same group found that patients taking 15 mg/day of folate (which is a super-large dose—the usual dose is 400–800 μg) found antidepressant medication to work significantly better, and much better when adding more pharmaceutical medications (Fava et al., 2010). Coppen and Bailey (2000), using much lower doses in 127 patients, also corroborate that 500 μg of folic acid taken daily with fluoxetine (Prozac) can greatly improve the therapeutic effect. The authors noted that higher levels of folic acid were required in men to optimally maintain folic acid levels.

These studies are showing us that a simple, water-soluble B vitamin support like folic acid may be a viable alternative to the vast array of adjunctive and add-on medications, including antipsychotic medications like Abilify or even antiepileptic meds like Lamictal. These drugs are often prescribed for nonresponders and treatment resistance – a situation which most clients on antidepressants experience sooner or later.

For patients taking antidepressant medications and looking for better support, they may start with 1 mg/day of folate and work up to a total of 15 mg/day. A prospective community study looking at 400 μg/day of folic acid along with 100 μg vitamin B12 did not see benefit (Christensen et al., 2011), so higher doses are likely better or possibly using a more natural form of folate would have worked better. It is best to use the methylfolate version of this nutrient, which is the more natural version. In my experience, 1mg doses are enough when used together with other holistic care discussed in this book. More about folate can be found in Chapter 4 and in the section about the *MTHFR* gene mutation in Chapter 3.

### Vitamin B12 (Methylcobalamin)

In a study by Hintikka et al. (2013), serum vitamin B12 levels were looked at in 115 people with major depressive disorder—all the patients were in normal range for the vitamin. In the subgroup of 40 patients that did not respond to medication, the average vitamin B12 level was 470.5 pg/ml (normal range is ~200–1,100 pg/ml). Among 34 people who had a partial response, average baseline vitamin B12 was 536.6 pg/ml. The 41 people who had a full response group had an average baseline vitamin B12 measurement of 594.9 pg/ml. This implies that the higher baseline vitamin B12 levels, the better the patient outcome. This suggests to me that patients with depression should have a B12 level of at least about 600 pg/ml, even though most doctors would be happy with a level over 200 pg/mL. Many blood tests even state that people with low levels, between 200 and 400 pg/mL, may show neuropsychiatric problems, so looking for 600 pg/mL or higher makes a lot of sense. I know of no reason to worry about B12 toxicity, even at levels of 1,200 pg/ml or more.

Anyone taking antidepressant medication should check their B12 levels. Patients can ask their doctor for intramuscular B12 shots once a week, or the methylcobalamin version of this vitamin can be taken orally, starting at a dose of 10,000 µg once a day, which is about 10 times the daily maintenance daily dose recommended in Chapter 4. If there is no change in blood levels after taking this for 1–2 months, increased dosage may be indicated. If levels do not change, consider working on digestion and absorption by improving foods and diet (see steps for a leaky gut in Chapter 3), for the main reason B12 stores are low is poor absorption by the digestive tract. For more about vitamin B12, see Chapter 4.

## Zinc

Like B vitamins, zinc may be a valuable ally if a patient is prescribed antidepressant medications that simply aren't working. Mlyniec, Oboszewska, & Nowak (2011) looked at the effect of zinc deprivation on the beneficial effect of antidepressant drugs. The researchers gave some mice a zinc-deficient diet, which significantly lowered the levels of this mineral in their body. The control mice had a normal diet. Then the animals were subjected to a stressor (the forced swim test) to induce depression. The animals that were zinc deprived had a minimal response to antidepressant medication support, whereas the animals with plenty of zinc in their body responded more positively when given medication. This suggests antidepressants could possibly work much better but that they may not work for so many people because we are a nutrient-depleted society.

Human studies also support this hypothesis. Nowak et al. (2003) ran a placebo-controlled, double-blind pilot human trial. One group of 6 patients with depression was given 25 mg zinc once a day with standard antidepressant drug therapy, while a control group of 8 patients were given standard antidepressant drug therapy only. Each patient's sense of well-being was evaluated before the treatment, and also 2, 6 and 12 weeks after the treatment started. Although the zinc treatment did not take effect until week 6, a very strong benefit was conferred on the mood of the patients taking the zinc over those who did not take the extra zinc. This was a small study, but given the safety of zinc and possible benefit, it may make sense to try. For zinc supplementation more than 2 months, it is helpful to take are taking 2 mg/day of copper, too (often found in a good multiple vitamin), for sometimes extra zinc can decrease copper levels in the body. More about zinc can be found in Chapter 3.

## SAMe

SAMe is a methionine compound helpful in supporting the methylation pathways needed to create optimal neurotransmitter balance. It is discussed Chapter 3, along with several studies. In addition, a study by De Beradis et al. (2013) examined 33 patients with second-stage treatment-resistant depressive disorder, meaning the pharmaceutical medications were not working after 8 weeks of two different antidepressants. These patients had depression for an average of 8 years. They were then openly given SAMe at 800 mg/day for 8 weeks in addition to their current medication. Hamilton Rating Scale for Depression scores at 8 weeks showed significant decreases, with response achieved by 60 percent of the patients and remission by 36 percent. Additionally, most responders demonstrated a 50 percent or greater reduction of total score within the first 5 weeks of treatment, which is quite rapid improvement in depressive symptoms, especially over the usual effect of antidepressant drugs when they do work (which is a minimum of 6 weeks). The most frequently observed side effects were mild constipation and nausea with decreased appetite. Another trial, called the STAR*D (Sequenced Treatment Alternatives to Relieve Depression), looking at multiple medications for treatment-resistant patients showed a remission rate of only 12.3 percent and 19.8 percent (Fava et al., 2006), far below the results seen with the SAMe.

## Rhodiola and Eleutherococcus

These herbal adaptogens have been observed to be a clinically effective adjunct when administered with tricyclic antidepressant medications. Twenty-one subjects took 150 mg/day of tricyclic antidepressants along with a noontime dose of 15–20 drops/day of a rhodiola tincture, while another 46 patients took the same dose of another adaptogen called eleutherococcus, which has similar properties to rhodiola (Brichenko, Kupriyanova, & Skorokhodova, 1986). Thirty-one patients served as a control and took only the antidepressant. Both herbs along with tricyclic antidepressant treatment showed a positive effect on psychopathologic symptoms with reduced affective, ideamotor (involuntary movement due to a thought), and motor components of the depression. The depressed patients who also had anxiety and hypochondria symptoms fared the best. Patients enjoyed increased general activity as well as greater intellectual and physical productivity. Side effects from the tricyclics (e.g., constipation, sinus tachycardia (fast heart beat), extremity tremors and headache) were fewer. However, disorders of extreme emotional issues and phobia fared worse.

## Lavender

One a double-blind randomized control trial looking at a combination of lavender with the antidepressant imipramine (Tofranil) found the herbal addition to be more effective than the drug alone in the treatment of depression (Akhondzadeh et al., 2003). This study's double treatment group took 100 mg/day of imipramine plus 60 drops/day of a lavender tincture. The findings suggested that taking a moderate amount of lavender may help reduce the amount of tricyclic antidepressants needed to treat depression, leading to fewer side effects. While there are no studies specifically using lavender with antianxiety medications, clinically I have seen benefit of adjunctive lavender, helping to decrease use of antianxiety medications.

## Acupuncture

Research using acupuncture alongside conventional medications is just starting to surface. One double-blind study looked at acupuncture in combination with Prozac for major depression. Zhang et al. (2009)

divided 80 patients into two groups: one received acupuncture plus 10 mg/day of Prozac and the second group received sham acupuncture plus 20–30 mg/day of Prozac. Acupuncture was administered five times a week for 6 weeks. Both groups showed similar responses (80 percent for the true acupuncture and 77.5 percent for the sham group), with the true acupuncture group showing lower medication side effects and anxiety. The overall rate of adverse events due to acupuncture from this study was 8.75 percent. In my clinical and research experience, this is a much higher adverse event rate than commonly encountered.

Table 6.1 reviews the best supports for patients on pharmaceutical medications for anxiety and depression.

## AVOIDING THE SEXUAL SIDE EFFECTS OF ANTIDEPRESSANT MEDICATION

Antidepressants are well known to cause sexual dysfunction. These symptoms include delayed orgasm, decrease sex drive, erectile dysfunction, and dyspareunia (pain with intercourse). Prevalence rates in medicated patients are as high as 50–90 percent. These side effects may be safely and adequately addressed with natural remedies gingko, yohimbe, and acupuncture. Table 6.2 reviews herbal supports for antidepressant sexual side effects.

### Ginkgo (*Ginkgo biloba*)

Ginkgo is a wonderful plant with a great hardiness and vitality. It was the first plant to grow after the bombing of Hiroshima and Nagasaki and has been used medicinally for thousands of years. Beneficial for both anxiety and depression, as well as memory and fatigue (Ernst, 2002), the flavonoids in ginkgo are strong antioxidants, which protect nerves, decrease clotting, help memory, and can help the body and brain balance stress hormones and normalize serotonin (Shah, Sharma, & Vohora,

Table 6.1. Support for Patients on Pharmaceutical Medications for Anxiety and Depression

| Medication support | Indication | Dosage |
|---|---|---|
| Exercise | Antianxiety and antidepressant support | Walking outside or more intense if preferable to the client |
| Thyroid hormone | Antidepressant medication support | |
| Estrogen | Antianxiety and antidepressant medication support | Dosing based on form of hormone used and lab work<br>*Watch for anxiety manifestations, along with other symptoms of excess thyroid (palpitations, fast heart rate, etc.) |
| Progesterone | • Antianxiety and antidepressant medication support<br>• To balance estrogen prescription | Dosing based on form of hormone used and lab work<br>*Can make some depression worse<br>*Concern of increasing tendency of addiction to benzodiazepines |
| Testosterone | Antianxiety and antidepressant medication support | |
| Fish oil | Antianxiety and antidepressant medication support | About 2 g/day of regular fish oil (to achieve 1,000 mg/day of EPA and ~800 mg/day of DHA)<br>OR<br>1 g/day ethyl-EPA |

| Supplement | Use | Dosage |
|---|---|---|
| Tryptophan and 5-HTP | For antidepressant medication support | With an SSRI: 500 mg up to 2 g L-tryptophan<br>With tricyclic antidepressant: 50 mg up to 300 mg/day of 5-HTP |
| Folic acid | For antidepressant medication support | With SSRI medications: 1 mg up to 15 mg/day |
| Vitamin B12 (methyl-cobalamin) | Antidepressant medication support | Intramuscular: B12 shots once a week<br>Oral: 10,000 µg doses once a day until levels rise, then 1,000 µg/day for maintenance |
| Zinc | Antidepressant medication support | 25 mg/day with food.<br>*Balance with 2 mg of copper/day if taking for more than 2 months, unless blood copper levels are high. |
| SAMe | Antidepressant medication support | 800 mg/day for 8 weeks |
| Rhodiola or eleutherococcus | Patients with depression or depression and anxiety on tricyclic antidepressants | • 15–20 drops/day of a rhodiola tincture before noontime<br>*People with severe emotional swings and phobias fare worse |

Table 6.2. Herbal Supports for Sexual Side Effects of Antidepressants

| Herbal support | Dosage |
| --- | --- |
| Ginkgo (*Ginkgo biloba*) | 40–80 mg three times a day, with a standardization of 24 percent gingko flavonglycosides<br>*May be especially useful for women<br>*Should be avoided if taking diabetes medications, anti-clotting medications, or antiepileptic drugs |
| Yohimbe (*Pausinystalia yohimbe*) | 5–20 drops of liquid tincture up to three times a day<br>OR<br>2.7–16.2 mg daily of the alkaloid yohimbine<br>*Best to try ginkgo first due to possible side effect profile of yohimbe<br>*May cause anxiety, wound up feelings, and excessive sweating<br>*Contraindicated with high blood pressure |

2003). Although reviews are mixed for Alzheimer's and non-Alzheimer's dementia, some report benefit for mood and cognition (Yancheva et al., 2009; Bachinskaya, Hoerr, & Ihl, 2011).

In an open trial, Cohen and Bartlik (1998) found ginkgo extract to be 84 percent effective in treating antidepressant-induced sexual dysfunction predominately caused by SSRIs. In this study of 96 people, women had more response to the sex-enhancing effects of ginkgo than the men, although both saw benefit. The relative success rates for women were 91 percent and for men were 76 percent. Ginkgo generally had a positive effect on all four phases of the sexual response cycle: desire, excitement (including erection and lubrication), orgasm, and resolution (the "afterglow" or good feeling immediately following orgasm). A triple-blind study by Wheatley (2004) of 240 mg gingko given to eight men and five women found some excellent individual responses in both groups, but as a whole there were no statistically significant differences suggesting benefit overall. While these studies are promising, more research is welcome to understand exactly who may benefit best from ginkgo.

### Ginkgo dosage and toxicity

*Gingko biloba* extract may be used at a dosage of 40–80 mg three times a day, standardized at 24 percent gingko flavonglycosides. Although levels the flavonglycosides are important, remember to use a preparation that includes the whole ginkgo leaf with it, for we do not know exactly what part or parts of the gingko are actually helping with mood and sexual side effects.

Ginkgo biloba leaf extract is quite low in toxicity, but this supplement should be avoided if a patient is taking diabetes medications (Kudolo, 2001), anticlotting medications (Kim et al., 1998), or antiepileptic drugs (Granger, 2001).

## Yohimbe (*Pausinystalia yohimbe*)

Hailing from the coffee family of plants, *Pausinystalia yohimbe* contains an alkaloid, named yohimbine, which is well known in the botanical medicine world for the treatment of erectile problems and impotence.

Medical science is starting to look into this herbal for depression. The National Institute of Mental Health has completed a trial on the effect of yohimbine as an antidepressant (Zarate, 2013), although analysis of this study has not been completed as of the time of this writing. This study is looking at the efficacy of a single intravenous dose of yohimbine compared with placebo in improving overall depression symptoms when administered during REM sleep. Yohimbe may be helpful with the sexual side effects of antidepressant medications. Its efficacy in treating sexual difficulties may be due to its ability to block presynaptic alpha-2 adrenergic receptors, which enhances adrenergic tone needed for a robust sexual response (Nelson, 1988).

Yohimbe also seems to help medicated patients respond quicker and better to SSRIs (Cappiello, 1995). A randomized controlled trial by Sanacora et al. (2004) of 50 patients with a diagnosis of major depressive disorder showed that subjects who took Prozac plus yohimbine responded more rapidly than those who took Prozac and a placebo. The subjects were randomly assigned to receive 20 mg of Prozac plus either placebo or a titrated dose of yohimbine. (Titration means the dose was slowly adjusted higher while monitoring a person for any safety problems.) In these cases, the yohimbine dose was titrated based on blood pressure changes over the treatment period. Keep note that one real concern about yohimbine and the plant yohimbe is that its powerful effect on the adrenal system not only improves mood and sexual feeling but also can raise blood pressure, so dosage needs to be watched carefully. Right now, we do not know who is more inclined to experience high blood pressure as a result, so each person taking this plant needs to be monitored closely.

Like ginkgo (described above), yohimbe has been studied as an adjunct to lower the sexual side effects of antidepressant medications. A study by Hollander and McCarley (1992) of six patients with obsessive-compulsive disorder, trichotillomania (obsessive hair pulling), anxiety, or affective disorders like depression who suffered sexual side effects after treatment with SSRIs were given yohimbine on an as-needed basis in an open clinical trial. Because of the concern about effects on blood pressure discussed above, different doses of yohimbine were employed to figure out which would be ideal for each patient. Five of the six patients experienced improved sexual functioning after taking yohimbine. The other patient did not take the doses as asked. In the largest study of this kind, 17 of 21 patients showed improvement of sexual side effects when treated with yohimbine at an average dose of 16.2 mg, as needed, for an 81 percent response rate.

### Pausinystalia yohimbe dosage and toxicity

A variety of sexual side effects, including low libido, have been reported to be alleviated by yohimbine (the drug component derived from the whole plant yohimbe) in doses ranging from 2.7 to 16.2 mg daily, usually divided into three daily doses. Typically, it has been prescribed either as 5.4 mg up to three times a day or on an as-needed basis with single doses up to 16.2 mg (Sanacora et al., 2004). Another choice is to use the whole plant herb itself instead of a prescription form of yohimbine. In this case, it may be easiest to use a liquid herbal tincture in a concentration of 1:5, taking a range of 5–20 drops three times a day. The amounts of yohimbine in these liquid preparations may vary.

For my patients with sexual side effects, I recommend trying gingko first (see above). If they do not show improvement with gingko after 2 months, herbal yohimbe may be a reasonable second choice. If you have a client who wants to work with yohimbe, then it important to work with a naturopathic physician, qualified herbalist, or other practitioner experienced with this herb—and critical to advise the prescribing medical doctor as well. It is best to start at low doses and titrate to therapeutic dose to avoid side effects, while monitoring blood pressure before starting and then daily while taking the herb.

My first experience hearing about yohimbine was as a researcher at Yale in the Department of Pharmacology. A postdoctoral fellow in whose lab I was assisting had taken some yohimbine while participating in a trial of the drug. The poor fellow suffered a full erection for over 24 hours and I believe needed a procedure to drain the penis. The potency of the drug yohimbine is much higher than that of the whole herb yohimbe. Possible side effects of yohimbe include higher blood pressures, excessive sweating, increased anxiety, and a wound-up feeling in some patients. This is not an herb to use lightly, so please be respectful of this one. It should not be used by anyone with high blood pressure or glaucoma, and may be contraindicated in anxiety disorders.

## Acupuncture

Acupuncture has a potential role in treating the sexual side effects of antidepressant medications. In a pilot study by Khamba et al. (2013), 35 patients (18 men and 17 women) experiencing antidepressant sexual side effects received a traditional Chinese medicine (TCM) assessment, followed by an acupuncture treatment protocol for 12 consecutive weeks. The treatment protocol used TCM theory and addressed what was called "heart yin deficiency" and "kidney qi deficiency," two diagnoses that relate to sexual dysfunction and mood issues. Acupuncture points were kidney 3, governing vessel 4, bladder 23, pericardium 6, and heart 7. Male participants reported significant improvement all areas of sexual functioning, as well as in both anxiety and depressive symptoms, while female participants reported a significant improvement in libido and vaginal lubrication and a nonsignificant trend toward improvement in several other areas of function.

Limiting this study was the fact that it was an open-label, noncontrolled study. Additionally, in TCM, chosen acupuncture points are typically individualized for the particular patient, which was not the case here. Individualized selection of point for the patients might have increased effectiveness. Nevertheless, this study corroborates what I see clinically in my practice regarding the benefit of using acupuncture alongside medications for helping with sexual side effects. With virtually no risk to the patient, it is worth trying.

## USING NATURAL MEDICINES TO HELP PATIENTS WEAN OFF MEDICATIONS

Patients who have moved through the steps of holistic care outlined in this book may be ready to work with their doctors to safely wean off medications. This section explains, step by step, how to do this. Table 6.3 provides a quick reference highlighting which supplements to consider with individual medications.

Stopping antianxiety and antidepressant medications is like stopping any other drug: there is the possibility of withdrawal that will have its own set of symptoms. While the drug companies and the medical community call it "discontinuation syndrome," it really is drug withdrawal. With antianxiety and antidepressant medications, withdrawal symptoms can include confusion, irritability, dizziness, lack of coordination, sleeping problems, crying spells, panic attacks, and blurry vision. In my office, I commonly see digestive upset, headaches, electrical "zaps," and the return of some familiar (but uncomfortable) feelings.

Research shows that antidepressant withdrawal evokes a major behav-

**Table 6.3 Natural Supports for Weaning Off Medication**

| Prescription Drug | Supplement support dosage |
|---|---|
| **SSRIs:**<br>Citalopram (Celexa)<br>Escitalopram (Lexapro)<br>Fluoxetine (Prozac, Prozac Weekly, Sarafem)<br>Paroxetine (Paxil, Paxil CR, Pexeva)<br>Sertraline (Zoloft) | **5-HTP:** before weaning the medication, start with 50 mg each day for 1 month, then start tapering off medication while adding 50 mg more a day once a week for the next 3 weeks.<br>OR<br>**Tryptophan:** 500 mg once a day in the evening for the first week, then start tapering medication while adding 500 mg both in the late afternoon and before bed. Add up 1,000 mg in the late afternoon and evening while tapering. |
| **SSRI/SSNRI Drugs:**<br>Venlafaxine (Effexor)<br>Desvenlafaxine (Pristiq)<br>Duloxetine (Cymbalta)<br>Milnacipran (Savella, Ixel) | **Tyrosine:** 500 mg once a day for 1 week, *THEN ADD* **5-HTP:** 50 mg/day for the second week. Start tapering medication, while adding 500 mg of tyrosine for week 3, then adding 50 mg of 5-HTP for week 4 while continuing the medication taper. |
| **Tricyclic Antidepressants:**<br>Amitriptyline (Elavil, Endep, Vanatrip)<br>Amoxapine (Asendin)<br>Desipramine (Norpramin)<br>Doxepin (Adapin, Silenor, Sinequan)<br>Imipramine (Tofranil, Tofranil-PM)<br>Maprotiline (Ludiomil)<br>Nortriptyline (Pamelor)<br>Protriptyline (Vivactil)<br>Trimipramine (Surmontil) | **Tyrosine:** 500 mg once a day for one week *THEN ADD* **5-HTP:** 50 mg/day for the second week. Start tapering medication, while adding 500 mg of tyrosine for week three, then 50 mg of 5-HTP for week four while continuing the medication taper. |

*(continued)*

239

**Table 6.3 Continued**

| Prescription Drug | Supplement support dosage |
|---|---|
| **Others** | |
| Bupropion (Wellbutrin, Zyban) | **Mucuna:** 200 mg extract once a day for 2 weeks, then start tapering medication while increasing to 200 mg twice/day. Once the patient is off the medication completely and feeling good for 2 weeks, 200 mg once a day for 1 month, then 200 mg every other day for 1 month, then discontinue. |
| Aripiprazole (Abilify) | **Mucuna:** 200 mg extract once a day for 2 weeks, *THEN ADD* **5-HTP:** 50 mg once a day for 2 weeks. Start medication taper. |
| Mirtazapine (Remeron) | **Tyrosine:** 500 mg once a day for 1 week *THEN ADD* **5-HTP:** 50 mg/day for the second week. Start tapering medication, while adding 500 mg tyrosine for week 3, and adding then 50 mg of 5-HTP for week 4 while continuing the medication taper. |
| Benzodiazepines (Xanax, Klonopin, Rivotril, Librium, Ativan) | *For sleep issues* <br> **Valerian:** 100 mg/day while weaning off benzodiazepines. <br> For general anxiety <br> **Kava:** 50 mg/day to start, moving up to 300 mg/day while tapering the benzodiazepine over 2 weeks, with a subsequent 3 weeks of 300 mg of kava/day. |

240

ioral stress response itself and can cause neurologic damage through pathways that create overexcitement in the system. Through these pathways, improper withdrawal of medications will cause greater neurologic damage and may create a great inability to respond well to future treatment options of any kind (Waxman, 2005).

One thing any patient using these medications should remember is that stopping the medication can be hard to do. The brain and body do become dependent on them.

If a patient has done the work recommended in the rest of this book (psychotherapy, sleep, diet, lifestyle, exercise, supplements, mind-body work) and believes he or she is ready to reduce medication, three steps will help organize this process: (1) talk to the prescribing doctor and assure monitoring, (2) follow the naturopathic path, and (3) prescribe supplements to support the medication weaning process.

## 1. Talk to the Prescribing Doctor and Assure Monitoring

Safety is the number one issue for any patient. As a naturopathic physician, I certainly prefer patients not take medications if they are not needed. However, weaning needs proper monitoring. Thus, the prescribing doctor should always be centrally involved. As I do in my office, working with a doctor open to CAM approaches is preferable. Also, patients with other issues beyond anxiety and depression, such as schizophrenia, bipolar, or other medical issues, may not be able to stop taking medications at this time. So please, ensure your client is checking with his or her prescribing doctor.

Also, this is a time to make sure the "support team" for the patient is available and scheduled. Depending on the patient, this would include his or her psychotherapist or psychologist, acupuncturist, naturopathic or other holistic doctor, and ideally the patient's home community of family or friends, if available. Keeping close tabs on the patient and alerting the prescribing doctor if there are withdrawal symptoms are important.

## 2. Follow the Naturopathic Path

This book goes over diet, lifestyle, laboratory testing, stress, sleep, gender factors, nutrients, botanicals—a range of issues to consider in CAM. If these factors have not been worked on and are not in place as a cohesive plan, a crucial supportive factor might be overlooked and the weaning process may suffer. As a general rule, I recommend the holistic plan this book outlines be in place for at least 4 months, and the patient should be feeling very well for at least 2 full months—maybe longer if the medication has been used for more than 2 years.

I try not to emphasize the notion of weaning off medications when first working with holistic options. I typically find, though, that after a few months working with holistic care, my patients who are still on medications will bring up the question of whether medications are still needed. This is an important moment: it tells me there has been some shift in their body and mind, and we can get start down the road to safely weaning off the medications. This shift is not always tangible, but when it happens, the patient often recognizes it first. Once that shift is noticed, it is best to wait at least another month or two to make sure that shift holds, and then consider step 3 below.

## 3. Supplements to Support the Medication Weaning Process

In this step we add a few supplemental supports to help the body get up to neurotransmitter speed. The general idea is to review the medications your client is taking and then gently support the body by feeding it the precursors to the neurotransmitters that the drugs already support. Table 6.3 lists the amino acid or herbal supports to help the body create its own neurotransmitters for weaning off each medication. An analogy to this would be like creating little stairs to go down a steep incline, instead of using an icy ramp. These amino acids and herbs are little steps for the nervous and hormonal systems to take as they move down the path to a medication-free life.

Please note that many of these supplements have not been backed by double-blind randomized placebo controlled trials for use in medication weaning. This work is instead based on my last 10 years of clinical practice, the evidenced-based research I reviewed elsewhere in this book, and common sense. More studies on this type of work are most welcome, and one of my hopes is that this book will stimulate further research, so we can refine and create an evidence base and safety parameters for this kind of truly integrative medicine.

# SEVEN

# Making Recommendations and
# Designing Treatment Plans

---

Integrative thinking is the ability to constructively face the
tensions of opposing models, and, instead of choosing one at
the expense of the other, generating a creative resolution of
the tension in the form of a new model that contains elements of the individual models, but is superior to each.
—Rotman School of Management, 2012

Chapters 1–6 discussed a wide range of topics: conventional medicine,
the brain, hormones, sleep, blood sugar, foods, amino acids, herbs, exercise, environment, toxins, homeopathy, and probably way more research
than you were interested in.

The million dollar question is, How does a practitioner select from
among the many choices to help our client? There is no possible way a
client can do them all—nor would that be useful. So, how do we distill
all this to meet the needs of the person with anxiety or depression?

Thinking integratively and creating an effective treatment plan
generally require consideration of more variables than would be considered in conventional care. It requires using intuition and imagination
along with reason and scientific research. Paul Rosch, current chairman
of the board of the American Institute of Stress and clinical professor of
medicine and psychiatry at New York Medical College, applies the con-

cept of integration to medicine and suggests that integrative medicine implies "the ability to extract bits of information from seemingly disparate disciplines and synthesize them into something that is meaningful" (Rosh, 1997).

In this spirit, Figure 7.1 is a flow chart that helps guide integrative thinking, to help you sense where all these moving parts fit in a cogent and cohesive plan for your client.

Below are six steps to help the practitioner gather the right information and drill down to what will be most important to guide the patient:

1. Listen to the patient and take a good history
2. Assure the lifestyle basics

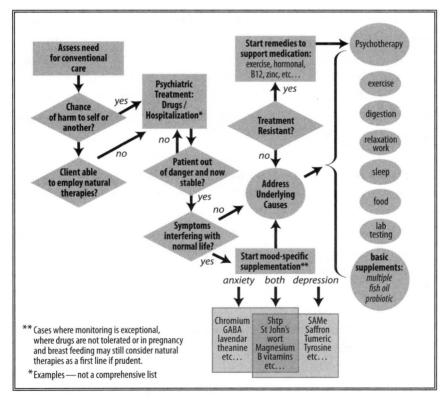

Figure 7.1. A decision flow chart for the integrative care of anxiety and depression.

3. Get some tests
4. Add basic supplementation
5. Add specific supplements that match the patient profile
6. Print out a clear and simple plan of action

## 1. LISTEN TO THE PATIENT AND TAKE A GOOD HISTORY

Undoubtedly, this is something you as a therapist are doing quite well. You are the expert in listening carefully. This section is not here to teach you another method but to place this into the context of holistic and integrative care.

Twentieth-century theologian Paul Tillich said: "The first duty of love is to listen." Sir William Osler, a founding professor of Johns Hopkins Hospital, is quoted to say: "The good physician knows the disease the patient has. The great physician knows the patient who has the disease." Together, these thoughts may sum up the spirit of effective integrative and holistic care: to listen to your patient and learn who your patient truly is. When you know your patient well in terms of hopes, dreams, sensitivities, physical predispositions, preferences, schedule, real and perceived limitations, and so on, you will find ways to work with that person in order to start making good decisions that will bring back balance.

Treatment options draw from a multitude of recommendations, including food changes, lifestyle work, spiritual work, vitamins, herbs, acupuncture, drugs, and sometimes even surgery. The best physician knows these tools are all valuable, and the strongest integrative physician strives to understand which will be most valuable at a given moment.

I consider the first visit I have with my patient as very important. It is my first opportunity to show *agape* (love of humankind), to listen closely and to get to know the person. The first visit may also be the most important in terms of earning the trust needed to share the intimacy that is that person's life and help make decisions to change its trajectory. As a therapist, you are keenly aware the critical nature of meeting each person where he or she is in terms of speaking tone, communication style, and vocabulary, which will be invaluable in creating a therapeutic relationship that both is professional and feels safe for your client. To create a holistic plan, this therapeutic relationship is key.

The first two questions I typically ask a patient are these:

*I know you are here to work on having a better mood. If I could wave a magic wand, is there any particular feeling, thought, or symptom that you would like to see go away or balance out first?*

This is not a standard question, but I find this helps me understand what is really bothering the patient. For example, I may know a patient is diagnosed with generalized anxiety disorder, but I don't know what bothers that person most—is it the sweating in their palms, the fear someone will touch them, the tingling in their feet? This can give a strong clue as to what treatment modality will help the most.

*When was the last time you felt well?*

This question helps me ascertain if the patient remembers or can visualize what it was like to feel well at some point. Patients who can remember this well typically get better quicker—the others may be more challenging. Patients who respond "I always felt this way" or "I cannot remember the last time I felt well" typically need a longer course, closer monitoring, and possibly more rigorous treatment regimens.

Following these two questions, I will ask about the mood issue itself.

## Mood Concern Onset and Chronology

*When is the very first time these mood issues came on?*

*What was going on in your life when you first noticed these feelings? Did you get sick or have a change in your health before or around that time? Were there any traumatic events or losses in your life at that time?*

247

It is key to understand what life events were happening for a particular patient when it all started. Sometimes difficult sickness can contribute to feeling depressed, and sometimes it can clue a practitioner in to possible underlying causes.

## Family History

*Do mood disorders appear in your family?*

Establishing family history may clue the clinician in that healing and balance may be a longer-term and more neurotransmitter-based endeavor than someone without family history. In my clinical experience, those patients with a strong family history often have more neurotransmitter imbalances, and typically need a longer duration of care for healing. Of course, there are exceptions, as thoughts and messages are learned from our family environment the same way genetics are passed on.

## Medications

*What medications are you now taking?*

*Have any medications been helpful to you? Which ones?*

*Have any medications made you feel worse?*

Knowing what medications a patient is taking can alert you to other conditions present, as well as how to watch out for interactions with natural treatments. The last two questions can help you ascertain what mechanisms are more salient, which can help you decide which natural supplements would be more effective or possibly make a patient feel worse.

## Supplements

*Are you currently taking any natural supplements?*

*Have any supplements helped you?*

*Have any supplements made you feel worse?*

Patients typically visit a holistic practitioner after hitting the health food store a few times and trying things themselves outside of a comprehensive treatment plan. If any supplement may have helped or made the patient worse, this may aide in future supplement choices.

## Better/Worse and Associated Symptoms

*What makes your symptoms better or worse?*

*Foods?* You may suggest certain food allergies or sensitivities

*Time of day?* You can suggest circadian rhythm or blood sugar relationship. A diet and lifestyle diary that outlines diet and symptomology can be very helpful to further elucidate food, activities, and other factors in your client's life that may play a role in triggering mood changes (see appendix VI).

*Time of year or season?* This ascertains whether there is seasonal affective disorder or circadian disruption that needs adjustment.

*Do these feelings go away when you are on vacation?* If yes, they are more acute stress related.

*Does exercise make it better or worse?* If the patient is fatigued after exercise, this may be more a sign of "adrenal fatigue," HPA dysregulation, or overall depletion. Often in these cases blood pressure will be lower as well and may need support.

*Does being alone make it better or worse?* This helps the practitioner to understand the patient's experience of relating to other people or inclination to separate from the world.

*Is it worse or better during certain parts of your menstrual cycle?* If yes, this may suggest elevation or depression of certain hormones that contribute to mood issues.

## Review of Systems/Physical Examination

This is a basic tool used by primary care physicians, where questions are asked about the different symptoms, and the body is checked for physical signs. Instead of recreating the full review and examination, below is a summary of those items I have found most pertinent to ask about in working with anxiety and depression.

### Skin/Integument

- Rashes, itching may indicate inflammation, digestive issues, poor toxin elimination.
- Pale skin may be a sign of iron deficiency or vitamin D deficiency due to little sunlight.
- Pale crevices in hands may be a sign of iron deficiency.
- Purple or darkness under the eyes may be a sign of inadequate sleep or food allergies.
- Nail cracks, ridges, furrows may be a sign of general nutrition deficiency.
- Lower leg swelling not associated with kidney or heart problems is often a sign of hypothyroidism or circulation challenges.
- Dry skin—consider fatty acid deficiency, inadequate hydration, or low thyroid function.

### Tongue

In Chinese medicine, the tongue has a lot to offer regarding understanding the body and digestion. Here is a quick summary of main ones features to look for:

Thick white coat—slow digestion
Think yellow coat—slow digestion with excess heat, that may represent anger or low acid production
Large deep crack in middle of tongue—deep emotional issues
Red tipped tongue—low yin energy
Oversized and pale tongue—spleen qi deficiency (digestive weakness) or blood deficiency (often caused by low nutrient status)

Lateral sides darkened—liver qi stagnated (often a sign of high stress)

### Lungs

In traditional Chinese medicine, lung issues are correlated with grief. Anyone with lung issues may be asked if they have experienced unusual grief or grief that has not dissipated with time.

### Cardiovascular system

Low blood pressure can be a sign of adrenal fatigue.

### Nervous system

- *Tingling in hands and feet?* This can be a sign of blood sugar instability. In Chinese medicine it also suggests "phlegm" or stuck energy in the middle of the body not moving out to the periphery. Diabetes and neurological issues should be ruled out.
- *Excess sweating?* This can be a sign of hyperthyroid function. In Chinese medicine it may be a sign of "yang deficiency."

### Hormonal system

- Problems with the thyroid (either hypo- or hyperthyroid) will affect mood.
- Menstrual irregularities change both serotonin levels and receptivity in the brain to affect mood.
- Problems with the parathyroid gland will also affect mood via suppression of vitamin D.

### Digestion and bowel habits

- *Any digestive problems?*
- *How often do you have a bowel movement?*

Digestive issues of many kinds may be a sign of food allergies or sensitivities, inflammation, and poor ability to balance neurotransmitters. It may also suggest an imbalance in bowel flora.

*Musculoskeletal system*

Poor muscle tone—consider lack of exercise.

Back or joint pain—may hinder a person's ability for mood to improve due to excess pain, or from lack of exercise. In either case, a plan to address pain may be needed as a first step even before fully addressing mood issues.

## History of Toxic Exposure

History of exposure to toxins may suggest a detoxification protocol to be appropriate:

> *Have you ever been exposed to any toxic chemicals or lived in an industrial areas?*
>
> *Have you ever lived close to a highway or major street for a period of time?*
>
> *Has your home been checked for toxic mold, lead paint, or water impurities?*
>
> *Is there anything you are allergic to?*
>
> *Can you tolerate perfume and smells? Can you tolerate coffee or alcohol?*

Often, yes answers to these questions (except the last) suggest the liver is challenged with detoxifying environmental chemicals.

## 2. ASSURE LIFESTYLE BASICS ARE IN ORDER

Below is a summary of lifestyle items I have found most pertinent to ask about while working with anxiety and depression.

Schedule: *What time do you eat your meals, have bowel movements, go to work, come home, and so on?*

This is a key piece of information, for this will help you understand what you reasonably can ask a patient to do. For instance, if a patient works

12 hours a day, it may not be physically possible to ask her to exercise. In which case, you may need to be creative as to what you suggest.

Sleep: *What time do you go to bed and wake up?*
*Any trouble falling or staying asleep?*
*Any history of sleep apnea? Has a partner ever mentioned*
*that you snore, or stop breathing while sleeping?*

Any sleep deficit can cause or exacerbate mood problems. Difficulty falling asleep would suggest melatonin may be useful. Difficulty staying asleep would point to using 5-HTP, tryptophan, or sustained-released melatonin. If sleep apnea is present, it should be treated.

Exercise: *Do you exercise? What is your routine? After you exercise,*
*do you feel better, or worse?*

Exercise, in virtually any form, is beneficial for mood. It is also helpful to get a sense of a patient's constitution and energy reserves. Some equate inability to feel energetic after exercise as an issue of "adrenal fatigue" requiring support.

Food intake: *What did you eat for breakfast, lunch, and dinner yesterday?*
I recommend having each patient, if possible, complete a diet and lifestyle diary that tracks what a patient eats, their activities, and their emotions for 7 days. (See appendix VI.) Often, patients themselves will make connections between their food, activity, and their emotions

*How do you feel if you don't eat for a few hours?*

Both anxiety and depression can be related to hypoglycemia and low blood sugar. Generally, people who get symptoms when they haven't eaten will benefit from blood-sugar-related work, such as eating more protein at breakfast, frequent meals, and chromium supplementation.

Recreational drugs and smoking
*Number of alcohol drinks per day? Past or current history of alcohol*
*abuse?*

253

*Do you smoke? If yes, how much?*

*Is there current recreational drug use, or a history of substantial recreational drug use or abuse?*

Current use of cigarettes, alcohol, and recreational drugs may hinder the effort for healing. Substantial past use may indicate toxicity and the need for a detoxification protocol as well.

Stress reduction rituals. *Do you have a daily stress reduction ritual?* Everyone should have some daily ritual that helps process or mitigate the effects of stress: meditation, prayer, massage, acupuncture, journaling, and so forth. If this is not in place in your client's schedule, this is an opportunity to learn what your client might enjoy.

## 3. GET THE RIGHT BLOOD TESTS

Ask your patient to get the blood tests listed in Appendix II.

## 4. ADD BASIC SUPPLEMENTATION

Chapter 4 discusses the use and benefit of the following:
- A high-quality general multiple vitamin. Take with meals.
- Fish oil (assuring 1,000 mg EPA).
- A high-quality probiotic (I use a combination of *Lactobacillus* and *Bifidus* strains).

## 5. ADD SPECIFIC SUPPLEMENTS THAT MATCH THE PATIENT PROFILE

Consider such supplements as 5-HTP, tryptophan, valerian, and SAMe, based on the patient's constitution, profile, medication use, and symptomology. Chapter 4 explains the different supplements and gives clues to suggest which specific supplements might best support a particular patient. These are summarized in Appendix IV. Testing results will also suggest which nutrients would be of value.

## 6. PRINT OUT A CLEAR AND SIMPLE PLAN OF ACTION

When a patient comes for a visit, I tell them they are welcome to write down any notes they want—but they don't have to. As I talk with them and listen, I am preparing their treatment plan. This will be a clear printout of steps that will be our individualized plan of action.

---

### Sample First Visit: Chart Notes

The following composite will take you through a truncated form that first highlights pertinent notes charted for a composite patient and then show you the accompanying recommendation plan. While the patient is a composite, these are all common notes and plans.

Patient: Carla Composite        Date: 03-21-2014
DOB: 1-19-1966

### S//:
#### Chief Concern: Depression with Anxiety
- Onset: started with depression at age 31 during divorce, in strong relationship now. Depression "comes and goes" but anxiety persists. Symptoms do not stop patient from working, or taking care of her two children.
- Previous history: experienced some great anxiety after boyfriend breakup during college; used medications for 5 years, and then stopped due to pregnancy consideration.

---

- Current symptoms: functional but always worried. When really tired, sometimes she prefers not to get out of bed at all.
- Never suicidal: "would never do that to my kids."
- Working with therapist on relationship issues and sense that "I will always be alone."

### Second Concern: Fatigue

- Wakes up exhausted
- Some energy during the end of the day into the evening
- "When I don't eat, I get a little crazy and I feel cold."
- Worse fatigue: after exercise in the AM. "I try to work out hard so I don't disappoint my trainer, but, sometimes I can't— I'm just exhausted."
- "Doctor says I'm anemic, but I stopped taking iron two years ago for it was making me more constipated."

### Other concerns:

- Patient would like to lose some weight.

### Review of Systems and Lifestyle Factors:

*Digestion:*

- Bowel movement every third day—"been like this since high school. MD says it's normal for me."

*Foods/Water*

- No time for breakfast, sandwich for lunch and "healthy dinner" of chicken, some vegetable and quinoa. Tend to overeat late night.
- Water intake—"not great."
- Coffee: "Need it. Starbucks venti with milk and 3 sugars twice a day. Only thing that keeps me up, but makes me more anxious."
- No alcohol or recreational drug use.

*Sleep:*
- In bed by 12:30 a.m. and up by 6:30 a.m.
- Trouble falling asleep every night, so "I like to stay up and watch late night with Conan. He is so hilarious and it helps me stay calm until I am finally sleepy." Once asleep, I tend to stay asleep.
- Sometimes I can't fall asleep because my mind is bouncing all over the place. The klonopin helps this by knocking me out.

*Relaxation Work:*
- "I tried to meditate, but it makes me crazy."

*Medications:*
- Zoloft: helps the anxiety a little, but no change in the depression.
- Klonopin at night when needed (once a week, usually).

*Supplements:*
- Centrum, "sometimes."
- CoQ10 (friend told her would be good for energy), hasn't helped.

**O//:**
- Patient appears well nourished and not in distressed.
- Height: 5' 9"
- Weight: 142 lbs
- Blood pressure, left arm 92/58

**A//:**
Depression, Anxiety

**P//:**
See recommendation plan below

Patient: Carla Composite                    Date: 03-21-2014
DOB: 1-19-1966

### Sample First Visit: Treatment Plan

**1. FOLLOW-UP TESTS:**
- Adrenal saliva test and blood work (see attached list)—this way we can see how your stress hormones are running, and if there are any nutrient deficiencies or hormonal issues contributing to how you are feeling.

**2. THERAPY WORK:**
- Continue your work with your therapist, and have her contact me so we can coordinate care.

**3. EXERCISE**
- Please keep this gentle—gentle walking in the sun every morning as it feels good for you. For now, do not push your body with heavy duty exercise.

**4. SLEEP:**
- Shut any bright lights/computer/TV/cell phone by 10 p.m. and sit and read. Sip some chamomile tea with a dropperful of *Passiflora* tincture in the tea to help calm the mind.
- If you enjoy Conan, then DVR it to watch earlier the next night.
- Take one capsule of melatonin (1 mg per capsule) at 10:30 p.m. to be in bed at 11 p.m. If you are not falling asleep easily, please add one capsule (300 mg) of GABA to help the mind shut down.
- Before shutting the light, write down in bullet point form any thoughts you are having.

**5. WATER:**
- Drink water in the morning: one big glass, room temperature. You can squeeze half a lemon if you like.

## 6. FOODS:

- Eat breakfast every morning, here are some ideas:
    - Two hard-boiled eggs with Ezekiel toast and butter
    - Ezekiel bread with natural peanut butter
    - Rice protein powder with half a frozen banana and blueberries
    - Turkey bacon with scrambled eggs
    - Oatmeal with walnuts, butter, and cinnamon
- For constipation help, add these to your daily diet:
    - 5 organic prunes
    - 1 cup of dark greens
    - 1 tablespoon of flax meal—can add to oatmeal, a salad, or a shake
- For your coffee, ask for "¾ caf" for 2 weeks, then go to "½ caf."

## 7. SUPPLEMENTS:

- Discontinue Centrum and start a higher-potency multiple vitamin: 3 capsules a day with food.
- Fish oil: one teaspoon a day, with or away from food, for overall brain support.
- Probiotic: one capsule at bedtime, to support digestion.
- You can discontinue the CoQ10 for now if you feel it is not helping.

## 8. ACUPUNCTURE:

- Once a week to support energy, relax, and help lift mood.

NOTE: Please do not change any medications without speaking to your prescribing doctor.

*Next Visit Follow-up in One Month:*
- Check on recommendations above.
- Review saliva test blood tests: consider herbs and supplements for adrenal/circadian support and gentle iron or other nutrients depending on blood tests.
- Consider direct mood-supporting supplements.
- Longer term: weight loss work.

*Rationale for this treatment plan*

Carla's picture is a common one—she's a functional anxiously depressed person. While she is clearly anxious, from my perspective, it is hard to tell if she is depressed or simply too tired. Anemia alone can create a low mood/fatigue picture. Constipation will also affect mood and keep it low. Blood tests will help decide if her anemia may be due to low iron, or low oxygenation of her blood, or low B12 status. Then we can supplement appropriately. The adrenal tests will help us understand if her cortisol is very low, or is up and down at different times a day, contributing to anxiety and the nighttime wakefulness. Her blood pressure, low for her height, suggests to me her adrenal function is waning.

This first treatment plan focuses on some basics:

1. Better sleep
2. Improving bowel movements
3. Supporting morning blood sugar and eating breakfast

Sometimes these alone will go a long way to improving how she is feeling.

I encourage my patients to have their therapists contact me, so I can better understand a patient's challenges, as well as coordinate care, for even better results.

Shutting the bright lights earlier will help Carla's own melatonin secretion and support her natural evening circadian rhythm. The supplemental melatonin should also help Carla fall asleep, and the GABA works like a natural klonopin to support GABA if she still needs a little of that but doesn't want to rely on the drug. The herb *Passiflora* (passionflower) is a wonderful and gentle way to calm an overactive mind. The morning walk in bright light can also help establish her morning circadian pattern.

Drinking water will help bowel movements, as well as usher amino acids into her brain to support neurotransmitter function. Lowering caffeine will help the insomnia. It is best to wean slowly—especially because constipation and depression may get worse if coffee is removed quickly.

Breakfast is the first step to balancing blood sugar issues. We might consider adding supplemental chromium at a later date as well, if blood sugar needs further work or the blood tests show poor blood sugar control.

We are starting with the three general supplements: a good-quality multiple vitamin (store-bought tablets are usually very poor quality, the reason we switched this), a fish oil, and a probiotic.

While we are working on things and getting more information, starting acupuncture should help Carla start to feel less anxious, as well as pick up her energy and mood.

I like to place a follow-up plan at the end in order to explain to my patient what we will be doing at our next visit and what longer term options may be considered. This mentions that we will review the current plan, to see what was accomplished and helpful, and look further at what wasn't accomplished and understand the challenges to these. Also, I mention to the patient that we haven't actually used any "mood supplements" yet (e.g., 5-HTP or St. John's wort) but that we may discuss using these if needed. Many times, an executed plan like this precludes the need for direct mood supplementation. Finally, I mention addressing the weight loss. In truth, working on diet, bowels, and healthy exercise will probably have some positive effects on weight, but I want my patient to know that we are keeping all the things important to her in sight.

Finally, as I walk my patient out of my office into the waiting area, I ask permission to give her a hug, and tell her I look forward to our follow-up visit.

The namesake for my medical school, Bastyr University in Seattle, is John Bastyr, ND, DC. He recommended to his students to "always touch your patients—let them know you care" (Grimes, 2005, p. 58). At the end of the visit, this can take the shape of a two-handed deliberate handshake, or asking the patient, "Is it OK if I give you a hug?" In my 10 years of practice, only one person has ever said no—stating that he would not be comfortable. A gentle hug is a powerful expression of care and will relay to your patients your heartfelt interest in their well-being. Plus, it is very healthy for me to get a few hugs every day—a win-win for everyone involved.

# Appendices

# Top Seven CAM Recommendations You Can Offer Your Clients

1. Remain on medication, if you are taking medications. Consider medication if there are safety issues due to mental illness.
2. Have some blood tests (Appendix II).
3. Begin taking these supplements:
   - A high-quality multiple vitamin (full dose, with food)
   - Vitamin D (1000 IU/day with food)
   - Magnesium supplement (250 mg twice a day)
   - Fish oil (1,000 mg/day EPA)
4. Try to get out in the sun in the morning and begin an exercise program, if able.
5. Add specific foods to the diet that have proved beneficial for mood disorder:
   - Protein every morning (boiled eggs, protein shake)
   - Salmon, catfish, or other low-mercury fish 3 times a week
   - 1 cup of green vegetables every day
   - One tablespoon of olive oil every day
   - Handful of raw nuts every day
   - Handful of baby carrots every day
   - 1 probiotic food a day: 1 yogurt, 1/2 cup sauerkraut (freshly made if possible), miso soup

6. Get to bed by 11 p.m. and create a consistent sleep schedule.
7. Add specific supplements if not on medication:
   - Anxiety: a B complex and ashwagandha (300 mg twice a day)
   - Depression: rhodiola (100 mg three times a day)
8. Consider referral to a holistic practitioner (see Appendix III).

In most cases, the above simple steps are backed by evidenced-based medicine and alone can substantially impact the course of both anxiety and depression.

# Blood Test Recommendations

Below is a list of blood tests to check with anyone suffering from anxiety or depression. Please note that many conventional doctors may not find it necessary to run these. Or they may be uncomfortable running a test that is outside the purview of their specific specialty. For example, a psychiatrist may not feel comfortable running a celiac panel, which is usually under the jurisdiction of a gastroenterologist, even though inflammation from the gut can be a strong contributor to mood disorder. Also, most conventional doctors do not look at saliva adrenal testing. In my experience, even endocrinologists who work regularly with hormones usually do not look at this test. Nevertheless, from a holistic perspective, these tests may provide useful information regarding the underlying factors that contribute to a person's mood condition. While not all may be run for your client, whichever ones can be run will be of help for the long-term goal of understanding the underlying cause.

A few companies provide saliva testing for adrenal hormones. Here are two I have used (I have no financial relationship with these laboratories):

BioHealth Laboratory: http://www.Biohealthlab.com
Diagnostechs: http://www.diagnostechs.com

## *Recommended Blood Tests*

Suggested Blood Tests for:

Date of Birth:

Today's Date:

Fasting blood sugar

HgbA1C

Serum insulin

Complete metabolic panel

Lipid panel

Homocysteine

hsCRP

CBC (complete blood count)

Iron panel:

   Ferritin

   TIBC

   Transferrin

   Serum iron

Hormonal panel:

   TSH

   Free and total T3, T4

   PTH

DHEA

DHEAs

Testosterone: free and total

Serum estrogen (if female)

Serum progesterone (if female)

Celiac panel:

   Anti-gliadin IgG antibodies

   Anti-gliadin IgM antibodies

   TTG

   Secretory IgA

Serum carnitine

Serum folic acid

Serum B12

*MTHFR* gene test

Serum 25(OH)vitamin D

Serum mercury

# CAM Referrals and Resources

## PROFESSIONAL HOLISTIC COLLABORATION

As I have mentioned throughout the book, I have the honor of collaborating on my patient care with many psychotherapists, social workers, and open-minded psychiatrists. It is a pleasure to work together—I learn a great deal, and the patient receives a "team care" approach that offers the best of all worlds.

Health can be thought of like standing and balancing on a big ball. Most of the time we can keep ourselves standing, but when a disease comes in, we then begin to fall too easily. When appropriately used, medication itself can help push the person back up to the top. However, this position can prove temporary and often can push the person too far—even to the point of going off the other side in the process.

Using talk therapy, CAM medicines, and psychiatry in a team care approach can offer not just one hand pushing up from one direction but many hands gently propping-up the patient, adjusting the direction and force of these taps as we go, thus allowing patients to rebalance themselves for good and learning to use the resources we can offer as needed in the future.

It is a rare practitioner who has all the tools necessary to create health for any individual patient. I encourage you, as your client's often main and most trusted resource, to help him or her find other practitioners who can keep in communication with you and each other, to create the best care possible. Below is a resource list to help you find practitioners and more information.

## Holistic Practitioners and Conference Opportunities

*American Association of Naturopathic Physicians: www.naturopathic.org/*
This is the national association for naturopathic physicians, and their website offers information on naturopathic medicine, becoming a naturopathic doctor, and conferences and continuing education in naturopathy. Also, each state has its own state association. If you decide to refer to a naturopathic physician, this organization contains only credentialed physicians who went to federally recognized naturopathic medical colleges.

*The American Holistic Medical Association:*
*http://www.holisticmedicine.org*
The American Holistic Medical Association (AHMA) was founded in July 1978 by medical doctors who had an interest in natural and holistic medicine but had no support from their medical community. Today, members include medical doctors, naturopathic doctors, and many other practitioners. The AHMA runs excellent conferences, continuing education events, and retreats and is a source of community for holistic medical doctors.

*Institute of Functional Medicine: www.functionalmedicine.org*
The Institute of Functional Medicine consists of medical doctors, osteopathic physicians, and naturopathic doctors who espouse a systems-based approach. Besides having a practitioner base, they also offer resources and conferences geared towards medical doctors interested in learning about a more integrative approach.

## Journals

*Journal of Alternative and Complementary Medicine:*
*http://www.liebertpub.com/acm*
This well-respected peer-reviewed journal publishes research on a variety of CAM topics, including acupuncture, nutrition, massage, botanical medicine, Ayurveda, yoga, and many other modalities.

*Natural Medicine Journal: http://www.naturalmedicinejournal.com/*
This is the official journal of the American Association of Naturopathic Physicians. It is an e-journal offering peer-reviewed research on integrative and naturopathic medicine.

*Alternative and Complementary Therapies: http://www.liebertpub.com/*
*overview/alternative-and-complementary-therapies*
This is an evidence-based journal that includes articles on many different CAM modalities and integrative medicine topics, such as building a holistic practice and integrating CAM into a clinical practice.

*Evidence-Based Complementary and Alternative Medicine:*
*http://www.hindawi.com/journals/ecam/*
This is an international, peer-reviewed journal founded in 2004 with information on CAM and integrative medicine.

*Naturopathic Doctor News and Reviews: http://www.ndnr.com*
This publication provides clinical information for naturopathic physicians in North America. It informs and educates physicians in the recent developments of the practice of natural medicine. It includes protocols, practice management, business development, marketing, clinical research, news, and more.

*Holistic Primary Care: http://holisticprimarycare.net*
Provides health professionals with a credible source for natural and holistic medicine.

*Townsend Letter: http://townsendletter.com*
Since 1983, providing practitioners with a wide variety of alternative medicine topics.

# Supplements for Anxiety and Depression

Table IV.1. General supplementation That Should Be Considered for All Patients with Anxiety or Depression

| Supplement | Best use | Typical dose | Possible side effects | Toxicity/ contraindication/ interactions | Food sources |
|---|---|---|---|---|---|
| Multiple vitamin | • General anxiety and depression support | • Follow dosage on bottle. High-quality versions usually are in capsule form and dose between 4 and 6 capsules a day, with food, in divided doses | • Some patients experience nausea with minerals | • None known | • All vegetables and fruits |
| Fish oil | • Anxiety<br>• Depression<br>• High CRP | • About 2 g/day in total, looking for 1,000 mg/day of EPA and ~800 mg DHA | • Possible reflux | • None known<br>• Contraindicated if allergic to fish<br>• Monitor clotting times if on anti-clotting medications | • Fish |
| Probiotics | • General anxiety and depression support | • 4–8 billion *Lactobacillus acidophilus* and *Bifidobacterium lactis* one to three times a day | • None known | • None known | • Natto, kimchi, miso, sauerkraut |

## Table IV.2. Most Commonly Used Vitamins for Anxiety and Depression

| Supplement | Best use | Typical dose |
| --- | --- | --- |
| Vitamin C | • High CRP | • 500 mg twice a day |
| Vitamin D | • Low levels of vitamin D with depression or anxiety | • 1,000–5,000 IU/day taken with food and retest levels in 3 months |
| Vitamin B3 (niacinamide form) | • Panic and obsessive compulsive types of anxieties<br>• Benefits for staying asleep when used with tryptophan | • 100 mg three times a day |
| Vitamin B6 (pyridoxine or pyridine 5-phosphate) | • Anxiety and depression | • 25–50 mg/day<br>• May work best when taken with magnesium |
| Vitamin B12 (methylcobalamin) | • Anxiety and depression<br>• Support for treatment-resistant depression | • 1 mg daily |
| Folic acid (methylfolate) | • Depression<br>• Treatment-resistant depression<br>• Can help antidepressants work better | • 400–1,000 μg for depression or 5–15 mg daily in treatment-resistant depression cases |

| Possible side effects | Toxicity/ contraindication/ interactions | Food sources |
|---|---|---|
| • Runny stools and diarrhea at high doses | • Large amounts may contribute to kidney stones | Papaya, bell peppers, broccoli, strawberries, pineapple, kiwi |
| • None known at physiologic doses | • Fat-soluble vitamin can build up to toxic levels<br>• Overdosing can raise calcium absorption, leading to heart abnormalities<br>• May help antidepressants work better | Small amounts in salmon, tuna, mackerel, beef, liver, egg yolk |
| • None known | • Long-term use should include precautionary monitoring of liver enzymes<br>• Use may increase effectiveness of tryptophan<br>• Avoid with anticonvulsant medication | Chicken, turkey, beef, liver, peanuts, sunflower seeds, mushrooms, avocado, green peas |
| • 200 mg or more a day may cause reversible hand and food tingling and/or fatigue | • Birth control pills can lower B6 status | Bell peppers, spinach, potatoes, bananas, turnip greens |
| • Occasionally will cause insomnia if taken too late in the day | • Metformin can lower B12 status | Snapper, calf's liver, venison, shrimp, scallops, salmon, beef |
| • No side effects | • Avoid when taking methotrexate for cancer treatment<br>• Avoid with epilepsy medications | Spinach, asparagus, romaine lettuce, turnip greens, mustard greens, calf's liver, collard greens, cauliflower, broccoli, parsley, lentils, beets |

(continued)

## Table IV.2. Continued

| Supplement | Best use | Typical dose |
|---|---|---|
| Inositol | • Panic disorder | • 6–18 g/day |
| B complex: vitamins B1, B2, B5, B6, B12, folate, and inositol | • General daily stress support for nonanxious people and to support depression and anxiety<br>• High homocysteine | 40 mg vitamin B6, 1.2 mg B12 (methylcobalamin form), 1 g folate (l-methyltetrahydrofolate form) per day |
| Betaine (trimethyl-glycine) | • High homocysteine | • 3,600 mg/day |

| Possible side effects | Toxicity/ contraindication/ interactions | Food sources |
|---|---|---|
| • Minor gastric discomfort | • None known | Most vegetables, nuts, wheat germ, brewers yeast, bananas, liver, brown rice, oat flakes, unrefined molasses, raisins |
| • High levels of B6 can cause reversible neuropathy symptoms | • No known toxicities | Vegetables, whole grains, beans |
| • Rare transient gastrointestinal upset | • None known | Beets, whole wheat, wheat germ, shellfish |

## Table IV.3. Supplementation Supportive in Specific Cases of Mood Dyregulation Due to Hormonal Imbalance

| Supplement | Best use | Typical dose |
|---|---|---|
| Armour Thyroid or Nature-Throid | • Low thyroid function | • Depends on individual needs |
| DHEA | • Anxiety and depression<br>• Consider for low levels, midlife-onset depression, autoimmunity, and addiction recovery for anxiety with withdrawal | • 5–10 mg for women, up to 25 mg for men; monitor levels with blood tests. Higher dose per individual need. |
| Testosterone | • Anxiety and depression<br>• May help antidepressants work better | • Depends on preparation |
| Estrogen | • Depression<br>• May help antidepressants work better | • Depends on preparation |
| Progesterone | • Anxiety or with depression<br>• As low dose when given estrogen<br>• Poor sleep | • Depends on preparation and needs |

| Possible side effects | Toxicity/ contraindication/ interactions | Food sources |
|---|---|---|
| • Racing heart<br>• Excess sweating<br>• Shakiness<br>• Anxiety<br>• Fast-paced thought patterns | • Use under physician supervision | Thyroid organ meat |
| • Excess hair<br>• Greasy skin and hair, acne<br>• Scalp itching, hair loss | • Use with physician guidance<br>• May be contraindicated in prostate cancer | None known |
| • Dermal patch can cause rash | • Use with physician guidance<br>• May be contraindicated due to heart disease and prostate cancer concerns | Zinc-containing foods may help boost testosterone (oysters, eggs, bananas, broccoli) |
| • Irritability<br>• Leg swelling<br>• Blood clots | • Higher risk of blood clots in smokers | Foods with gentle phytoestrogens: soy, kidney, pinto, and navy beans; flaxseeds; sunflower seeds |
| • Increased feelings of sadness and weepiness<br>• Vaginal bleeding | • Depression<br>• Sleepiness | Raw nuts and seeds may help increase progesterone production |

### Table IV.4. Plant-Derived Oils That Can Be Helpful for Mood

| Supplement | Best use | Typical dose |
|---|---|---|
| Gamma-linolenic acid (GLA) or primrose oil | • Heavy drinking and alcoholism with depression<br>• Premenstrual symptoms with depression | • GLA: 1,000–2,500 mg once a day<br>• Primrose oil: 4,000–8,000 mg daily |
| Vegan oils | • General anxiety and depression support | • ~4 g/day alpha-linolenic acid (ALA) |

### Table IV.5 Minerals Most Commonly Used to Support Anxiety and Depression

| Supplement | Best use | Typical dose |
|---|---|---|
| Chromium | • Anxiety and/or depression that correlates with hypo- or hyperglycemia, atypical depression | • 200–600 µg/day, taken in divided doses with meals |
| Zinc | • Treatment-resistant depression<br>• Leaky gut<br>• Helps support the immune system and the skin | • 15 mg twice a day<br>• Use zinc carnosine for leaky gut<br>• Balance with 2 mg/day copper if taken for >2 months (unless blood copper levels are high) |
| Iron | • Low iron anemia | • 25 mg one to three times a day<br>• Take with 500 mg of vitamin C for best absorption<br>• Use succinate or fumarate forms |

| Possible side effects | Toxicity/ contraindication / interactions | Food sources |
|---|---|---|
| • Occasional reflux | • Doses of GLA > 3,000 mg/day should be avoided<br>• Not be used in patients with epileptic history, in those with prostate cancer risk, or during pregnancy | Black currants |
| • None known | • None known | Flaxseed, rape seed oil, walnuts, tofu |

| Possible side effects | Toxicity/ contraindication / interactions | Food sources |
|---|---|---|
| • None known at recommended dosages | • Monitor for lowering of blood sugar in patients using diabetic medications<br>• Helps prevent glucocorticoid-induced chromium deficiency | Onions, romaine lettuce, tomatoes, Brewer's yeast, eggs, liver, bran cereal |
| • Can cause nausea when taken on an empty stomach or in sensitive individuals | • Large doses (>150 mg/ day) can cause vomiting and appetite loss<br>• Long-term zinc supplementation may deplete copper | Beef, lamb, turkey, chicken, pork, crabmeat, lobster, clams, salmon, pumpkin seeds |
| • Can be constipating in higher doses<br>• May turn stools black | • Contraindicated in postmenopausal women and in men except for clear iron deficiency unexplained by other medical issues | Dark turkey meat, red meat, cast iron pot cooking, lesser absorbable iron in dark green vegetables |

(continued)

## Table IV.5 Continued

| Supplement | Best use | Typical dose |
|---|---|---|
| Magnesium (glycinate or taurate form) | • Sleep issues<br>• Anxiety<br>• Depression plus anxiety | *For sleep issues or anxiety:*<br>• 250 mg glycinate form twice a day<br>*For depression plus anxiety:*<br>• 300–700 mg of either form<br>• One to two cups Epsom salts in a warm bath |
| Selenium | • Anxiety and/or depression with low thyroid function or low T3 | • 100–200 µg/day |
| Lithium orotate | • Anxiety or depression, especially in patients who benefit from oxytocin-related treatments like a massage | • 5–20 mg/day of elemental lithium |

| Possible side effects | Toxicity/ contraindication / interactions | Food sources |
|---|---|---|
| • Possible loose stools if sensitive<br>• Taurate form can cause diarrhea | • None known<br>• Avoid taurate form with kidney disease or diarrhea | Mineral water<br>Swiss chard, summer squash, blackstrap molasses, spinach, mustard greens, halibut, turnip greens, seeds (pumpkin, sunflower, flax) |
| • Doses >400 µg may cause symptoms of dermatitis, hair loss, and brittle nails | | Tuna, meat, fish, nuts (especially Brazil nuts), garlic |
| • Common supplemental doses show no toxicity<br>• High doses can cause muscle weakness, loss of appetite, mild apathy, tremors, nausea and vomiting | • Impaired kidney function | Mustard, sardines, whole grains, blue corn, vegetables |

Table IV.6. Top Supplemental Amino Acids Used for Anxiety and Depression

| Supplement | Best use | Typical dose |
|---|---|---|
| Glutamine | • Leaky gut | • 1 teaspoon twice a day |
| Carnitine | • Depression and possible antianxiety benefits<br>• Cognitive support in seniors | • 500–1,500 mg L-carnitine form twice a day to raise serum carnitine<br>*For cognitive support*<br>• 1–3 g acetyl-L-carnitine form |
| GABA | • Anxiety ("natural Xanax")<br>• To help calm mind to fall asleep | • 100–200 mg up to three times daily away from food<br>• Take no more than 1,000 mg within a 4-hour period and no more than 3,000 mg within a 24-hour period |
| Glycine | • Anxiety<br>• 30 minutes before anticipated panic situations | • 5–10 g (one to two teaspoons) a day or before an anticipated panic attack.<br>• Can be mixed with passionflower |
| Lysine and arginine | • Anxiety in stress situations | • 2–3 grams of each twice a day, away from food |
| L-Theanine | • Anxiety with chronic running or obsessive thoughts<br>• High cortisol:DHEA ratio<br>• Anxiety with blood pressure increases | • 200–400 mg/day, away from food |

| Possible side effects | Toxicity/ contraindication / interactions | Food sources |
|---|---|---|
| • None known | • May prevent chemotherapy-induced side effects<br>• May not be appropriate with liver or kidney disease | Cabbage, chicken, beef, fish |
| • None known | • May be beneficial to prevent deficiencies with anticonvulsant drugs | Beef, chicken, turkey, pork, lamb, fish |
| • Dizziness and sleepy feeling | • Rare increased bruising and bleeding at high doses | Tea (green, black, oolong) fermented foods (yogurt, kimchi, sauerkraut); whole grains (oats, brown rice) |
| • None known | • Check with a doctor before using if liver or kidney disease is present<br>• May be beneficial in schizophrenia | Fish, meat, beans, dairy |
| • High doses (20–30 g) of arginine may cause diarrhea | • Arginine is contraindicated if there is a heart attack history<br>• Arginine may be contraindicated with type 1 herpetic sores | Nuts, red meat, spinach, lentils, whole grains, chocolate, eggs, seafood, soy |
| • None known | • May increase effects of some chemotherapy | Green tea |

*(continued)*

## Table IV.6. Continued

| Supplement | Best use | Typical dose |
|---|---|---|
| L-Tryptophan | • Trouble staying asleep | • 500–2,500 mg<br>• Take away from food, but with a high glycemic simple carbohydrate (e.g., cracker) |
| 5-HTP | • Anxiety, especially agoraphobia and panic<br>• Expression with a social anxiety or panic component | • 100–200 mg three times a day, on an empty stomach<br>• 200 mg 90 minutes before anticipated panic attack |
| Tyrosine | • Depression with apathy and despair<br>• Supportive with physical stressors and sleep deprivation<br>• Tobacco withdrawal<br>• Low thyroid function | • *For depression or tobacco withdrawal support:* 500–1,000 mg two or three times a day up to 6,000 mg total<br>• *For tobacco withdrawal support:* Add chromium, 200 mg/three times a day<br>• *For low thyroid function:* 300 mg/day |
| Phenylalanine | • Same as for Tyrosine, above, with concomitant pain symptoms | • Up to 14 g/day L-form in divided doses<br>• 350 mg/day D-form |

| Possible side effects | Toxicity/ contraindication / interactions | Food sources |
|---|---|---|
| • Sleepy in the morning | • None known<br>• Studies with Prozac showed benefit, without interaction<br>• Monitor for serotonin syndrome when used with SSRIs and tricyclics | Small amounts in pumpkin seeds, bananas, turkey |
| • Nausea and occasional vomiting | • May increase diarrhea symptoms in prone individuals<br>• Monitor for serotonin syndrome when used with SSRIs and tricyclics | None |
| • With higher dosing: nausea, diarrhea, headache, vomiting, or excessive nervousness<br>• Consider avoiding night supplementation or use with tryptophan at night if night wakefulness results | • Not recommended with anxiety, high blood pressure, multiple myeloma, Grave's disease, or MAOIs | Fish, soy, chicken, almonds, avocados, bananas, dairy products, lima beans, sesame seeds |
| • Same as for Tyrosine, above | • Same as for Tyrosine, above<br>• Phenylketonuria | Torula yeast, soybean protein isolate and concentrate, peanut flour, dried spirulina, seaweed, defatted and low-fat soybean flour, dried and salted cod, tofu, Parmesan cheese, almond meal, dry roasted soybean nuts, dried watermelon seeds, fenugreek seeds |

(continued)

## Table IV.6. Continued

| Supplement | Best use | Typical dose |
|---|---|---|
| Phosphatidylserine | • Anxiety and depression<br>• Chronically high or low cortisol<br>• Chronic high stress | • 200–800 mg/day in divided doses on an empty stomach—combines well with essential fatty acids |
| N-Acetyl-cysteine | • Obsessive-compulsive disorder<br>• Gambling issues<br>• Trichotillomania<br>• Possibly bipolar disorder<br>• Adjunct to respiridone, for irritability symptoms | • 500–600 mg two or three times a day |
| Taurine | • Anxiety with low energy and cardiovascular concerns | • 500 mg taurine up to three times daily |
| SAMe | • Mild to moderate depression, especially with low energy and little motivation | • 200 mg twice daily to start; 400 mg twice daily on day 3; 400 mg three times daily on day 10; 400mg four times daily on day 14 |

| Possible side effects | Toxicity/ contraindication / interactions | Food sources |
|---|---|---|
| • None known | • May benefit high liver enzymes | Organ meats (liver and kidney), mackerel, herring, tuna, soft-shelled clams, white beans |
| • Occasional headache or stomach discomfort | • None | Cysteine precursor found in high-protein foods (meats, tofu, eggs, dairy products) |
| • Headaches <br> • Nausea <br> • Nosebleeding <br> • Temporary balance disturbance | • Possible blood pressure-lowering effect: monitor with blood pressure medications | Meats, eggs |
| • Anxiety <br> • Mild nausea <br> • Mild diarrhea | • Contraindicated in bipolar disorder | None |

## Table IV.7 Top Botanical Medicines for Anxiety and Depression

| Supplement | Best use | Typical dose |
|---|---|---|
| Psyllium (*Plantago ovata*) | • High CRP | • One teaspoon twice a day |
| Cinnamon (*Cinnamomum cassia*) | • Blood sugar imbalance with mood issues | • One teaspoon a day |
| Curcumin (from *Curcuma longa*) | • Inflammation<br>• Gut inflammation and leaky gut issues<br>• Depression<br>• Possible anxiety benefit<br>• Studied for its benefits as adjunct with fluoxetine and imipramine | • 1,000 mg/day of the BCM-95 form of curcumin away from meals<br>• Turmeric spice has small, non-therapeutic amounts |
| Robert's formula | • Leaky gut<br>• Inflammation | • 2 capsules three times a day between meals |
| Passionflower (*Passiflora incarnata*) | • Anxiety<br>• Generalized anxiety disorder<br>• Anticipated stressors<br>• "Spinning thoughts" | • 1 dropperful of tincture (about 30 drops) three times a day<br>• Can be taken 90 minutes before anticipated stressors |
| Kava (*Piper methysticum*) | • Anxiety, especially with muscle tension<br>• Women with interstitial cystitis<br>• To help wean off benzodiazepine medications | • 30 drops tincture two or three times a day in water or as a tea<br><br>• 400 mg/day of extract<br>*For weaning:*<br>• 50 mg/day to start<br>• Move up to 300 mg/day while tapering the benzodiazepine over 2 weeks<br>• Subsequent 300 mg/day for 3 weeks |

| Possible side effects | Toxicity/contraindication /interactions |
|---|---|
| • Can cause transient bloating as flora adjust to higher fiber levels | • Diarrhea at high doses<br>• Contraindicated in gastroparesis or other conditions involved poor digestive tract movement |
| • None known | • Excessive quantities can increase coumarin intake and cause liver damage |
| • Nausea and gastritis are rare | • None known |
| • None known | • None known |
| • Unlikely, but possible minor dizziness, drowsiness, and confusion | • Do not combine with alcohol<br>• If using sedatives, work with a health care practitioner<br>• Avoid with MAOI antidepressant drugs |
| • Paradoxical increase in anxiety symptoms in small percentage of users | • May be best avoided with liver disease |

*(continued)*

## Table IV.7 Continued

| Supplement | Best use | Typical dose |
|---|---|---|
| Lavender (*Lavendula angustfolium*) | • Anxiety, especially with "nervous stomach" <br> • Studied for benefit when used with SSRIs and tricy-clics for depression | • One 80 mg capsule of immediate-release oil <br> • One or two teaspoons per cup of tea <br> • 30 drops of tincture three times a day <br> • Essential oil on the pillow at night or in a warm bath |
| Ashwagandha (*Withania somnifera*) | • Chronic anxiety <br> • Alopecia <br> • Low sperm count | • 300 mg once or twice a day, standardized for ≥1–5% witha-nolide |
| Rhodiola (*Rhodiola rosea*) | • Anxiety, generalized anxiety, depression <br> • Helpful for feelings of burn-out and self-esteem chal-lenges | • 340–680 mg/day, standardized for 1% rosavin |
| St. John's wort (*Hypericum per-foratum*) | • Depression and depression with anxiety <br> • Postmenopausal depression <br> • May help lower blood sugar levels in diabetics <br> • Improves effectiveness of clopidogrel (Plavix) | • 900 to 1,800 mg/day of an extract standardized to contain 0.3% hypericin |
| Saffron (*Crocus sativus*) | • Depression, especially if asso-ciated with digestive tract issues | • 5 mg of petal or stigma (saf-fron) twice a day |
| Macuna (*Macuna pruriens*) | • Depression, especially in patients who do well with dopamine-boosting drugs (e.g., Bupropion, Aripipra-zole | • 200 mg extract once per day, increasing to twice a day after 2 weeks |

| Possible side effects | Toxicity/contraindication /interactions |
|---|---|
| • May cause mild "lavender burp" after ingestion | • None |
| • Vomiting and gastric distress in minority of users | • Watch for excessive hair growth and check DHEA levels if supplementing in women |
| • Possible dry mouth and dizziness | • None known |
| • Photosensitivity | • Can enhance or reduce effectiveness of many drugs metabolized by the P450 system: check with pharmacist when patient is on other medications |
| • Rare reports of mild gastric discomfort | • Caution with kidney or liver issues are present |
| • Bloating and nausea<br>• High doses can cause vomiting, palpitations, difficulty in falling asleep, delusions, or confusion | • Avoid with anticoagulant medications<br>• Contraindicated in PCOS<br>• Use with knowledgeable practitioner if patient is on antidepressant medications |

# Homeopathics Commonly Used
# for Depression and Anxiety

---

Homeopathy is useful in anxiety and depression, as described in the two tables below. Dosages vary with the type of homeopathic used. They have no known typical side effects, but check for aggravation of symptoms after first dosage.

Table V.1. Homeopathics Commonly Used for Depression

| Homeopathic remedy | Mental/emotional symptoms | Physical and special symptoms |
|---|---|---|
| Arsenicum album | • Insecure and anxious with low mood and depression<br>• Perfectionistic expectations (in both self and others) are not met<br>• Demanding<br>• Type A' person: impatient, interrupts others, walks and talk sat a fast pace<br>• Has a short fuse and can be curt or rude<br>• Enjoys company | • Very neat and clean<br>• Feels better in warm weather<br>• Shortness of breath |
| Aurum metallicum | • "Type A" person: impatient, interrupts others<br>• Walks and talks at a fast pace<br>• Short fuse<br>• Can be curt or rude<br>• Depressed when performing poorly, or when not living up to expectations and sense of ability<br>• Very serious and believes self is worthless<br>• Strong sense of despair about life<br>• Easily offended<br>• Sense of humiliation and anger that can lead to feelings of emptiness and worthlessness<br>• Extreme cases are suicidal | • Nightmares or insomnia<br>• Nighttime head pain and high blood pressure<br>• Sensitivity to noise and light<br>• Physical and emotional symptoms worse at night |

(continued)

**Table V.1. Continued**

| Homeopathic remedy | Mental/emotional symptoms | Physical and special symptoms |
|---|---|---|
| *Calcarea carbonica* | • If female, depression is worse before or during menstruation<br>• Dependable and industrious person—overwhelmed from too much worry, work, or physical illness<br>• Brought to tears rather easy<br>• Experiences anxiety, fatigue, confusion, discouragement, self-pity, and mood swings<br>• Dread of disaster is in consciousness<br>• Can be childlike and often enjoys being consoled and gaining sympathy, especially when given by a mother or in a mother-like manner<br>• Overall personality is mild and gentle<br>• Avoids conflict and argument<br>• Decision making is a slow and arduous process | • Perspires easily, especially while eating and working<br>• Feels chilly and sluggish and easily tired with exertion<br>• Desires the open air and the outdoors, which can make client feel better, while stuffy rooms will make symptoms worse<br>• Crave rich and fatty foods and eggs |
| *Causticum* | • Sense of loss and continually experiencing grief<br>• Frequently crying<br>• Mentally dullness and forgetful<br>• Severely discouraged<br>• Sees great injustice and feels sympathy toward those who are wronged<br>• Can be angry and irritable | • Burning symptoms: urinary tract infections, joints<br>• Pale white look to skin<br>• Worse with relationships |

| Remedy | | |
|---|---|---|
| *Cimicifuga* | • Energetic and talkative when feeling well, but upset and gloomy when depressed<br>• Under a dark cloud<br>• Exaggerated fears (of things like going insane, of being attacked or of disaster)<br>• May dream of impending doom | • Experience painful menstrual periods<br>• Headaches that involve the neck |
| *Ignatia amara* | • Sensitive person who has suffered grief, loss of loved ones, and/or disappointment and tries to keep the hurt inside<br>• Guarded, defensive, and moody in order to avoid showing hurt<br>• Laugh or cry inappropriately | • Feeling of a lump in the throat and having a heaviness in the chest<br>• Insomnia (or excessive sleeping), headaches, and cramping pains in the abdomen and back are common<br>• Frequently sighing or yawning |
| *Kali phosphoricum* | • More depressed after stressors: excess work, illness, emotional stress, or excitement<br>• Ability to concentrate is low, and as a result becomes discouraged and loses confidence | • Exhausted as well as nervous and jumpy<br>• Experiences headaches from mental effort, with easy perspiration<br>• Anemic<br>• Insomnia and indigestion are common complaints<br>• Sensitive to cold |
| *Natrum carbonicum* | • Depression is experienced after hurt, disappointment, or illness<br>• Mild, gentle, and selfless—makes an effort to be cheerful and helpful<br>• Avoids conflict<br>• Keeps feelings to self<br>• When feeling lonely, withdraws to rest or listen to sad music, which can increase isolation | • Emotionally and physically sensitive (sun, weather changes, and many foods, especially milk) |

*(continued)*

297

**Table V.1. Continued**

| Homeopathic remedy | Mental/emotional symptoms | Physical and special symptoms |
|---|---|---|
| *Natrum muriaticum* | • Experience feelings of betrayal from trusted persons<br>• If female, depressed prior to or during menstruation<br>• Private with strong inner feelings (grief, romantic attachment, anger, or fear of misfortune) that rarely show<br>• Generally quite reserved and responsible<br>• Angered by consolation from another<br>• Cry only when alone, with heavy sobbing<br>• Anxious along with depression<br>• Dwells on past grievance | • May get migraines, back pain, and insomnia when depressed<br>• Craves salt<br>• Tired with sun exposure<br>• Generally worse during hot weather<br>• Inadequate bonding with or nurture from mother and/or father or feel a lack of nurturing from them |
| *Phosphorum acidicum* | • Gets tired when depressed<br>• Depression drains emotional and physical energy<br>• Anhedonia<br>• Exercise increases fatigue and depression<br>• Feels emotionally numb or indifferent<br>• Feels empty inside<br>• Can't concentrate<br>• Doesn't feel as intelligent as usual<br>• Lost motivation at work and no longer interested in business matters<br>• Past disappointments like lost love are hard to get over | • Noticed hair turned gray or fallen out after an episode of severe depression or grief<br>• Oversensitive to light, sound, and odors<br>• Feels physically weak, especially in the morning<br>• Exposure to the cold outdoors and to drafts makes mood worse |

*Pulsatilla*
- Depression brings tears, with desire for consolation and hugs
- Childlike softness and sensitivity
- Sometimes whiny, jealous, and moody
- Crying, fresh air, and gentle exercise usually improves mood
- Anxiety can get worse with warmth or being in a stuffy room
- If female: experienced more depression around the time of hormonal changes (e.g., puberty, menstrual periods, menopause)
- Childlike behavior and clinging

*Sepia*
- Depression comes with great fatigue and feeling worn out from daily life
- Prefer to be left alone and not be consoled
- Feel better with vigorous exercise and with crying
- If female: menstrual problems are common
- Sense of organ prolapse (the falling or slipping down of an organ, e.g., the uterus)
- Digestion is very slow
- Indifferent to family members

*Staphysagria*
- Depressed and feel shame, resentment, and humiliation because of an insult or loss of pride
- Suppressed emotions can lead to depression
- Depression comes after a bout of anger
- Feel the need to keep dignity when feeling beaten down
- Can easily fly into fits of anger when pressured
- Easily offended
- Tremble with strong emotions
- Experience a lot of self-pity
- Quiet, sensitive, and emotional person who has difficulty standing up for oneself
- Circadian rhythms are off: feel sleepy all day but are unable to sleep at night
- Pains manifesting as toothaches, headaches, stomachaches, or bladder infections that are stress related
- Have strong sexual desires and are prone to masturbate

## Table V.2. Homeopathics Commonly Used for Anxiety

| Homeopathic remedy | Mental/emotional symptoms | Physical and special symptoms |
| --- | --- | --- |
| Aconite napellus | • Panic and anxiety attacks that come out of nowhere<br>• Sense of doom or impending death<br>• Sense of shock that affects a person at their core | • Symptoms come on suddenly<br>• Fever may come on suddenly |
| Argentum nitricum | • Generalized anxiety disorder<br>• Chronic anxiety<br>• Chronic worrier<br>• Fear of heights | • Sense of palpitations |
| Arsenicum album | • Anxiety about safety<br>• Concerned with being robbed<br>• Perfectionistic expectations (in both self and others) are not met<br>• Demanding<br>• "Type A" person: impatient, interrupts others, walks and talks at a fast pace<br>• Has a short fuse and can be curt or rude<br>• Enjoys company | • Feels better in warm weather<br>• Shortness of breath |
| Calcarea carbonica | • Fear of changes<br>• Feeling overwhelmed by physical illness<br>• Afraid of losing control<br>• Afraid of animals and insects | • Perspires easily, especially while eating and working<br>• Feels chilly and sluggish and easily tired with exertion<br>• Desires the open air and the outdoors, which can make client feel better, while stuffy rooms will make symptoms worse<br>• Crave rich and fatty foods and eggs |
| Gelsemium | • Agoraphobia | • Muscular weakness from performance anxiety<br>• Overall fatigued<br>• Muscular shakiness |

| Homeopathic remedy | Mental/emotional symptoms | Physical and special symptoms |
| --- | --- | --- |
| Ignatia amara | • Anxiety with mood swings leading to low mood<br>• Anxiety with menopause | • Feeling of a lump in the throat and have a heaviness in the chest<br>• Insomnia (or excessive sleeping), headaches, and cramping pains in the abdomen and back<br>• Frequently sighing or yawning |
| Kali arsenicosum | • Anxiety, especially about cardiovascular problems | • Often feels cold<br>• Symptoms worse at night<br>• Might sleep holding hand over the heart area |
| Lycopodium | • Low self-esteem and confidence<br>• Anxiety with being in front of an audience<br>• Little self-confidence and may talk too much to compensate | • Loves sweets<br>• Flatulence and stomach upset<br>• Bed-wetting as a child |
| Phosphorus | • Greatest fear is being alone with anxiety compounded by loneliness<br>• Loves company<br>• Highly social and likeable person<br>• Highly imaginative person | • Affected by odors and noise<br>• Prefers cold |
| Pulsatilla | • Childlike sweetness<br>• Clingy and teary anxiousness<br>• Loves to be consoled | • Often a women's remedy for premenstrual symptoms and painful menses<br>• Thick mucus discharge (nasal, vaginal) |
| Silica | • Oversensitivity brings on sense of dread<br>• New task or situation can bring anxiety easily | • Thin frame and osteoporosis<br>• Frailty<br>• Responsible and diligent people<br>• Low stamina and easily sickened from overwork |

# Example Diet and Lifestyle Diary

| Date | Time | Foods Eaten – Include fluids, vitamins and medications | Physical Symptoms (Rate 1 to 10) : 1= little 10= worst possible describe |
|------|------|------|------|
|      |      |      |      |

| Feelings: emotions, stress levels (Rate 1 to 10) : 1= little 10= worst possible describe | Bowel movement, Urination, Gas, Bloating | Major Activities |
|---|---|---|
| | | |

# Information about Dr. Peter Bongiorno

Inner Source Natural Health and Acupuncture in New York is the clinic of husband-and-wife team and co-medical directors Dr. Peter Bongiorno and Dr. Pina LoGiudice, where they practice as naturopathic doctors and licensed acupuncturists. With clinics in New York City and Long Island, Inner Source Health is compromised of the top naturopathic, acupuncture and integrative practitioners.

Please sign up for the free InnerSource newsletter, which contains the latest information regarding research, natural medicine, and health.

Website: www.InnerSourceHealth.com
Facebook: http://www.facebook.com/pages/InnerSource-Health /200391990434—or search for "InnerSource Health"
Twitter: search for "InnerSource Health" or @InnerSourceIt
Dr. Peter Bongiorno's personal twitter: @drbongiorno
Dr. Peter Bongiorno's personal webpage: http://www.drpeter bongiorno.com

Other Books by Dr. Bongiorno:

*Healing Depression: Integrated Naturopathic and Conventional Treatments* (CCNM Press, 2010; www.InnerSourceHealth. com/depression). This is Dr. Bongiorno's textbook, written to teach physicians how to work with patients suffering from depression using natural and integrative treatments. It is very detailed and a great source for someone in the medical profession or anyone who would like to read about this information at a higher level of scientific discussion.

*How Come They're Happy and I'm Not? The Complete Natural Program for Healing Depression for Good* (Red Wheel/Weiser/Conari Press, 2012) http://www.drpeterbongiorno.com/books/how-come-theyre-happy-and-im-not). Written for a lay audience, this book offers Dr. Bongiorno's approach to the treatment of depression, as well as a way to safely wean off medication without relapsing or side effects. Many of Dr. Bongiorno's mental health colleagues recommend this work to their clients in order to learn how to use holistic care in a safe and effective manner.

*How Come I'm Anxious, and They're Not? The Complete Natural Program for Healing Anxiety for Good* (Red Wheel/Weiser/Conari Press, *in press*) Written for a lay audience, this upcoming book offers Dr. Bongiorno's approach to the treatment of anxiety.

# References

AACE. (2002) Medical Guidelines for Clinical Practice for the Evaluation and Treatment of Hyperthyroidism and Hypothyroidism. *Endocrine Practice*; 8,6, Nov/Dec.

Abbasi, B., Kimiagar, M., Sadeghniiat, K., Shirazi, M. M., Hedayati, M., & Rashidkhani, B. (2012). The effect of magnesium supplementation on primary insomnia in elderly: A double-blind placebo-controlled clinical trial. *Journal of Research in Medical Sciences, 17*, 1161–1169.

Abdou, A. M., Higashiguchim S., Horie, K., Kim, M., Hatta, H., Yokogoshi, H. (2006). Relaxation and immunity enhancement effects of gamma-aminobutyric acid (GABA) administration in humans. *Biofactors, 26*, 201–8.

Adams, P. B., Lawson, S., & Sanigorski, A. (1996). Arachidonic acid to eicosapentaenoic acid ratio in blood correlates positively with clinical symptoms of depression. *Lipids, 31* (Suppl.), S157–S161.

Agazzi, A., De Ponti, F., De Giorgio, R., Candura, S. M., Anselmi, L., Cervio, E., . . . Tonini, M. (2003). Review of the implications of dietary tryptophan intake in patients with irritable bowel syndrome and psychiatric disorders. *Digestive & Liver Disease, 35*, 590–595.

Akçay, M. N., & Akçay, G. (2003). The presence of the antigliadin antibodies in autoimmune thyroid diseases. *Hepatogastroenterology, 50* (Suppl. 2), cclxxix–cclxxx.

Akhondzadeh, B., A., Moshiri, E., Noorbala, A. A., Jamshidi, A. H., Abbasi, S. H., & Akhondzadeh, S. (2007). Comparison of petal of *Crocus sativus* L. and fluoxetine in the treatment of depressed outpatients: A pilot double-blind randomized trial. *Progress in Neuro-Psychopharmacology & Biological Psychiatry, 31*, 439–442.

Akhondzadeh, S., Fallah-Pour, H., Afkham, K., Jamshidi, A. H., & Khalighi-Cigaroudi, F. (2004). Comparison of *Crocus sativus* L. and imipramine in the treatment of mild to moderate depression: A pilot double-blind randomized trial [ISRCTN 45683816]. *BMC Complementary & Alternative Medicine, 4*, 12.

Akhondzadeh, S., Kashani, L., Fotouhi, A., Jarvandi, S., Mobaseri, M., Moin, M., . . . Taghizadeh, M. (2003). Comparison of *Lavandula angustifolia* Mill. tincture and imipramine in the treatment of mild to moderate depression: A double-blind, randomized trial. *Progress in Neuropsychopharmacology & Biological Psychiatry, 27,* 123–127.

Akhondzadeh, S., Naghavi, H. R., Vazirian, M., Shayeganpour, A., Rashidi, H., & Khani, M. (2001). Passionflower in the treatment of generalized anxiety: A pilot double-blind randomized controlled trial with oxazepam. *Journal of Clinical Pharmacy & Therapy, 26,* 363–367.

Akhondzadeh, S., Tamacebi-Pour, N., Noorbala, A. A., Amini, H., Fallah Pour, H., Jamshidi, A. H., & Khani, M. (2005). *Crocus sativus* L. in the treatment of mild to moderate depression: A double-blind, randomized and placebo controlled trial. *Phytotherapy Research, 19,* 25–29.

Alhaj, H. A., Massey, A. E., & McAllister-Williams, R. H. (2006). Effects of DHEA administration on episodic memory, cortisol and mood in healthy young men: A double-blind, placebo-controlled study. *Psychopharmacology, 188,* 541–551.

Alkatib, A. A., Cosma, M., Elamin, M. B., Erickson, D., Swiglo, B. A., Erwin, P. J., & Montori, V. M. (2009). A systematic review and meta-analysis of randomized placebo-controlled trials of DHEA treatment effects on quality of life in women with adrenal insufficiency. *Journal of Endocrinology & Metabolism, 94,* 3676–3681.

Alldredge, B. K., Corelli, R. L., Ernst, M. E., Guglielmo, B. J., Jr., Jacobson, P. A., Kradjan, W. A., & Williams, B. R. (2012). Pediatric insomnia. In M. A. Koda-Kimble & B. K. Alldredge (Eds.), *Koda-Kimble & Young's applied therapeutics: The clinical use of drugs* (10th ed.), pp. 1900–1921. Baltimore, MD: Wolters Kluwer Health/Lippincott Williams & Wilkins.

Allen, J. J., Schnyer, R. N., Chambers, A. S., Hitt, S. K., Moreno, F. A., & Manber, R. (2006). Acupuncture for depression: A randomized controlled trial. *Journal of Clinical Psychiatry, 67,* 1665–1673.

Allen, J. M. (2002). The consequences on methyl mercury exposure on interactive function between astrocytes and neurons. *Neurotoxicology, 23,* 755–759.

Almeida, O. P., Flicker, L., Lautenschlager, N. T., Leedman, P., Vasikaran, S., & van Bockxmeer, F. M. (2005). Contribution of the MTHFR gene to the causal pathway for depression, anxiety and cognitive impairment in later life. *Neurobiology of Aging, 26,* 251–257.

Almeida, O. P., Lautenschlager, N. T., Vasikaran, S., Leedman, P., Gelavis, A., & Flicker L. A. (2006). Twenty-week randomized controlled trial of estradiol replacement therapy for women aged 70 years and older: Effect on mood, cognition and quality of life. *Neurobiology of Aging, 27*, 141–149.

Almeida, O. P., McCaul, K., Hankey, G. J., Norman, P., Jamrozik, K., & Flicker, L. (2008). Homocysteine and depression in later life. *Archives of General Psychiatry, 65*, 1286–1294.

Al-Omary, F. A. (2013). Melatonin: Comprehensive profile. *Profiles of Drug Substances, Excipients, & Related Methodology, 38*, 159–226.

American Psychiatric Association. (2013). *Diagnostic and statistical manual of mental disorders* (5th ed.). Arlington, VA: American Psychiatric Publishing.

Anders, H. J., Andersen, K., & Stecher, B. (2013). The intestinal microbiota, a leaky gut, and abnormal immunity in kidney disease. *Kidney International, 83*, 1010–1016.

Anderson, R. A. (1998). Chromium, glucose intolerance and diabetes. *Journal of the American College of Nutrition, 17*, 548–555.

Andreatini, R., & Leite, J. R. (1994). Effect of valepotriates on the behaviour of rats on the elevated plus maze during benzodiazepine withdrawal. *European Journal of Pharmacology, 260*, 233–235.

Andrews, G., Cuijpers, P., Craske, M. G., McEvoy, P., & Titov, N. (2010). Computer therapy for the anxiety and depressive disorders is effective, acceptable and practical health care: A meta-analysis. *PLoS One, 5*, e13196.

Anisman, H., & Merali Z. (2003). Cytokines, stress and depressive illness: Brain-immune interactions. *Annals of Medicine, 35*, 2–11.

American Psychiatric Association. (2010). *Practice guideline for the treatment of patients with major depressive disorder.* (3rd ed.). Arlington, VA: American Psychiatric Association.

Antony, B., Merina, B., Iyer, V. S., Judy, N., Lennertz, K., & Joyal S. (2008). A pilot cross-over study to evaluate human oral bioavailability of BCM-95CG (Biocurcumax), a novel bioenhanced preparation of curcumin. *Indian Journal of Pharmaceutical Sciences, 70*, 445–449.

Araghiniknam, M., Chung, S., Nelson-White, T., Eskelson, C., & Watson, R. R. (1996). Antioxidant activity of dioscorea and dehydroepiandrosterone (DHEA) in older humans. *Life Sciences, 59*, PL147–PL157.

Arias, A. J., Steinberg, K., Banga, A., & Trestman, R. L. (2006). Systematic review of the efficacy of meditation techniques as treatment for medical illness. *Journal of Alternative & Complementary Medicine, 12*, 817–832.

Armstrong, D. J., Meenagh, G. K., Bickle, I., Lee, A. S., Curran, E. S., Finch, M. B. (2007). Vitamin D deficiency is associated with anxiety and depression in fibromyalgia. *Clinical Rheumatology, 26*, 551–554.

Aschner, M., Syversen, T., Souza, D. O., Rocha, J. B., & Farina, M. (2007). Involvement of glutamate and reactive oxygen species in methyl mercury neurotoxicity. *Brazilian Journal of Medical & Biological Research, 40*, 285–289.

Attenburrow, M. J., Odontiadis, J., Murray, B. J., Cowen, P. J., & Franklin, M. (2002). Chromium treatment decreases the sensitivity of 5HT2A receptors. *Psychopharmacology, 159*, 432–436.

Auger, C. J., & Forbes-Lorman, R. M. (2008). Progestin receptor-mediated reduction of anxiety-like behavior in male rats. *PLoS One, 3*, e3606.

Augustsson, K., Michaud, D. S., Rimm, E. B., Leitzmann, M. F., Stampfer, M. J., Willett, W. C., & Giovannucci, E. (2003). A prospective study of intake of fish and marine fatty acids and prostate cancer. *Cancer Epidemiology, Biomarkers & Prevention, 12*, 64–67.

Autier, P., & Gandini, S. (2007). Vitamin D supplementation and total mortality: A meta-analysis of randomized controlled trials. *Archives of Internal Medicine, 167*, 1730–1737.

Babalonis, S., Lile, J. A., Martin, C. A., Kelly, T. H. (2011). Physiological doses of progesterone potentiate the effects of triazolam in healthy, premenopausal women. *Psychopharmacology (Berlin), 215*, 429–439.

Babyak, M. (2000). Exercise treatment for major depression: Maintenance of therapeutic benefit at 10 months. *Psychosomatic Medicine, 62*, 633–638.

Bachinskaya, N., Hoerr, R., & Ihl, R. (2011). Alleviating neuropsychiatric symptoms in dementia: The effects of *Ginkgo biloba* extract EGb 761. Findings from a randomized controlled trial. *Neuropsychiatric Disease & Treatment, 7*, 209–215.

Badawy, A. A., & Evans, M. (1976). The regulation of rat liver tryptophan pyrrolase activity by reduced nicotinamide-adenine dinucleotide (phosphate). Experiments with glucose and nicotinamide. *Biochemical Journal, 156*, 381–390.

Banderet, L. E., & Lieberman, H. R. (1989). Treatment with tyrosine, a neurotransmitter precursor, reduces environmental stress in humans. *Brain Research Bulletin, 22*, 759–762.

Banki, C. M., Vojnik, M., Papp, Z., Balla, K. Z., & Arató, M. (1985). Cerebrospinal fluid magnesium and calcium related to amine metabolites, diagnosis, and suicide attempts. *Biological Psychiatry, 20*, 163–171.

Barbadoro, P., Annino, I., Ponzio, E., Romanelli, R. M., D'Errico, M. M., Prospero, E., & Minelli, A. (2013). Fish oil supplementation reduces cortisol basal levels and perceived stress: A randomized, placebo-controlled trial in abstinent alcoholics. *Molecular Nutrition & Food Research, 57*, 1110–1114.

Barbagallo, M., & Resnick, L. M. (1994). The role of glucose in diabetic hypertension: Effects on intracellular cation metabolism. *American Journal of the Medical Sciences, 307* (Suppl. 1), S60–S65.

Barbara, G., Zecchi, L., Barbaro, R., Cremon, C., Bellacosa, L., Marcellini, M., . . . Stanghellini, V. (2012). Mucosal permeability and immune activation as potential therapeutic targets of probiotics in irritable bowel syndrome. *Journal of Clinical Gastroenterology, 46* (Suppl.), S52–S5.

Barendsen, K. (1996, November/December). Low-dog T. *Yoga Journal.* Retrieved from http://www.natural-connection.com/resource/yoga_journal/self_care .html.

Barnes, P. M., Bloom, B., & Nahin, R. L. (2008). Complementary and alternative medicine use among adults and children: United States, 2007. National Health Statistics Reports 12. Hyattsville, MD: National Center for Health Statistics.

Barowsky, J., & Schwartz, T. L. (2006). An evidence-based approach to augmentation and combination strategies for treatment-resistant depression. *Psychiatry (Edgmont), 3,* 42–61.

Barragán-Rodríguez, L., Rodríguez-Morán, M., & Guerrero-Romero, F. (2008). Efficacy and safety of oral magnesium supplementation in the treatment of depression in the elderly with type 2 diabetes: A randomized, equivalent trial. *Magnesium Research, 21,* 218–223.

Barry, R., & Lewis, D. (2006). Hydrotherapy. In J. E. Pizzorno & M. T. Murray (Eds.), *The textbook of natural medicine* (3rd ed.), pp. 401–416. New York: Elsevier/Churchill Livingstone.

Baskin, M., Cobin, R. H., Duick, D. S., Gharib, H., Guttler, R. B., Kaplan, M. M., American Association of Clinical Endocrinologists. (2002). American Association of Clinical Endocrinologists medical guidelines for clinical practice for the evaluation and treatment of hyperthyroidism and hypothyroidism. *Endocrine Practice, 8.* Retrieved from https://www.aace .com/files/hypo_hyper.pdf.

Baumel, S. (2000). *Dealing with depression naturally* (2nd ed.).Keats.Lincolnwood, Illinois, p. 50

Becker, M., Alzahabi, R., & Hopwood, C. (2013). Media multitasking is associated with symptoms of depression and social anxiety. *Cyberpsychology, Behavior & Social Networking, 16,*132–135.

Beck-Friis, J., von Rosen, D., Kjellman, B. F., Ljunggren, J. G., & Wetterberg, L. (1984). Melatonin in relation to body measures, sex, age, season and the use of drugs in patients with major affective disorders and healthy subjects. *Psychoneuroendocrinology, 9,* 261–277.

Beddoe, A., & Lee, K. (2008). Mind-body interventions during pregnancy. *Journal of Obstetric, Gynecolic and Neonatal Nursing*, Mar–Apr; 37(2), 165–175.

Beers M. H., & Berkow, R. (Eds.). (1999). *Merck manual* (17th ed.).West Point, PA.

Beghi E., Pupillo, E., Bonito, V., Buzzi, P., Caponnetto, C., Chiò, A., Corbo, M., Giannini, F., Inghilleri, M., Bella, V., Logroscino, G., Lorusso, L., Lunetta, C., Mazzini, L., Messina, P., Mora, G., Perini, M, Quadrelli, M., Silani, V., Simone, I., Tremolizzo, L.; Italian ALS Study Group (2013). Randomized double-blind placebo-controlled trial of acetyl-L-carnitine for ALS. *Amyotroph Lateral Scler Frontotemporal Degener*. 14(5–6), 397–405.

Belleville, G. (2010). Mortality hazard associated with anxiolytic and hypnotic drug use in the National Population Health Survey. *Canadian Journal of Psychiatry*, 55, 558–567.

Belongia, E. A., Hedberg, C. W., Gleich, G. J., White, K. E., Mayeno, A. N., Loegering, D. A, Dunnette, S. L., Pirie, P. L., MacDonald, K. L., Osterholm, M. T. (1990). An investigation of the cause of the eosinophilia-myalgia syndrome associated with tryptophan use. *New England Journal of Medicine*. 9, 323, 357–365.

Benammi, H., El Hiba, O., Romane, A., & Gamrani, H. (2014). A blunted anxiolytic like effect of curcumin against acute lead induced anxiety in rat: Involvement of serotonin. *Acta Histochemica*, doi: 10.1016/j.acthis.2014.03.002.

Benton, D. (2002). Selenium Intake, mood and other aspects of psychological functioning. *Nutritional Neuroscience*, 5, 363–374.

Benton, D., & Brock, H. (2010). Mood and the macro-nutrient composition of breakfast and the mid-day meal. *Appetite*, 55, 436–440.

Benton, D., Williams, C., & Brown, A. (2007). Impact of consuming a milk drink containing a probiotic on mood and cognition. *European Journal of Clinical Nutrition*, 61, 355–361.

Bercik, P., Verdu, E. F., Foster, J. A., Macri, J., Potter, M., Huang, X., . . . Collins, S. M. (2010). Chronic gastrointestinal inflammation induces anxiety-like behavior and alters central nervous system biochemistry in mice. *Gastroenterology*, 139, 2102–2112.

Berger, M., Lund, R., Bronisch, T., & von Zerssen, D. (1983). REM latency in neurotic and endogenous depression and the cholinergic REM induction test. *Psychiatry Research*, 10, 113–123.

Berk, M., Dean, O. M., Cotton, S. M., Gama, C. S., Kapczinski, F., Fernandes, B., . . . Malhi, G. S. (2012). Maintenance N-acetyl cysteine treatment for bipolar disorder: A double-blind randomized placebo controlled trial. *BMC Medicine, 10,* 91.

Berman, R. M., Cappiello, A., Anand, A., Oren, D. A., Heninger, G. R., Charney, D. S., & Krystal, J. H. (2000). Antidepressant effects of ketamine in depressed patients. *Biological Psychiatry, 47,* 351–354.

Bermond, P. (1982). Therapy of side effects of oral contraceptive agents with vitamin B6. *Acta Vitaminologica et Enzymologica, 4,* 45–54.

Bernard, S., Enayati, A., Redwood, L., Roger, H., Binstock, T., et al. (2001). Autism: a novel form of mercury poisoning.*Medical Hypotheses, 56,* 4,462-7.

Bhattacharya, S. K., Bhattacharya, A., Sairam, K., & Ghosal, S. (2000). Anxiolytic-antidepressant activity of *Withania somnifera* glycowithanolides: An experimental study. *Phytomedicine, 7,* 463–469.

Bhatti, S. K., O'Keefe, J. H., & Lavie, C. J. (2013). Coffee and tea: Perks for health and longevity? *Current Opinion in Clinical Nutrition & Metabolic Care, 16,* 688–697.

Bilbo, S. D., & Tsang, V. (2010). Enduring consequences of maternal obesity for brain inflammation and behavior of offspring. *FASEB Journal, 24,* 2104–2115.

Binder, G., Weber, S., Ehrismann, M., Zaiser, N., Meisner, C., Ranke, M. B., . . . South German Working Group for Pediatric Endocrinology. (2009). *Journal of Endocrinology & Metabolism, 94,* 1182–1190.

Bjelland, I., Tell, G. S., Vollset, S. E., Refsum, H., & Ueland, P. M. (2003). Folate, vitamin B12, homocysteine, and the MTHFR 677C→T polymorphism in anxiety and depression: The Hordaland Homocysteine Study. *Archives of General Psychiatry, 60,* 618–626.

Bjorntorp, P., & Rosmond, R. (2000), The metabolic syndrome—a neuroendocrine disorder? *British Journal of Nutrition, 83* (Suppl. 1), S49–S57.

Bland, J. (2002). Slowing the aging process through individualized nutrition. *Chiropractic Economics.*accessed online at: http://www.chiroeco.com/article/2002/Mar/Nutrition3.php

Block, G., Jensen, C. D., Dalvi, T. B., Norkus, E. P., Hudes, M., Crawford, P. B, Holland, N., Fung, E. B., Schumacher, L., Harmatz, P. (2008). Vitamin C treatment reduces elevated C-reactive protein. *Free Radical Biology & Medicine. 46,* 70–77.

Blumenthal, J. A., Babyak, M. A., Moore, K. A., Craighead, W. E., Herman, S., Khatri, P., . . . Krishnan, K. R. (1999). Effects of exercise training on older patients with major depression. *Archives of Internal Medicine, 159,* 2349–2356.

Bokemeyer, C., & Foubert, J. (2004). Anemia impact and management: Focus on patient needs and the use of erythropoietic agents. *Seminars in Oncology, 31*, 4–11.

Bongiorno, P. B. (2010). *Healing depression: Integrated naturopathic and conventional treatments.* Toronto: CCNM Press.

Boschert, S. (2011, June). Web-based CBT appears effective for depression. *Clinical Psychiatry News, 1*, 23.

Bottiglieri, T. (2002). S-Adenosyl-L-methionine (SAMe): From the bench to the bedside—molecular basis of a pleiotrophic molecule. *American Journal of Clinical Nutrition, 76*, 1151S–1157S.

Bowden, R. G., Wilson, R. L., Deike, E., & Gentile, M. (2009). Fish oil supplementation lowers C-reactive protein levels independent of triglyceride reduction in patients with end-stage renal disease. *Nutrition in Clinical Practice, 24*, 508–512.

Brasky T. M., Darke, A. K., Song, X., Tangen, C. M., Goodman, P. J., Thompson, I. M., Meyskens, F. L., Jr., Goodman, G. E., Minasian, L. M., Parnes, H. L., Klein, E. A., & Kristal, A. R. ( 2013). Plasma phospholipid fatty acids and prostate cancer risk in the SELECT trial. *Journal of the National Cancer Institute. 105*, 1132–1141

Bravo, J. A., Forsythe, P., Chew, M. V., Escaravage, E., Savignac, H. M., Dinan, T. G., . . . Cryan, J. F. (2011). Ingestion of *Lactobacillus* strain regulates emotional behavior and central GABA receptor expression in a mouse via the vagus nerve. *Proceedings of the National Academy of Sciences of the USA, 108*, 16050–16055.

Brichenko, V. S., Kupriyanova, I. E., & Skorokhodova, T. F. (1986). The use of herbal adaptogens together with tricyclic antidepressants in patients with psychogenic depressions. *Modern Problems of Pharmacology & Search for New Medicines, 2*, 58–60.

Brink, C. B., Viljoen, S. L., de Kock, S. E., Stein, D. J., Harvey, & B. H. (2004). Effects of myo-inositol versus fluoxetine and imipramine pretreatments on serotonin 5HT2A and muscarinic acetylcholine receptors in human neuroblastoma cells. *Metabolic Brain Disease, 19*, 51–70.

Brocardo, P. S., Budni, J., Lobato, K. R., Santos, A. R., & Rodrigues, A. L. (2009). Evidence for the involvement of the opioid system in the antidepressant-like effect of folic acid in the mouse forced swimming test. *Behavioral Brain Research, 200*, 122–127.

Brocke, B., Armbruster, D., Muller, J., Hensch, T., Jacob, C. P., Lesch, K. P., . . . & Strobel, A. (2006). Serotonin transporter gene variation impacts innate fear processing: Acoustic startle response and emotional startle. *Molecular Psychiatry, 11*, 1106–1112.

Broota, A., & Dhir, R. (1990). Efficacy of two relaxation techniques in depression. *Journal of Personality & Clinical Studies, 6*, 83–90.

Brown, M. A., Goldstein-Shirley, J., Robinson, J., Casey, S.. (2001). The effects of multi-modal intervention trial on light, exercise, and vitamins on women's mood. *Women & Health, 34*, 93–112.

Burton, J. (2009, April). Safety Trial of High Dose Oral Vitamin D3 With Calcium in Multiple Sclerosis. Annual Meeting of the American Academy of Neurology. Seattle, WA.

Butchko, H. H., Stargel, W. W., Comer, C. P., Mayhew, D. A., Benninger, C., Blackburn, G. L., . . . Trefz, F. K. (2002). Aspartame: Review of safety. *Regulatory Toxicology & Pharmacology, 35* (Suppl.), S1–S93.

Buydens-Branchey, L., Branchey, M., & Hibbeln, J. R. (2008). Associations between increases in plasma n-3 polyunsaturated fatty acids following supplementation and decreases in anger and anxiety in substance abusers. *Progress in Neuropsychopharmacology & Biological Psychiatry, 32*, 568–575.

Buysse, D. J., Frank, E., Lowe, K. K., Cherry, C. R., & Kupfer, D. J. (1997). Electroencephalographic sleep correlates of episode and vulnerability to recurrence in depression. *Biological Psychiatry, 41*, 406–418.

Bystritsky, A., Kerwin, L., & Feusner, J. D. (2008). A pilot study of *Rhodiola rosea* (Rhodax) for generalized anxiety disorder (GAD). *Journal of Alternative & Complementary Medicine, 14*, 175–180.

Callaghan, P. (2004). Exercise: A neglected intervention in mental health care? *Journal of Psychiatric & Mental Health Nursing, 11*, 476–483.

Camacho, A., & Dimsdale, J. E. (2000). Platelets and psychiatry: Lessons learned from old and new studies. *Psychosomatic Medicine, 62*, 326–336.

Campanella, J., Biagi, F., Bianchi, P. I., Zanellati, G., Marchese, A., & Corazza, G. R. (2008). Clinical response to gluten withdrawal is not an indicator of coeliac disease. *Scandinavia Journal of Gastroenterology, 43*, 1311–1314.

Cappiello, A., McDougle, C. J., Malison, R. T., Heninger, G. R., & Price, L. H. (1995). Yohimbine augmentation of fluvoxamine in refractory depression: A single-blind study. *Biological Psychiatry, 38*, 765–767.

Carey, B. (2013, November 18). Treating insomnia to may help cure depression. *New York Times*. Retrieved from http://www.nytimes.com/2013/11/19/health/treating-insomnia-to-heal-depression.html?hp.

Carnahan, R. M., & Perry, P. J. (2004). Depression in aging men: The role of testosterone. *Drugs & Aging, 21*, 361–376.

Carrasco, G. A., Barker, S. A., Zhang, Y., Damjanoska, K. J., Sullivan, N. R., Garcia, F., . . . Van De Kar, L. D. (2004). Estrogen treatment increases the levels of regulator of G protein signaling-Z1 in the hypothalamic paraventricular nucleus: possible role in desensitization of 5-hydroxytryptamine(1A) receptors. *Neuroscience, 127,* 261–267.

Casper, R. C., Redmond, D. Z., Katz, M. M., Schaffer, C.B., Davis, J.M., Koslow, S.H.. (1985). Somatic symptoms in primary affective disorder. *Archives of General Psychiatry, 42,* 1098–1104.

Caspi, A., Sugden, K., Moffitt, T. E., Taylor, A., Craig, I. W., Harrington, H., . . . Poulton, R. (2003). Influence of life stress on depression: Moderation by a polymorphism in the 5-HTT gene. *Science, 301,* 386–389.

Cayer, C., Ahmed, F., Filion, V., Saleem, A., Cuerrier, A., Allard, M., . . . Arnason, J. T. (2013). Characterization of the anxiolytic activity of Nunavik *Rhodiola rosea. Planta Medica, 79,* 1385–1391.

Razin A, Cedar H. 1994. DNA methylation and genomic imprinting. *Cell.* 20, 77(4), 473-6.

Centers for Disease Control and Prevention. (2010). Current depression among adults—United States, 2006 and 2008. *Morbidity & Mortality Weekly Report, 59,* 1229–1235.

Chandrasekhar, K., Kapoor, J., & Anishetty, S. (2012). A prospective, randomized double-blind, placebo-controlled study of safety and efficacy of a high-concentration full-spectrum extract of ashwagandha root in reducing stress and anxiety in adults. *Indian Journal of Psychological Medicine, 34,* 255–262.

Chiesa, A., & Serretti, A. (2009). Mindfulness-based stress reduction for stress management in healthy people: A review and meta-analysis. *Journal of Alternative & Complementary Medicine, 15,* 593–600.

Choi, L. J., & Huang, J. S. (2013). A pilot study of S-adenosylmethionine in treatment of functional abdominal pain in children. *Alternative Therapies in Health & Medicine, 19,* 61–64.

Christakis, D. A., & Zimmerman, F. J. (2007). Violent television viewing during preschool is associated with antisocial behavior during school age. *Pediatrics, 120,* 993–939.

Christensen, H., Aiken, A., Batterham, P. J., Walker, J., Mackinnon, A. J., Fenech, M., & Hickie, I. B. (2011). No clear potentiation of antidepressant medication effects by folic acid + vitamin B12 in a large community sample. *Journal of Affective Disorders, 130,* 37–45.

Church, D., De Asis, M., & Brooks, A. J. (2012). Brief group intervention using EFT (emotional freedom techniques) for depression in college students: A randomized controlled trial. *Depression Research & Treatment.* 2012, 257172

Cizza, G., Eskandari, F., Coyle, M., Krishnamurthy, P., Wright, E. C., Mistry, S., . . . POWER (Premenopausal, Osteoporosis Women, Alendronate, Depression) Study Group. (2009). Plasma CRP levels in premenopausal women with major depression: A 12-month controlled study. *Hormone & Metabolic Research, 41*, 641–648.

Cohen, A. J., & Bartlik, B. (1998). *Ginkgo biloba* for antidepressant-induced sexual dysfunction. *Journal of Sexual & Marital Therapy, 24*, 139–143.

Cohen, S., Doyle, W. J., Alper, C. M., Janicki-Deverts, D., & Turner, R. B. (2009). Sleep habits and susceptibility to the common cold. *Archives of Internal Medicine, 169*, 62–67.

Committee on the Review of Medicines (1980). Systematic review of the benzodiazepines. Guidelines for data sheets on diazepam, chlordiazepoxide, medazepam, clorazepate, lorazepam, oxazepam, temazepam, triazolam, nitrazepam, and flurazepam. Committee on the Review of Medicines. *British Medical Journal, 280*, 6218, 910–912.

Connor, K. M., & Davidson, J. R. (2002). A placebo-controlled study of kava kava in generalized anxiety disorder. *International Clinical Psychopharmacology, 17*, 185–188.

Cooley, K., Szczurko, O., Perri, D., Mills, E. J., Bernhardt, B., Zhou, Q., & Seely, D. (2009). Naturopathic care for anxiety: A randomized controlled trial ISRCTN78958974. *PLoS One, 4*, e6628.

Copeland, W. E., Shanahan, L., Worthman, C., Angold, A., & Costello, E. J. (2012a). Cumulative depression episodes predict later C-reactive protein levels: A prospective analysis. *Biological Psychiatry, 71*, 15–21.

Copeland, W. E., Shanahan, L., Worthman, C., Angold, A., & Costello, E. J. (2012b). Generalized anxiety and C-reactive protein levels: a prospective, longitudinal analysis. *Psychological Medicine, 42*, 2641–2650.

Coppen, A., & Bailey, J. (2000). Enhancement of the antidepressant action of fluoxetine by folic acid: A randomised, placebo controlled trial. *Journal of Affective Disorders, 60*, 121–130.

Coppen, A., & Bolander-Gouaille, C. (2005). Treatment of depression: time to consider folic acid and vitamin B12. *Journal of Psychopharmacology, 19*, 59–65.

Coppen, A., Chaudhry, S., & Swade, C. (1986). Folic acid enhances lithium prophylaxis. *Journal of Affective Disorders, 10*, 9–13.

Coppen, A., Shaw, D. M., Malleson, A., Eccleston, E., & Gundy, G. (1965). Tryptamine metabolism in depression. *British Journal of Psychiatry, 111*, 993–998.

Cotman, C. W., & Berchtold, N. C. (2002). Exercise: A behavioral intervention to enhance brain health and plasticity. *Trends in Neuroscience, 25,* 295–301.

Coventry, P. A., Bower, P., Keyworth, C., Kenning, C., Knopp, J., Garrett, C., . . . Dickens, C. (2013). The effect of complex interventions on depression and anxiety in chronic obstructive pulmonary disease: Systematic review and meta-analysis. *PLoS One, 8,* e60532.

Cox, D. J., Gonder-Frederick, L., Polonsky, W., Schlundt, D., Kovatchev, B., & Clarke, W. (2001). Blood glucose awareness training (BGAT-2): long-term benefits. *Diabetes Care, 24,* 637–642.

Crinnion, W. (2000). Environmental medicine, part 1: The human burden of environmental toxins and their common health effects. *Alternative Medicine Review, 5,* 52–63.

Crinnion, W. (2009). The benefits of pre and post challenge urine heavy metal testing: Part 1. *Alternative Medicine Review, 14,* 3.

Cromie, W. J. (2006). Meditation found to increase brain size—mental calisthenics bulk up some layers. Harvard News Office. Retrieved from http://www.news.harvard.edu/gazette/daily/2006/01/23-meditation.html.

Cruciani, R. A., Dvorkin, E., Homel, P., Malamud, S., Culliney, B., Lapin, J., Portenoy, R., Esteban-Cruciani, N. (2006). Safety, tolerability and symptom outcomes associated with l-carnitine supplementation in patients with cancer, fatigue, and carnitine deficiency: A phase I/II study. *Journal of Pain Symptom Management, 32,* 551–559.

Cui, S. S., Bowen, R. C., Gu, G. B., Hannesson, D. K., Yu, P. H., & Zhang, X. (2001). Prevention of cannabinoid withdrawal syndrome by lithium: involvement of oxytocinergic neuronal activation. *Journal of Neuroscience, 21,* 9867–9876.

Cuijpers, P., Sijbrandij, M., Koole, S. L., Andersson, G., Beekman, A. T., & Reynolds CF 3rd. (2013). The efficacy of psychotherapy and pharmacotherapy in treating depressive and anxiety disorders: A meta-analysis of direct comparisons. *World Psychiatry, 12,* 137–148.

Czekalla, J., Gastpar, M., Hubner, W. D., & Jager, D. (1997). The effect of *Hypericum* extract on cardiac conduction as seen in the electrocardiogram compared to that of imipramine. *Pharmacopsychiatry, 30* (Suppl. 2), 86–88.

Czyzewski, A. (2007). Glutamate elevated in brains of mood disorder patients. *Biological Psychiatry, 62,* 1310–1316.

Danner, M., Kasl, S. V., Abramson, J. L., & Vaccarino, V. (2003). Association between depression and elevated C-reactive protein. *Psychosomatic Medicine, 65,* 347–356.

Darbinyan, V., Aslanyan, G., Amroyan, E., Gabrielyan, E., Malmstroumlm, C.,

& Panossian, A. (2007). Clinical trial of *Rhodiola* and *Rosea*, L. extract SHR-5 in the treatment of mild to moderate depression. *Nordic Journal of Psychiatry, 61*, 343–348.

Das, U. N. (2007). Vagus nerve stimulation, depression, and inflammation. *Neuropsychopharmacology, 32*, 2053–2054.

Das, Y. T., Bagchi, M., Bagchi, D., & Preuss, H. G. (2004). Safety of 5-hydroxy-l-tryptophan. *Toxicology Letters, 150*, 111–122.

da Silva, T. M., Munhoz, R. P., Alvarez, C., Naliwaiko, K., Kiss, A., Andreatini, R., & Ferraz, A. C. (2008). Depression in Parkinson's disease: A double-blind, randomized, placebo-controlled pilot study of omega-3 fatty-acid supplementation. *Journal of Affective Disorders, 111*, 351–359.

Davidson, J. R., Abraham, K., Connor, K. M., McLeod, M. N. (2003). Effectiveness of chromium in atypical depression: A placebo-controlled trial. *Biological Psychiatry, 53*, 261–264.

Davidson, J. R., Crawford, C., Ives, J. A., & Jonas, W. B. (2011). Homeopathic treatments in psychiatry: A systematic review of randomized placebo-controlled studies. *Journal of Clinical Psychiatry, 72*, 795–805.

Davidson, J. R., Morrison, R. M., Shore, J., Davidson, R. T., & Bedayn, G. (1997). Homeopathic treatment of depression and anxiety. *Alternative Therapies in Health & Medicine, 3*, 46–49.

Davies, B. (2008) Successful treatment of depression with IV glutathione. *Naturopathic Doctor News and Reviews.4*, 6, 1, 6-7.

Davis, J. D., & Tremont, G. (2007). Neuropsychiatric aspects of hypothyroidism and treatment reversibility. *Minerva Endocrinologica, 32*, 953–959.

Davis, S. R. (2002). When to suspect androgen deficiency other than at menopause. *Fertility & Sterility, 77* (Suppl. 4), 68–71.

Davison, K. M., & Kaplan, B. J. (2012). Nutrient intakes are correlated with overall psychiatric functioning in adults with mood disorders. *Canadian Journal of Psychiatry. 57*, 85–92.

De Assis, S., Cruz, M. I., Warri, A., & Hilakivi-Clarke, L. (2010). Exposure of rat dams to a high-fat or estradiol-supplemented diet during pregnancy alters mammary gland morphology and increases mammary cancer risk in their daughters and granddaughters. Abstract 2931 in: *Proceedings of the 101st Annual Meeting of the American Association for Cancer Research;* Apr 17–21; Washington, DC. Philadelphia: American Association for Cancer Research.

De Berardis, D., Marini, S., Serroni, N., Rapini, G., Iasevoli, F., Valchera, A., . . . Di Giannantonio M. (2013). S-Adenosyl-L-methionine augmentation in patients with stage II treatment-resistant major depressive disorder: An open label, fixed dose, single-blind study. *Scientific World Journal*, 2013, 204649.

De Kloet, E. R. (2004). Hormones and the stressed brain. *Annals of the New York Academy of Sciences, 1018*, 1–15.

de la Mora, M. P., Gallegos-Cari, A., Arizmendi-García, Y., Marcellino, D., & Fuxe, K. (2010). Role of dopamine receptor mechanisms in the amygdaloid modulation of fear and anxiety: Structural and functional analysis. *Progress in Neurobiology, 90*, 198–216.

Delarue, J., Matzinger, O., Binnert, C., Schneiter, P., Chiolero, R., & Tappy, L. (2003). Fish oil prevents the adrenal activation elicited by mental stress in healthy men. *Diabetes & Metabolism, 29*, 289–295.

Delle Chiaie, R., Pancheri, P., & Scapicchio, P. (2002). Efficacy and tolerability of oral and intramuscular S-adenosyl-L-methionine 1,4-butanedisulfonate (SAMe) in the treatment of major depression: Comparison with imipramine in 2 multicenter studies. *American Journal of Clinical Nutrition, 76*, 1172S–1176S.

Demetrio, F. N., Rennó J., Jr., Gianfaldoni, A., Gonçalves, M., Halbe, H. W., Filho, A. H., & Gorenstein, C. (2011). Effect of estrogen replacement therapy on symptoms of depression and anxiety in non-depressive menopausal women: A randomized double-blind, controlled study. *Archives of Women's Mental Health, 14*, 479–486.

Dubois, O., Salamon, R., Germain, C., Poirier, M. F., Vaugeois, C., Banwarth, B., . . . Olié, J. P. (2010). Balneotherapy versus paroxetine in the treatment of generalized anxiety disorder. *Complementary Therapies in Medicine, 18*, 1–7.

Denou, E., Jackson, W., Jun, L. U., Blennerhassett, P. McCoy, K, Verdu, E. F., . . . Bercik, P. (2011). The intestinal microbiota determines mouse behavior and brain BDNF levels. *Gastroenterology, 140* (Suppl. 1), S57.

De Souza, M. C., Walker, A. F., Robinson, P. A., & Bolland, K. (2000). A synergistic effect of a daily supplement for 1 month of 200 mg magnesium plus 50 mg vitamin B6 for the relief of anxiety-related premenstrual symptoms: A randomized, double-blind, crossover study. *Journal of Women's Health & Gender-Based Medicine, 9*, 131–139.

Devinsky, O., Morrell, M. J., & Vogt, B. A. (1995). Contributions of anterior cingulate cortex to behaviour. *Brain, 118*, 279–306.

Dinan, T. G. (2009). Inflammatory markers in depression. *Current Opinion in Psychiatry, 22*, 32–36.

Dinan T. G., Stanton, C., & Cryan, J. F. (2013). Psychobiotics: a novel class of psychotropic. *Biol Psychiatry, 74*,10,720-6.

D'Mello, D. (2011, May). The Immediate Efficacy of Computer-Assisted CBT in Patients Hospitalized with Major Depressive Disorder. Poster abstract. Annual Meeting of the American Psychiatric Association. Honolulu, HA.

Donaldson, Z. R., Piel, D. A., Santos, T. L., Richardson-Jones, J., Leonardo, E. D., Beck, . . . Hen R. (2014). Developmental effects of serotonin 1a autoreceptors on anxiety and social behavior. *Neuropsychopharmacology.* 9,291-302

Dowdy, D. W., Dinglas, V., Mendez-Tellez, P. A., Bienvenu, O. J., Sevransky, J., Dennison, C. R., . . . , D. M. (2008). Intensive care unit hypoglycemia predicts depression during early recovery from acute lung injury. *Critical Care Medicine, 36*, 2726–2733.

Duntas, L. H., Mantzou, E., & Koutras, E. A. (2003). Effects of a six month treatment with selenomethionine in patients with autoimmune thyroiditis. *European Journal of Endocrinology, 148*, 389–393.

Durlach, J., Pagès, N., Bac, P., Bara, M., & Guiet-Bara, A. (2002). Biorhythms and possible central regulation of magnesium status, phototherapy, darkness therapy and chronopathological forms of magnesium depletion. *Magnesium Research, 15*, 49–66.

Dwyer, J. H., Rieger-Ndakorerwa, G. E., Semmer, N. K., et al. (1988). Low-level cigarette smoking and longitudinal change in serum cholesterol among adolescents. *Journal of the American Medical Association, 259*, 2857–2862.

Ebbing, M., Bleie, Ø., Ueland, P. M., Nordrehaug, J. E., Nilsen, D. W., Vollset, S. E., . . . Nygård, O. (2008). Mortality and cardiovascular events in patients treated with homocysteine-lowering B vitamins after coronary angiography: A randomized controlled trial. *Journal of the American Medical Association, 300*, 795–804.

Eby, G. A., & Eby, K. L. (2006). Rapid recovery from major depression using magnesium treatment. *Medical Hypotheses, 67*, 362–367.

Einat, H., Clenet, F., Shaldubina, A., Belmaker, R. H., & Bourin, M. (2001). The antidepressant activity of inositol in the forced swim test involves 5-HT(2) receptors. *Behavioral Brain Research, 118*, 77–83.

Einat, H., Karbovski, H., Korik, J., Tsalah, D., & Belmaker, R. H. (1999). Inositol reduces depressive-like behaviors in two different animal models of depression. *Psychopharmacology, 144*, 158–162.

Eisele, L., Dürig, J., Broecker-Preuss, M., Dührsen, U., Bokhof, B., Erbel, R., . . . Heinz Nixdorf Recall Study Investigative Group. (2013). Prevalence and incidence of anemia in the German Heinz Nixdorf Recall Study. *Annals of Hematology, 92*, 731–737.

el Daly, E. S. (1998). Protective effect of cysteine and vitamin E, *Crocus sativus* and *Nigella sativa* extracts on cisplatin-induced toxicity in rats. *Journal de pharmacie de Belgique, 53,* 87–93.

El Idrissi, A., Boukarrou, L., Heany, W., Malliaros, G., Sangdee, C., & Neuwirth, L. (2009). Effects of taurine on anxiety-like and locomotor behavior of mice. *Advances in Experimental Medicine & Biology, 643,* 207–215.

Ellison, R. C., Zhang, Y., Qureshi, M. M., Knox, S., Arnett, D. K., & Province, M. A. (2004). Lifestyle determinants of high-density lipoprotein cholesterol: The National Heart, Lung, and Blood Institute Family Heart Study. *American Heart Journal, 147,* 529–535.

Elvevoll, E. O., Barstad, H., Breimo, E. S., Brox, J., Eilertsen, K. E., Lund, T., . . . Osterud, B. (2006). Enhanced incorporation of n-3 fatty acids from fish compared with fish oils. *Lipids, 41,* 1109–1114.

Emmanuel, A. V., Mason, H. J., & Kamm, M. A. (2001). Relationship between psychological state and level of activity of extrinsic gut innervation in patients with a functional gut disorder. *49,* 209-213.

Entringer, S., Kumsta, R., Hellhammer, D. H., Wadhwa, P. D., & Wüst, S. (2009). Prenatal exposure to maternal psychosocial stress and HPA axis regulation in young adults. *Hormones & Behavior, 55,* 292–298.

Erickson, K. I., Voss, M. W., Prakash, R. S., Basak, C., Szabo, A., Chaddock, L., . . . Kramer, A. F. (2011). Exercise training increases size of hippocampus and improves memory. *Proceedings of the National Academy of Sciences of the USA, 108,* 3017–3022.

Ernst, E. (2002). The risk-benefit profile of commonly used herbal therapies: Ginkgo, St. John's wort, ginseng, echinacea, saw palmetto, and kava. *Annals of Internal Medicine, 136,* 42–53.

Ernst, W., & Adrian, R. (2001). Prospective studies of the safety of acupuncture: A systematic review. *American Journal of Medicine, 110,* 481–485.

Eskelinen, M. H., Ngandu, T., Tuomilehto, J., Soininen, H., & Kivipelto, M. (2009). Midlife coffee and tea drinking and the risk of late-life dementia: a population-based CAIDE study. *Journal of Alzheimers Disease, 16,* 85–91.

Eyles, D. W., Smith, S., Kinobe, R., Hewison, M., & McGrath, J. J. (2005). Distribution of the vitamin D receptor and 1 alpha-hydroxylase in human brain. *Journal of Chemical Neuroanatomy, 29,* 21–30.

Fasano, A. (2012). Leaky gut and autoimmune diseases. *Clin Rev Allergy Immunol, 42*(1), 71–78.

Fasano, A., & Catassi, C. (2001). Current approaches to diagnosis and treatment of celiac disease: An evolving spectrum. *Gastroenterology, 120,* 636–651.

Fava, M., Borus, J. S., Alpert, J. E., Nierenberg, A. A., Rosenbaum, J. F., & Bottiglieri, T. (1997). Folate, vitamin B12, and homocysteine in major depressive disorder. *American Journal of Psychiatry, 154*, 426–428.

Fava, M., Rush, A. J., Wisniewski, S. R., Nierenberg, A. A., Alpert, J. E., McGrath, P. J., Thase, M. E., Warden, D., Biggs, M., Luther, J. F., Niederehe, G., Ritz, L., Trivedi, M. H. (2006). A comparison of mirtazapine and nortriptyline following two consecutive failed medication treatments for depressed outpatients: A STAR*D report. *American Journal of Psychiatry, 163*, 1161–1172.

Fava, M., Shelton, R. C., Zajecka, J. M., et al. (2010, December 5–9). L-Methylfolate as adjunctive therapy for selective serotonin reuptake inhibitor-resistant major depressive disorder: Results of two randomized, double-blind, parallel-sequential trials. Poster presented at the 49th annual meeting of the American College of Neuropsychopharmacology, Miami Beach, FL.

Feldman, S. R., Liguori, A., Kucenic, M., Rapp S. R., Fleischer A. B., Jr., Lang W., & Kaur, M. (2004). Ultraviolet exposure is a reinforcing stimulus in frequent indoor tanners. *Journal of the American Academy of Dermatologists, 51*, 45–51.

Fernández-San-Martín, M. I., Masa-Font, R., Palacios-Soler, L., Sancho-Gómez, P., Calbó-Caldentey, C., & Flores-Mateo, G. (2010). Effectiveness of Valerian on insomnia: a meta-analysis of randomized placebo-controlled trials. *Sleep Medicine, 11*, 505–511.

Ferrell-Torry, A. T., & Glick, O. J. (1993). The use of therapeutic massage as a nursing intervention to modify anxiety and the perception of cancer pain. *Cancer Nursing, 16*, 93–101.

Ferrari, A. J., Charlson, F. J., Norman, R. E., Patten, S. B., Freedman, G., Murray, C. J., . . . Whiteford, H. A. (2013). Burden of depressive disorders by country, sex, age, and year: Findings from the global burden of disease study 2010. *PLoS Medicine, 10*, e1001547.

Field, T., Diego, M., & Hernandez-Reif, M. (2006). Prenatal depression effects on the fetus and newborn: A review. *Infant Behavior & Development, 29*, 445–455.

Field, T., Grizzle, N., Scafidi, F., & Schanberg, S. (1996). Massage and relaxation therapies' effects on depressed adolescent mothers. *Adolescence, 31*, 903–911.

Field, T., Hernandez-Reif, M., Diego, M. Schanberg, S., Kuhn, C. (2005). Cortisol decrease and serotonin and dopamine increase following massage therapy. *International Journal of Neuroscience, 115*, 1397–1413.

Fischer, E., Heller, B., Nachon, M., & Spatz, H. (1975). Therapy of depression by phenylalanine. Preliminary note. *Arzneimittelforschung, 25*, 132.

Fisher, A. A., Purcell, P., & Le Couteur, D. G. (2000). Toxicity of *Passiflora incarnata*, L. *Journal of Clinical Toxicology, 38,* 63–66.

Fitzpatrick, L. A., Pace, C., & Wiita, B. (2000). Comparison of regimens containing oral micronized progesterone or medroxyprogesterone acetate on quality of life in postmenopausal women: A cross-sectional survey. *Journal of Women's Health & Gender-Based Medicine, 9,* 381–387.

Flora, S. J. S., Mehta, A., & Gupta, R. (2008). Prevention of arsenic induced hepatic apoptosis by concomitant administration of garlic extracts in mice. *Chemico-Biological Interactions. 177,* 227–233

Flora, S. J. S., Mittal, M., & Mehta, A. (2008). Heavy metal induced osidative stress and its possible reversal by chelation therapy. *Indian Journal of Medical Research, 128,* 501–523.

Ford, D. E., & Kamerow, D. B. (1989). Epidemiologic study of sleep disturbances and psychiatric disorders: An opportunity for prevention? *Journal of the American Medical Association, 262,* 1479–1484.

Fortmann, S. P., Burda, B. U., Senger, C. A., Lin, J. S., & Whitlock, E. P. (2013). Vitamin and mineral supplements in the primary prevention of cardiovascular disease and cancer: An updated systematic evidence review for the U.S. Preventive Services Task Force. *Annals of Internal Medicine. 159,* 824–834.

Foster, J. A., & McVey Neufeld, K. A. (2013). Gut-brain axis: How the microbiome influences anxiety and depression. *Trends in Neuroscience, 36,* 305–312.

Fournier, J. C., DeRubeis, R. J., Hollon, S. D., Dimidjian, S., Amsterdam, J. D., Shelton, R. C., & Fawcett, J. (2010). Antidepressant drug effects and depression severity: A patient-level meta-analysis. *Journal of the American Medical Association, 303,* 47–53.

Francis, A. J., & Dempster, R. J. (2002). Effect of valerian, *Valeriana edulis*, on sleep difficulties in children with intellectual deficits: Randomised trial. *Phytomedicine, 9,* 273–279.

Frangou, S., Lewis, M., & McCrone, P. (2006). Efficacy of ethyl-eicosapentaenoic acid in bipolar depression: Randomised double-blind placebo-controlled study. *British Journal of Psychiatry, 188,* 46–50.

Fraser, I. S., & Lobo, R. (Eds.). (1999). Update on progestogen therapy. *Journal of Reproductive Medicine, 44,* 139–232.

Fraser, L. A., Leslie, W. D., Targownik, L. E., Papaioannou, A., Adachi, J. D., & CaMos Research Group. (2013). The effect of proton pump inhibitors on fracture risk: Report from the Canadian Multicenter Osteoporosis Study. *Osteoporos International, 24,* 1161–1168.

Freeman, M. P. (2000). Omega-3 fatty acids in psychiatry: A review. *Annals of Clinical Psychiatry, 12*, 159–165.

Fu, A. L., Wu, S. P., Dong, Z. H., Sun, M. J. (2006). A novel therapeutic approach to depression via supplement with tyrosine hydroxylase. *Biochemical & Biophysical Research Communications, 351*, 140–145.

Fugh-Berman, A., & Cott, J. M. (1999). Dietary supplements and natural products as psychotherapeutic agents. *Psychosomatic Medicine, 61*, 712–728.

Furukawa, T., Watanabe, N., & Churchill, R. (2007). Combined psychotherapy plus antidepressants for panic disorder with or without agoraphobia. Retrieved from Cochrane Database of Systematic Reviews, CD004364.

Fux, M., Levine, J., Aviv, A., & Belmaker, R. H. (1996). Inositol treatment of obsessive-compulsive disorder. *American Journal of Psychiatry, 153*, 1219–1221.

Gaby, A. R. (2011). *Nutritional medicine.* Concord, NH: Fritz Perlberg Publishing.

Gaik, F. (2003). Merging East and West: A preliminary study applying spring forest qigong to depression as an alternative and complementary treatment (doctoral dissertation). *U.S. Dissertation Abstracts International: Section B: Sciences & Engineering, 63*, 6093.

Gallagher, P., Malik, N., Newham, J., Young, A. H., Ferrier, I. N., & Mackin, P. (2008). Antiglucocorticoid treatments for mood disorders. Retrieved from Cochrane Database of Systematic Reviews, CD005168.

Garcia, J. J., Reiter, R. J., Guerrero, J. M., Escamer, G., Yu, B. P., Oh, C. S., Muñoz-Hoyos, A. (1997). Melatonin prevents changes in microsomal membrane fluidity during induced lipid peroxidation. *FEBS Letters, 408*, 297–300.

Gareau, M. G., Jury, J., MacQueen, G., Sherman, P. M., & Perdue, M. H. (2007). Probiotic treatment of rat pups normalises corticosterone release and ameliorates colonic dysfunction induced by maternal separation. *Gut, 56*, 1522–1528.

Garland, C. F., Gorham, E. D., Mohr, S. B., Grant, W. B., Giovannucci, E. L., Lipkin, M., . . . Garland, F. C. (2007). Vitamin D and prevention of breast cancer: Pooled analysis. *Journal of Steroid Biochemistry & Molecular Biology, 103*, 708–711.

Gelenberg, A. J., & Gibson, C. J. (1984). Tyrosine for the treatment of depression *Nutrition & Health, 3*, 163–173.

Gelenberg, A. J., Wojcik, J. D., Falk, W. E., Baldessarini, R. J., Zeisel, S. H., Schoenfeld, D., & Mok, G. S. (1990). Tyrosine for depression: A double-blind trial. *Journal of Affective Disorders, 19*, 125–132.

Geller, S. E., & Studee, L. (2007). Botanical and dietary supplements for mood and anxiety in menopausal women. *Menopause, 14,* 541–549.

Gershon, M. (1999). *The second brain.* New York: Harper Collins.

Ghanizadeh, A., Derakhshan, N., & Berk, M. (2013). N-Acetylcysteine versus placebo for treating nail biting, a double blind randomized placebo controlled clinical trial. *Anti-inflammatory & Anti-allergy Agents in Medicinal Chemistry, 12,* 223–238.

Ghanizadeh, J., Hero, T., Franz, N., Contreras, C., & Schubert, M. (2012). Omega-3 fatty acids administered in phosphatidylserine improved certain aspects of high chronic stress in men. *Nutrition Research, 32,* 241–250.

Ghanizadeh, A., & Moghimi Sarani, E. (2013). A randomized double blind placebo controlled clinical trial of N-acetylcysteine added to risperidone for treating autistic disorders. *BMC Psychiatry, 13,* 196.

Gilhotra, N., & Dhingra, D. (2010). GABAergic and nitriergic modulation by curcumin for its antianxiety-like activity in mice. *Brain Research, 1352,* 167–175.

Gnanadesigan, N., Espinoza, R. T., Smith, R., Israel, M., & Reuben, D. B. (2005). Interaction of serotonergic antidepressants and opioid analgesics: Is serotonin syndrome going undetected? *Journal of the American Medical Directors Association, 6,* 265–269.

Goodyer, I. M., Herbert, J., Tamplin, A., & Altham, P. M. (2000). Recent life events, cortisol, dehydroepiandrosterone and the onset of major depression in high-risk adolescents. *British Journal of Psychiatry, 177,* 499–504.

Granger, A. S. (2001). *Ginkgo biloba* precipitating epileptic seizures. *Age & Ageing, 30,* 523–525.

Grant, J. E., Odlaug, B. L., & Kim, S. W. (2009). N-Acetylcysteine, a glutamate modulator, in the treatment of trichotillomania: A double-blind, placebo-controlled study. *Archives of General Psychiatry, 66,* 756–763.

Greeley, M. (2000). *Alcoholism as an allergy.* Bloomington, IN: Xlibris.

Green, T., Steingart, L., Frisch, A., Zarchi, O., Weizman, A., & Gothelf, D. (2012). The feasibility and safety of S-adenosyl-L-methionine (SAMe) for the treatment of neuropsychiatric symptoms in 22q11.2 deletion syndrome: A double-blind placebo-controlled trial. *Journal of Neural Transmission, 119,* 1417–1423.

Grimes, M. J. (2005). *Dr. John Bastyr: Philosophy and practice.* Seattle: Alethea Book Co.

Gulick, R., Lui, H., Anderson, R., Kollias. N., Hussey, S., & Crumpacker, C. (1992). Human hypericism. A photosensitivity reaction to hypericin (St John's wort ). *International Conference on AIDS, 8,* B90.

Gurguis, G. N., Vo, S. P., Griffith, J. M., & Rush, A. J. (1999). Platelet alpha2A-adrenoceptor function in major depression: GI coupling, effects of imipramine and relationship to treatment outcome. *Psychiatry Research, 89,* 73–95.

Guzmán, Y. F., Tronson, N. C., Jovasevic, V., Sato, K., Guedea, A. L., Mizukami, H., . . . Radulovic, J. (2013). Fear-enhancing effects of septal oxytocin receptors. *Nature Neuroscience, 16,* 1185–1187.

Hadjivassiliou, M., Sanders, D. S., Grünewald, R. A., Woodroofe, N., Boscolo, S., & Aeschlimann, D. (2010). Gluten sensitivity: From gut to brain. *Lancet Neurology, 9,* 318–330.

Hakanen, M., Luotola, K., Salmi, J., Laippala, P., Kaukinen, K., & Collin, P. (2001). Clinical and subclinical autoimmune thyroid disease in adult celiac disease. *Digestive Disease Science, 46,* 2631–2635.

Hall, S. D., Wang, Z., Huang, S. M., Hamman, M. A., Vasavada, N., Adigun, A. Q., . . . Gorski, J. C. (2003). The interaction between St John's wort and an oral contraceptive. *Clinical Pharmacology & Therapeutics, 74,* 525–535.

Hallert, C., Svensson, M., Tholstrup, J., & Hultberg, B. (2009). Clinical trial: B vitamins improve health in patients with coeliac disease living on a gluten-free diet. *Alimentary Pharmacology & Therapeutics, 29,* 811–816.

Hammerness, P., Ethan, B., Ulbricht, C., Barrette, E. P., Foppa, I., Basch, S., Bent, S., Boon, H., Ernst, E.; Natural Standard Research Collaboration. (2003). St. John's wort: A systematic review of adverse effects and drug interactions for the consultation psychiatrist. *Psychosomatics, 44,* 271–282.

Hanai, H., Iida, T., Takeuchi, K., Watanabe, F., Maruyama, Y., Andoh, A., Tsujikawa, T., Fujiyama, Y., Mitsuyama, K., Sata, M., Yamada, M., Iwaoka, Y., Kanke, K., Hiraishi, H., Hirayama, K., Arai, H., Yoshii, S., Uchijima, M., Nagata, T., Koide, Y. (2006). Curcumin maintenance therapy for ulcerative colitis: Randomized, multicenter, double-blind, placebo-controlled trial. *Clinical Gastroenterology & Hepatology, 4,* 1502–1506.

Hariri, A. R., Mattay, V. S., Tessitore, A., Kolachana, B., Fera, F., Goldman, D., . . . Weinberger, D. R. (2002). Serotonin transporter genetic variation and the response of the human amygdala. *Science, 297,* 400–403.

Harley, K. G., Gunier, R. B., Kogut, K., Johnson, C., Bradman, A., Calafat, A. M., & Eskenazi, B. (2013). Prenatal and early childhood bisphenol A concentrations and behavior in school-aged children. *Environmental Research, 126,* 43–50.

Harris, E., Kirk, J., Rowsell, R., Vitetta, L., Sali, A., Scholey, A. B., & Pipingas, A. (2011). The effect of multivitamin supplementation on mood and stress in healthy older men. *Human Psychopharmacology, 26,* 560–567.

Harris, W. S., Pottala, J. V., Sands, S. A., & Jones, P. G. (2007). Comparison of the effects of fish and fish-oil capsules on the n-3 fatty acid content of blood cells and plasma phospholipids. *American Journal of Clinical Nutrition*, 86, 1621—1625

Harvey, B. H., McEwen, B. S., & Stein, D. J. (2003). Neurobiology of antidepressant withdrawal: implications for the longitudinal outcome of depression. *Biological Psychiatry*, 54, 1105–1117.

Harvey, R., & Chompe, P. (2005). *Biochemistry* (3rd ed.). Baltimore: Lippincott.

Hata, Y., & Nakajima, K. (2000). Life-style and serum lipids and lipoproteins. *Journal of Atherosclerosis & Thrombosis*, 7, 177–197.

Hatcher, H., Planalp, R., Cho, J., Torti, F. M., & Torti, S. V. (2008). Curcumin: From ancient medicine to current clinical trials. *Cellular & Molecular Life Sciences*, 65, 1631–1652.

Hawkins, E. B., & Ehrlich, S. D. (2011). Gamma-linolenic acid (GLA). Retrieved from University of Maryland Medical Center website, http://www.umm.edu/altmed/articles/gamma-linolenic-000305.htm.

Heim, C., Young, L. J., Newport, D. J., Mletzko, T., Miller, A. H., & Nemeroff, C. B. (2009). Lower CSF oxytocin concentrations in women with a history of childhood abuse. *Molecular Psychiatry*, 14, 954–958.

Helgason, C. M., Wieseler F. J. L., Johnson, D. R., Frank, M. G., & Hendricks, S. E. (2000). The effects of St. John's wort (*Hypericum perforatum*) on NK cell activity in vitro. *Immunopharmacology*, 46, 247–251.

Hellhammer, J., & Schubert, M. (2013). Effects of a homeopathic combination remedy on the acute stress response, well-being, and sleep: A double-blind, randomized clinical trial. *Journal of Alternative & Complementary Medicine*, 19, 161–169.

Henry, J. A., Alexander, C. A., & Sener, E. K. (1995). Relative mortality from overdose of antidepressants. *British Medical Journal*, 310, 221–224.

Heresco-Levy, U., Javitt, D. C., Ermilov, M., Mordel, C., Silipo, G., & Lichtenstein, M. (1999). Efficacy of high-dose glycine in the treatment of enduring negative symptoms of schizophrenia. *Archives of General Psychiatry*, 56, 29–36.

Hernanz, A., & Polanco, I. (1991). Plasma precursor amino acids of central nervous system monoamines in children with coeliac disease. *Gut*, 32, 1478–1481.

Hibbeln, J. R. (1998). Fish consumption and major depression. *Lancet*, 351, 1213.

Hibbeln, J. R., & Salen, N. (1995). Dietary polyunsaturated fats and depression: When cholesterol does not satisfy. *American Journal of Clinical Nutrition*, 62, 1–9.

Hibbeln, J. R., Umhau, J. C., George, D. T., & Salem, N., Jr. (1997). Do plasma polyunsaturates predict hostility and depression? *World Review of Nutrition & Dietetics, 82,* 175–186.

Hintikka, J., Tolmunen, T., Tanskanen, A., & Viinamäki, H. (2003). High vitamin B12 level and good treatment outcome may be associated in major depressive disorder. *BMC Psychiatry, 3,* 17.

Hoch, T., Kreitz, S., Hess, A., & Pischetsrieder, M. (2013, April). Everyday desire: Influence of snack food on whole brain activity patterns. Presented at the Advances in the Generation and Integration of Food Sensation and Cognition 245th National Meeting and Exposition of the American Chemical Society. New Orleans, LA.

Hofman, S. (2013). Effect of oxytocin nasal sprays on social behavior in social anxiety disorder. Retrieved from http://clinicaltrials.gov/show/NCT6530.

Hofmann, S. G., Sawyer, A. T., Witt, A. A., & Oh, D. (2010). The effect of mindfulness-based therapy on anxiety and depression: A meta-analytic review. *Journal of Consulting & Clinical Psychology, 78,* 169–183.

Hollander, E., & McCarley, A. (1992). Yohimbine treatment of sexual side effects induced by serotonin reuptake blockers. *Journal of Clinical Psychiatry, 53,* 207–209.

Hollinrake, E., Abreu, A., Maifeld, M., Van Voorhis, B. J., & Dokras, A. (2007). Increased risk of depressive disorders in women with polycystic ovary syndrome. *Fertility & Sterility, 87,* 1369–1376.

Hollis, B. W., & Wagner, C. L. (2004). Assessment of dietary vitamin D requirements during pregnancy and lactation. *American Journal of Clinical Nutrition, 79,* 717–726.

Hollon, S., DeRubeis, R., Shelton, R., Amsterdam, J., Salomon, R., O'Reardon, J., Lovett, M., Young, P., Haman, K., Freeman, B., & Gallop, R. (2005). Cognitive therapy vs medications in the treatment of moderate to severe depression. *Archives of General Psychiatry, 62,* 417–422.

Holsboer, F. (2000). The corticosteroid receptor hypothesis of depression. *Neuropsychopharmacology, 23,* 477–501.

Hoogendijk, W. J. G , Lips, P., Dik, M. G., Deeg, D. J., Beekman, A. T., & Penninx, B. W. (2008). Depression is associated with decreased 25-hydroxyvitamin D and increased parathyroid hormone levels in older adults. *Archives of General Psychiatry, 65,* 508–512.

Horrobin, D. F. (1983). The role of essential fatty acids and prostaglandins in the premenstrual syndrome. *Journal of Reproductive Medicine, 28,* 465–468.

Horrobin, D. F. (1993). Fatty acid metabolism in health and disease: The role of delta-6-desaturase. *American Journal of Clinical Nutrition, 57,* 732S–736S.

Hossain S. J. 1, Aoshima, H., Koda, H., & Kiso, Y. (2004). Fragrances in oolong tea that enhance the response of GABAA receptors. *Bioscience, Biotechnology, & Biochemistry, 68*, 1842–1848.

Hosseinzadeh, H., Karimi, G., & Niapoor, M. (2004, May). Antidepressant effect of *Crocus sativus*, L. stigma extracts and their constituents, crocin and safranal, in mice. Presented at the 1st International Symposium on Saffron Biology and Biotechnology. Albacete, Spain.

Howren, M. B., Lamkin, D. M., & Suls, J. (2009). Associations of depression with C-reactive protein, IL-1, and IL-6: A meta-analysis. *Psychosomatic Medicine, 71*, 171–186.

HP-200 in Parkinson's Disease Study Group. (1995) An alternative medicine treatment for Parkinson's disease: results of a multicenter clinical trial. *Journal of Alternative and Complement ary Medicine, 1*, 249–55.

Hrnčič, D., Rašić-Marković, A., Mikić, J., Demchuk, G., Leković, J., Šušić, V., . . . Stanojlović, O. (2013). Anxiety-related behavior in adult rats after acute homocysteine thiolactone treatment. *Clinical Neurophysiology, 124*, e14–e15.

Hughes, J. W., Watkins, L., Blumenthal, J. A., Kuhn, C., & Sherwood, A. (2004). Depression and anxiety symptoms are related to increased 24-hour urinary norepinephrine excretion among healthy middle-aged women. *Journal of Psychosomatic Research, 57*, 353–358.

Hulsewe, K. W., van der Hulst, R. W., van Acker, B. A., von Meyenfeldt, M. F., & Soeters, P. B. (2004). Inflammation rather than nutritional depletion determines glutamine concentrations and intestinal permeability. *Clinical Nutrition, 23*, 1209–1216.

Hunt, P. W. (2012). Leaky gut, clotting, and vasculopathy in SIV. *Blood, 120*, 1350–1351.

Husain, G. M., Chatterjee, S. S., Singh, P. N., & Kumar, V. (2011). Beneficial effect of *Hypericum perforatum* on depression and anxiety in a type 2 diabetic rat model. *Acta Poloniae Pharmaceutica, 68*, 913–918.

Hyman, S., & Nestler, E. (1996). Initiation and adaptation: A paradigm for understanding psychotropic drug action. *American Journal of Psychiatry, 153*, 151–161.

Hyman, S., & Greenberger P. (2001, March 24). Depression in women and men: What's the difference? Smithsonian Resident Association Series National Institute of Mental Health and the Society for Women's Health Research. Meeting. THe NIH Record. May 15. http://nihrecord.nih.gov/newsletters/05_15_2001/story08.htm

Iggo, A., & Iggo, B. J. (1971). Impulse coding in primate cutaneous thermoreceptors in dynamic thermal conditions. *Journal of Physiology (Paris), 63,* 287–290.

Innes, K. E., Selfe, T. K., Brown, C., Rose, K., & Thompson-Heisterman, A. (2012). The effects of meditation on perceived stress and related indices of psychological status and sympathetic activation in persons with Alzheimer's disease and their caregivers: a pilot study. *Evid Based Complement Alternat Med, 92,* 7509.

Iowa State University Extension and Outreach. (2009). Food and nutrition melatonin. Retrieved from http://www.extension.iastate.edu/nutrition/sup plements/melatonin.php.

Izzo, A. A. (2004). Drug interactions with St. John's Wort (*Hypericum perforatum*): A review of the clinical evidence. *International Journal of Clinical Pharmacology & Therapeutics, 42,* 139–148.

Jacka, F. N., Overland, S., Stewart, R., Tell, G. S., Bjelland, I., & Mykletun, A. (2009). Association between magnesium intake and depression and anxiety in community-dwelling adults: The Hordaland Health Study. *Australia & New Zealand Journal of Psychiatry, 43,* 45–52.

Jacka, F. N., Pasco, J. A., Williams, L. J., Meyer, B. J., Digger, R., & Berk, M. (2013). Dietary intake of fish and PUFA, and clinical depressive and anxiety disorders in women. *British Journal of Nutrition, 109,* 2059–2066.

Jackson, J. R., Eaton, W. W., Cascella, N. G., Fasano, A., & Kelly, D. L. (2012). Neurologic and psychiatric manifestations of celiac disease and gluten sensitivity. *Psychiatric Quarterly, 83,* 91–102.

Jacobs, B. P., Bent, S., Tice, J. A., Blackwell, T., & Cummings, S. R. (2005). An internet-based randomized, placebo-controlled trial of kava and valerian for anxiety and insomnia. *Medicine (Baltimore), 84,* 197–207.

Jedema, P., Finlay, J. M., Sved, A. F., & Grace, A. A. (2001). Chronic cold exposure potentiates CRH-evoked increases in electrophysiologic activity of locus coeruleus neurons. *Biological Psychiatry, 49,* 351–359.

Jee, S. H., Miller, E. R., 3rd, Guallar, E., Singh, V. K., Appel, L. J., & Klag, M.J. (2002). The effect of magnesium supplementation on blood pressure: A meta-analysis of randomized clinical trials. *American Journal of Hypertension, 15,* 691–696.

Jelovsek, F. R. (2009). Progesterone—its uses and effects. Retrieved from http://www.wdxcyber.com/nmood11.htm.

Jezova, D., Makatsori, A., Smriga, M., Morinaga, Y., & Duncko, R. (2005). Subchronic treatment with amino acid mixture of L-lysine and L-arginine modifies neuroendocrine activation during psychosocial stress in subjects with high trait anxiety. *Nutritional Neuroscience, 8,* 155–160.

Joffe, R. (1992). Triiodothyronine potentiation of fluoxetine in depressed patients. *Canadian Journal of Psychiatry, 37,* 48–50.

Joffe, R. T., & Singer, W. (1990). A comparison of triiodothyronine and thyroxine in the potentiation of tricyclic antidepressants. *Psychiatry Research, 32,* 241–251.

Johnson, Kay M., Nelson, K. M., & Bradley, K. A. (2006). Television viewing practices and obesity among women veterans. *Journal of General & Internal Medicine, 21* (Suppl. 3), S76–S81.

Jones, N. A., & Field, T. (1999). Massage and music therapies attenuate frontal EEG asymmetry in depressed adolescents. *Adolescence, 34,* 529–534.

Jordea, R., Snevea, M., Figenschaua, Y., Svartberga, J., & Waterlooa, K. (2008). Effects of vitamin D supplementation on symptoms of depression in obese subjects: Randomized double blind trial. *Journal of Internal Medicine, 264,* 599–609.

Jorissen, B. L., Brouns, F., Van Boxtel, M. P., & Riedel, W. J. (2002). Safety of soy-derived phosphatidylserine in elderly people. *Nutritional Neuroscience, 5,* 337–343.

Kabat-Zinn, J. (2003). Mindfulness-based interventions in context: Past, present, and future. *Clinical Psychology: Science & Practice, 10,* 144–156.

Kabat-Zinn, J., Massion, A. O., Kristeller, J., Peterson, L. G., Fletcher, K. E., Pbert, L., . . . Santorelli, S. F. (1992). Effectiveness of a meditation-based stress reduction program in the treatment of anxiety disorders. *American Journal of Psychiatry, 149,* 936–943.

Kabra, N., & Nadkarni, A. (2013). Prevalence of depression and anxiety in irritable bowel syndrome: A clinic based study from India. *Indian Journal of Psychiatry, 55,* 77–80.

Kahn, R. S., Westenberg, H. G., Verhoeven, W. M., Gispen-de Wied, C. C., & Kamerbeek, W. D. (1987). Effect of a serotonin precursor and uptake inhibitor in anxiety disorders; a double-blind comparison of 5-hydroxytryptophan, clomipramine and placebo. *International Clinical Psychopharmacology, 2,* 33–45.

Kalani, A., Bahtiyar, G., & Sacerdote, A. (2012). Ashwagandha root in the treatment of non-classical adrenal hyperplasia. *BMJ Case Reports,* bcr201 2006989.

Kalueff, A. V., Lou, Y. R., Laaksi, I., & Tuohimaa, P. (2004). Increased anxiety in mice lacking vitamin D receptor gene. *Neuroreport, 15,* 1271–1274.

Karakuła, H., Opolska, A., Kowal, A., Domański, M., Płotka, A., & Perzyński, J. (2009). Does diet affect our mood? The significance of folic acid and homocysteine. *Polski Merkuriusz Lekarski, 26,* 136–141.

Karishma, K. K., & Herbert, J. (2002). Dehydroepiandrosterone (DHEA) stimulates neurogenesis in the hippocampus of the rat, promotes survival of newly formed neurons and prevents corticosterone-induced suppression. *European Journal of Neuroscience, 16,* 445–453.

Kapusta, N. D., Mossaheb, N., Etzersdorfer, E., Hlavin, G., Thau, K., Willeit, M., . . . Leithner-Dziubas, K. (1987). Lithium in drinking water and suicide mortality. *International Clinical Psychopharmacology, 2,* 33–45.

Kasper, S., Gastpar, M., Möller, H. J., Müller, W. E., Volz, H. P., Dienel, A., & Kieser, M. (2010a). Better tolerability of St. John's wort extract WS 5570 compared to treatment with SSRIs: a reanalysis of data from controlled clinical trials. *International Clinical Psychopharmacology, 25,* 204–213.

Kasper, S., Gastpar, M., Müller, W. E., Volz, H. P., Möller, H. J., Dienel, A., & Schläfke, S. (2010b). Silexan, an orally administered Lavandula oil preparation, is effective in the treatment of "subsyndromal" anxiety disorder: A randomized, double-blind, placebo controlled trial. *International Clinical Psychopharmacology, 25,* 277–287.

Katzenschlager, R., Evans, A., Manson, A., Patsalos, P. N., Ratnaraj, N., Watt, H., . . . Lees, A. J. (2004). *Mucuna pruriens* in Parkinson's disease: A double blind clinical and pharmacological study. *Journal of Neurology, Neurosurgery, & Psychiatry, 75,* 1672–1677.

Kelly, G. S. (2001). Rhodiola rosea: A Possible Plant Adaptogen. *Alternative Medicine Review, 6,* 293–302.

Kemel, M. M., & El-lethey, H. S. (2011). The potential health hazard of tartrazine and levels of hyperactivity, anxiety-like symptoms, depression and anti-social behaviour in rats. *Journal of American Science, 7,* 6. http://www.jofamericanscience.org/journals/am-sci/am0706/183_6181am0706_1211_1218.pdf

Kepler, C. K., Huang, R. C., Meredith, D., Kim, J. H., & Sharma, A. K. (2012). Omega-3 and fish oil supplements do not cause increased bleeding during spinal decompression surgery. *Journal of Spinal Disorders & Techniques, 25,* 129–132.

Kessler, D. (2009). *The end of overeating: Taking control of the insatiable American appetite.* Rodale. New York, NY

Kessler, R. C., Berglund, P., Demler, O., Jin, R., Merikangas, K. R., & Walters, E. E. (2005). Lifetime prevalence and age-of-onset distributions of DSM-IV disorders in the National Comorbidity Survey Replication. *Archives of General Psychiatry, 62,* 593–602.

Khaja, M., Thakur, C. S., Bharathan, T., Baccash, E., & Goldenberg, G. (2005). "Fiber 7" supplement as an alternative to laxatives in a nursing home. *Gerodontology, 22,* 106–108.

Khamba, B., Aucoin, M., Lytle, M., Vermani, M., Maldonado, A., Iorio, C., . . . Katzman, M. A. (2013). Efficacy of acupuncture treatment of sexual dysfunction secondary to antidepressants. *Journal of Alternative & Complementary Medicine, 19,* 862–869.

Kahn, R. S., Westenberg, H. G., Verhoeven, W. M., Gispen-de Wied, C. C., & Kamerbeek, W. D. (1987).Effect of a serotonin precursor and uptake inhibitor in anxiety disorders; a double-blind comparison of 5-hydroxytryptophan, clomipramine and placebo. *International Clinical Psychopharmacology, 2,* 33–45.

Khattab, K., Khattab, A. A., Ortak, J., Richardt, G., & Bonnemeier, H. (2007). Iyengar yoga increases cardiac parasympathetic nervous modulation among healthy yoga practitioners. *Evidence-Based Complementary & Alternative Medicine, 4,* 511–517.

Khumar, S., Kaur, P., & Kaur, S. (1993). Effectiveness of Shavasana on depression among university students. *Indian Journal of Clinical Psychology, 20,* 82–87.

Kienast, T., Hariri, A. R., Schlagenhauf, F., Wrase, J., Sterzer, P., Buchholz, H. G., . . . Heinz, A. (2008). Dopamine in amygdala gates limbic processing of aversive stimuli in humans. *Nature Neuroscience, 11,* 1381–1382.

Kim, J. S., Schmid-Burgk, W., Claus, D., & Kornhuber, H. H. (1982). Increased serum glutamate in depressed patients. *Archiv für Psychiatrie und Nervenkrankheiten, 232,* 299–304.

Kim, Y. S., Pyo, M. K., Park, K. M., Park, P. H., Hahn, B. S., Wu, S. J., Yun-Choi, H. S. (1998). Antiplatelet and antithrombotic effects of a combination of ticlopidine and *Ginkgo biloba* ext (EGb 761). *Thrombosis Research, 91,* 33–38.

King, D. E., Egan, B. M., Woolson, R. F., Mainous, A. G., 3rd, Al-Solaiman, Y., & Jesri, A. (2007). Effect of a high-fiber diet vs a fiber-supplemented diet on C-reactive protein. *Archives of Internal Medicine, 167,* 502–506. 17353499.

Kinnunen, O., Winblad, I., Koistinen, P., & Salokannel, J. (1993). Safety and efficacy of a bulk laxative containing senna versus lactulose in the treatment of chronic constipation in geriatric patients. *Pharmacology, 47* (Suppl. 1), 253–255.

Kirkwood, G., Rampes, H., Tuffrey, V, Richardson, J., & Pilkington, K. (2005). Yoga for anxiety, a systematic review of the research evidence. *British Journal of Sports Medicine, 39,* 884–891.

Kjaer, T. W., Bertelsen, C., Piccini, P., Brooks, D., Alving, J., Lou, H. C. (2002). Increased dopamine tone during meditation-induced change of consciousness. *Brain Research. Cognitive Brain Research, 13,* 255–259.

Klaassen, T., Klumperbeek, J., Deutz, N. E., van Praag, H. M., & Griez, E. (1998). Effects of tryptophan depletion on anxiety and on panic provoked by carbon dioxide challenge. *Psychiatry Research, 77,* 167–174.

Knippenberg, S., Damoiseaux, J., Bol, Y., Hupperts, R., Taylor, B. V., Ponsonby, A. L., . . . van der Mei, I. A. (2014). Higher levels of reported sun exposure, and not vitamin D status, are associated with less depressive symptoms and fatigue in multiple sclerosis. *Acta Neurologica Scandinavica. 129,* 123–131.

Ko, R. J. (1998). Adulterants in Asian patent medicines. *New England Journal of Medicine, 339,* 847.

Kobak, K. A., Taylor, L. V., Bystritsky, A., Kohlenberg, C. J., Greist, J. H., Tucker, P., Warner, G., Futterer, R., Vapnik, T. (2005). St John's wort versus placebo in obsessive-compulsive disorder: results from a double-blind study. *International Clinical Psychopharmacology, 20,* 299–304.

Koga, K1, & Iwasaki, Y. (2013, April). Psychological and physiological effect in humans of touching plant foliage - using the semantic differential method and cerebral activity as indicators. *J Physiol Anthropol, 15,* 32(1):7.

Korte, S. M. (2001). Corticosteroids in relation to fear, anxiety and psychopathology. *Neuroscience & Biobehavioral Reviews, 25,* 117–142.

Kosfeld, M., Heinrichs, M., Zak, P. J., Fischbacher, U., & Fehr, E. (2005). Oxytocin increases trust in humans. *Nature, 435,* 673–676.

Kotani, S., Sakaguchi, E., Warashina, S., Matsukawa, N., Ishikura, Y. Kiso, Y., . . . Yamashima, T. (2006). Dietary supplementation of arachidonic and docosahexaenoic acids improves cognitive dysfunction. *Neuroscience Research, 56,* 159–164.

Kroes, R., Schaefer, E. J., Squire, R. A., & Williams, G. M. (2003). A review of the safety of DHA45-oil. *Food & Chemical Toxicology, 41,* 1433–1446.

Kudolo, G. B. (2001). The effect of 3-month ingestion of *Ginkgo biloba* extract (EGb 761) on pancreatic beta-cell function in response to glucose loading in individuals with non-insulin-dependent diabetes mellitus. *Journal of Clinical Pharmacology, 41,* 600–611.

Kulkarni, S., Dhir, A., & Akula, K. K. (2009). Potentials of curcumin as an antidepressant. *Scientific World Journal, 9,* 1233–1241.

Kumar, A. M., Solano, M. P., Fernandez, J. B., & Kumar, M. (2005). Adrenocortical response to ovine corticotropin-releasing hormone in young men: Cortisol measurement in matched samples of saliva and plasma. *Hormone Research, 64,* 55–60.

Kutner, J. S., Smith, M. C., Corbin, L., Hemphill, L., Benton, K., Mellis, B. K., Beaty, B., Felton, S., Yamashita, T. E., Bryant, L. L., Fairclough, D. L. (2008). Massage therapy versus simple touch to improve pain and mood in patients with advanced cancer. *Annals of Internal Medicine, 149,* 369–380.

Lakhan, S. E., & Vieira, K. F. (2008). Nutritional therapies for mental disorders. *Nutrition Journal, 7,* 2.

Lamas, G. A., Goertz, C., Boineau, R., Mark, D. B., Rozema, T., Nahin, R. L., . . . TACT Investigators. (2013). Effect of disodium EDTA chelation regimen on cardiovascular events in patients with previous myocardial infarction: The TACT randomized trial. *Journal of the American Medical Association, 309,* 1241–1250.

Lambert, G. W., Reid, C., Kaye, D. M., Jennings, G. L., & Esler, M. D. (2002). Effect of sunlight and season on serotonin turnover in the brain. *Lancet, 360,* 1840–1842.

Lamina, S., & Okoye, G. C. (2012). Effect of interval exercise training programme on C-reactive protein in the non-pharmacological management of hypertension: A randomized controlled trial. *African Journal of Medicine & Medical Sciences, 41,* 379–386.

Lansdowne, A. T. G., & Provost, S. C. (1998). Vitamin D3 enhances mood in healthy subjects during winter. *Psychopharmacology (Berlin), 135,* 319–323.

Lau, W. C., Welch, T. D., Shields, T., Rubenfire, M., Tantry, U. S., & Gurbel, P. A. (2011). The effect of St John's Wort on the pharmacodynamic response of clopidogrel in hyporesponsive volunteers and patients: increased platelet inhibition by enhancement of CYP3A4 metabolic activity. *Jounal of Cardiovascular Pharmacology. 57,* 86–93.

Ledford. R. (2013) Cholesterol limits lose their lustre. *Nature 494,* 410–411. http://www.nature.com/news/cholesterol-limits-lose-their-lustre-1.12509

Lespérance, F., Frasure-Smith, N., St-André, E., Turecki, G., Lespérance, P., & Wisniewski, S. R. (2011). The efficacy of omega-3 supplementation for major depression: A randomized controlled trial. *Journal of Clinical Psychiatry, 72,* 1054–1062.

Leung, S., Croft, R. J., O'Neill, B. V., & Nathan, P. J. (2008). Acute high-dose glycine attenuates mismatch negativity (MMN) in healthy human controls. *Psychopharmacology (Berlin), 196,* 451–460.

Levin, R., De Simone, N., Slotkin, J., & Henson, B.. Incidence of thyroid cancer surrounding Three Mile Island nuclear facility: the 30-year follow-up. *Laryngoscope.* 2013 Aug;123(8):2064-71. doi: 10.1002/lary.23953. Epub 2013 Jan 31.

Levine, J., Barak, Y., Gonzalves, M., Szor, H., Elizur, A., Kofman, O., Belmaker, R. H. (1995). Double-blind, controlled trial of inositol treatment of depression. *American Journal of Psychiatry, 152,* 792–794.

Levine, J., Gonsalves, M., Babur, I., Stier, S., Elizur, A., Kofman, O., & Belmaker, R. H. (1993). Inositol 6gm daily may be effective in depression but not in schizophrenia. *Human Psychopharmacology*, 8, 49–53.

Levine, J., Kaplan, Z., Pettegrew, J. W., McClure, R. J., Gershon, S., Buriakovsky, I., & Cohen, H. (2005). Effect of intraperitoneal acetyl-L-carnitine (ALCAR) on anxiety-like behaviours in rats. *International Journal of Neuropsychopharmacology*, 8, 65–74.

Levitan, R. D., Shen, J. H., Jindal, R., Driver, H. S., Kennedy, S. H., & Shapiro, C. M. (2000). Preliminary randomized double-blind placebo-controlled trial of tryptophan combined with fluoxetine to treat major depressive disorder: antidepressant and hypnotic effects. *Journal of Psychiatry & Neuroscience*, 25, 337–346.

Lewis, J. E., Tiozzo, E., Melillo, A. B., Leonard, S., Chen, L., Mendez, A., . . . Konefal, J. (2013). The effect of methylated vitamin B complex on depressive and anxiety symptoms and quality of life in adults with depression. *ISRN Psychiatry*, 2013, 621453.

Li, Q., Morimoto, K., Nakadai, A., Inagaki, H., Katsumata, M., Shimizu, T., . . . Kawada, T. (2007). Forest bathing enhances human natural killer activity and expression of anti-cancer proteins. *International Journal of Immunopathology & Pharmacology*, 20, 3–8.

Lieberman, J. (2009, April). Assessing the symptomatic overlap between anxiety and depression: The rule rather than the exception. *Psychiatric Times* (Suppl.), 2–6.

Lin, P., Campbell, D., Chaney, E., Liu, C., Heagerty, P., Felker, B., & Hedrick, S. (2005). The influence of patient preference on depression treatment in primary care. *Annals of Behavioral Medicine*, 30, 164–173.

Linde, K., Berner, M. M., & Kriston, L. (2008). St John's wort for major depression. Retrieved from Cochrane Database of Systematic Reviews, CD000448.

Lissoni, P. (2007). Biochemotherapy with standard chemotherapies plus the pineal hormone melatonin in the treatment of advanced solid neoplasms. *Pathologie Biologie (Paris)*, 55, 201–204.

Liu, J. J., Galfalvy, H. C., Cooper, T. B., Oquendo, M. A., Grunebaum, M. F., Mann, J. J., & Sublette, M. E. (2013). Omega-3 polyunsaturated fatty acid (PUFA) status in major depressive disorder with comorbid anxiety disorders. *Journal of Clinical Psychiatry*, 74, 732–738.

Lohr, V. I., Pearson-Mims, C. H., & Goodwin, G. K. (1996). Interior plants may improve worker productivity and reduce stress in a windowless environment. *J. of Environmental Horticulture*, 14, 97–100.

Long, S. J., & Benton, D. (2013). Effects of vitamin and mineral supplementation on stress, mild psychiatric symptoms, and mood in nonclinical samples: A meta-analysis. *Psychosomatic Medicine, 75,* 144–153.

Lowry, F. (2011, May 12). More lithium in drinking water equals lower suicide rates. *Medscape News.* http://www.medscape.com/viewarticle/742589

L-Tyrosine. (2007). *Alternative Medicine Review, 12,* 364–368.

Lu, K., Gray, M. A., Oliver, C., Liley, D. T., Harrison, B. J., Bartholomeusz, C. F., Phan, K. L., Nathan, P. J. (2004). The acute effects of L-theanine in comparison with alprazolam on anticipatory anxiety in humans. *Human Psychopharmacology, 19,* 457–465.

Lucas, M., Mirzaei, F., Pan, A., Okereke, O. I., Willett, W. C., O'Reilly, É. J., . . . Ascherio, A. (2011). Coffee, caffeine, and risk of depression among women. *Archives of Internal Medicine, 171,* 1571–1578.

Luo, H. C., Ureil, H., Shen, Y. C., Meng, F. Q., Zhao, X. Y., Liang, W., . . . Deng, P. (2003). Comparative study of electroacupuncture and fluoxetine for treatment of depression. *Chinese Journal of Psychiatry, 36,* 215–219.

Lydiard, R. B. (2004). Anxiety disorders. In: R. D. Rakel & T. E. Bope (Eds.), *Conn's current therapy,* pp. 1151–1155. Philadelphia: Saunders.

Lyon, M. R., Kapoor, M. P., & Juneja, L. R. (2011). The effects of L-theanine (Suntheanine®) on objective sleep quality in boys with attention deficit hyperactivity disorder (ADHD): a randomized, double-blind, placebo-controlled clinical trial. *Alternative Medicine Review, 16,* 348–354.

Maas, J., Koslow, S., Katz. M., Bowden, C., Gibbons, R., Stokes, P., Robins, E., Davis, J. (1984). Pretreatment neurotransmitter metabolite levels and response to tricyclic antidepressant drugs. *American Journal of Psychiatry, 141,* 1158–1171.

Maayan, R., Touati-Werner, D., Shamir, D., Yadid, G., Friedman, A., Eisner, D., . . . Herman, I. (2008). The effect of DHEA complementary treatment on heroin addicts participating in a rehabilitation program: A preliminary study. *European Neuropsychopharmacology, 18,* 406–413.

Maes, M., D'Haese, P. C., Scharpe, S., D'Hondt, P., Cosyns, P., & De Broe, M. E. (1994a). Hypozincemia in depression. *Journal of Affective Disorders, 31,* 135–140.

Maes, M., Kubera, M., & Leunis, J. C. (2008). The gut-brain barrier in major depression: intestinal mucosal dysfunction with an increased translocation of LPS from gram negative enterobacteria (leaky gut) plays a role in the inflammatory pathophysiology of depression. *Neuroendocrinology Letters, 29,* 117–124.

Maes, M., Meltzer, H. Y., Cosyns, P., & Schotte, C. (1994b). Evidence for the existence of major depression with and without anxiety features. *Psychopathology, 27*, 1–13.

Maes, M., Smith, R., Christophe, A., Vandoolaeghe, E., Van Gastel, A., Neels, H., . . . Meltzer, H. Y. (1997a). Lower serum high-density lipoprotein cholesterol (HDL-C) in major depression and in depressed men with serious suicidal attempts: Relationship with immune-inflammatory markers. *Acta Psychiatrica Scandinavica, 95*, 212–221.

Maes, M., Vandoolaeghe, E., Neels, H., Demedts, P., Wauters, A., Meltzer, H. Y., . . . Desnyder, R. (1997b). Lower serum zinc in major depression is a sensitive marker of treatment resistance and of the immune/inflammatory response in that illness. *Biological Psychiatry, 42*, 349–358.

Maes, M., Verkerk, R., Vandoolaeghe, E., Van Hunsel, F., Neels, H., Wauters, A., . . . Scharpe, S. (1997c). Serotonin-immune interactions in major depression: Lower serum tryptophan as a marker of an immune-inflammatory response. *European Archives of Psychiatry & Clinical Neuroscience, 247*, 154–161.

Maes, M., Yirmyia, R., Noraberg, J., Brene, S., Hibbeln, J., Perini, G., . . . Maj M. (2009). The inflammatory and neurodegenerative (I&ND) hypothesis of depression: Leads for future research and new drug developments in depression. *Metabolic Brain Disease, 24*, 27–53.

Magalhães, P. V., Dean, O. M., Bush, A. I., Copolov, D. L., Malhi, G. S., Kohlmann, K., Jeavons, S., Schapkaitz, I., Anderson-Hunt, M., Berk, M. (2011). N-acetylcysteine for major depressive episodes in bipolar disorder. *Revista Brasileira de Psiquiatria, 33*, 374–378.

Magnesium. (2002). *Alternative Medicine Review Monographs.* 251–256.

Mahdi, A. A., Shukla, K. K., Ahmad, M. K., Rajender, S., Shankhwar, S. N., Singh, V., & Dalela, D. (2009). *Withania somnifera* improves semen quality in stress-related male fertility. *Evidence-Based Complementary & Alternative Medicine, 29.*

Mahoney, C. R., Castellani, J., Kramer, F. M., Young, A., & Lieberman, H. R. (2007). Tyrosine supplementation mitigates working memory decrements during cold exposure. *Physiology & Behavior, 92*, 575–582.

Mäki, M., & Collin, P. (1997). Coeliac disease. *Lancet, 349*, 1755–1759.

Malaguarnera, M., Bella, R., Vacante, M., Giordano, M., Malaguarnera, G., Gargante, M. P., . . . Pennisi, G. (2011). Acetyl-L-carnitine reduces depression and improves quality of life in patients with minimal hepatic encephalopathy. *Scandinavian Journal of Gastroenterology, 46*, 750–759.

Malsch, U., & Kieser, M. (2001). Efficacy of kava-kava in the treatment of nonpsychotic anxiety, following pretreatment with benzodiazepines. *Psychopharmacology (Berlin)*, *157*, 277–283.

Malvaez, M., Barrett, R. M., Wood, M. A., & Sanchis-Segura, C. (2009). Epigenetic mechanisms underlying extinction of memory and drug-seeking behavior. *Mammalian Genome*, *20*, 612–623.

Mandal, A. (2012). Anxiety and depression linked to computer games. Retrieved from http://www.news-medical.net/news/20120110/Anxiety-and-depression-linked-to-computer-games.aspx.

Mark, L. P., Prost, R. W., Ulmer, J. L., Smith, M. M., Daniels, D. L., Strottmann, J. M., Douglas Brown, W., Hacein-Bay, L. (2001). Pictorial review of glutamate excitotoxicity: Fundamental concepts for neuroimaging. *American Journal of Neuroradiology*, *22*, 1813–1824.

Mao, G. X., Cao, Y. B., Lan, X. G., He, Z. H., Chen, Z. M., Wang, Y. Z., . . . Yan, J. (2012). Therapeutic effect of forest bathing on human hypertension in the elderly. *Journal of Cardiology*, *60*, 495–502.

Marazziti, D., Baroni, G., Giannaccini, S., Catena Dell'Osso, M., Consoli, G., Picchetti, M., Carlini, M., Massimetti, G., Provenzano, S., Galassi A. (2007). Thermal balneotherapy induces changes of the platelet serotonin transporter in healthy subjects. *Progress in Neuro-Psychopharmacology & Biological Psychiatry*, *1*, 1436–1439.

Marcusson, J. A., Cederbrant, K., & Gunnarsson, L.-G. (2000). Serotonin production in lymphocytes and mercury intolerance. *Toxicology In Vitro*, *14*, 133–137.

Markopouloua, K., Papadopoulosa, A., Juruenaa, M. F., Poonb, L., Pariantec, C. M., & Cleare, A. J. (2009). The ratio of cortisol/DHEA in treatment resistant depression. *Psychoneuroendocrinology*, *34*, 19–26.

McCarty, M. F. (1982). Nutritional support of central catecholaminergic tone may aid smoking withdrawal. *Medical Hypotheses*, *8*, 95–102.

McLean, A., Rubinsztein, J. S., Robbins, T. W., & Sahakian, B. J. (2003). The effects of tyrosine depletion in normal healthy volunteers: Implications for unipolar depression. *Psychopharmacology (Berlin)*. *171*, 286–297.

Medicine.net. (2009). The definition of homeopathy. Retrieved from http://www.medterms.com/script/main/art.asp?articlekey=3775.

Meltzer, H., Bastani, B., Jayathilake, K., & Maes, M. (1997). Fluoxetine, but not tricyclic antidepressants, potentiates the 5-hydroxytryptophan-mediated increase in plasma cortisol and prolactin secretion in subjects with major depression or with obsessive compulsive disorder. *Neuropsychopharmacology*, *17*, 1–11.

Merlo, L. J., & Stone, A. M. (2007, March 6–9). Anxiety Linked with Cell

Phone Dependence Abuse Anxiety. Poster 55 presented at the Anxiety Disorders Association of America 28th annual meeting. Gainesville, FL.

Messaoudi, M., Lalonde, R., Violle, N., Javelot, H., Desor, D., Nejdi, A., . . . Cazaubiel, J. M. (2011). Assessment of psychotropic-like properties of a probiotic formulation (*Lactobacillus helveticus* R0052 and *Bifidobacterium longum* R0175) in rats and human subjects. *British Journal of Nutrition, 105,* 755–764.

Metso, S., Hyytiä-Ilmonen, H., Kaukinen, K., Huhtala, H., Jaatinen, P., Salmi, J., . . . Collin, P. (2012). Gluten-free diet and autoimmune thyroiditis in patients with celiac disease: A prospective controlled study. *Scandinavian Journal of Gastroenterology, 47,* 43–48.

Meyer, J. H., McNeely, H. E., Sagrati, S., Boovariwala, A., Martin, K., Verhoeff, N. P., Wilson, A. A., Houle, S. (2006). Elevated putamen D(2) receptor binding potential in major depression with motor retardation: an [11C] raclopride positron emission study. *American Journal of Psychiatry, 163,* 1594–1602.

Meynen, G., Unmehopa, U. A., Hofman, M. A., Swaab, D. F., & Hoogendijk, W. J. (2007). Hypothalamic oxytocin mRNA expression and melancholic depression. *Molecular Psychiatry, 12,* 118–119.

Michalsen, A., Grossman, P., Acil, A., Langhorst, J., Lüdtke, R., Esch, T., . . . Dobos, G. J. (2005). Rapid stress reduction and anxiolysis among distressed women as a consequence of a three-month intensive yoga program. *Medical Science Monitor, 11,* CR555–CR561.

Mild depression in general practice: Time for a rethink? (2003). *Drug & Therapeutics Bulletin, 41,* 60–64.

Millan, M. (2006). Multi-target strategies for the improved treatment of depressive states: conceptual foundations and neuronal substrates, drug discovery and therapeutic application. *Pharmacology and Therapeutics,* 110, 135–370.

Miller, A. (2008). The methylation, neurotransmitter, and antioxidant connections between folate and depression. *Alternative Medicine Review, 13,* 216–226.

Miller, H. E., Deakin, J. F., & Anderson, I. M. (2000). Effect of acute tryptophan depletion on $CO_2$-induced anxiety in patients with panic disorder and normal volunteers. *British Journal of Psychiatry, 176,* 182–188.

Miller, K. J., Conney, J. C., Rasgon, N. L., Fairbanks, L. A., Small, G. W. (2002). Mood symptoms and cognitive performance in women estrogen users and nonusers and men. *Journal of the American Geriatric Society, 50,* 1826–1830.

Milleron, O., Pilliere, R., Foucher, A., de Roquefeuil, F., Aegerter, P., Jondeau,

G., . . . Dubourg, O. (2004). Benefits of obstructive sleep apnoea treatment in coronary artery disease: a long-term follow-up study. *European Heart Journal, 25*, 709–711, 728–734.

Mills, K. C. (1997). Serotonin syndrome. *Medical Toxicology, 13*, 763–783.

Miodownik, C., Maayan, R., Ratner, Y., Lerner, V., Pintov, L., Mar, M., . . . Ritsner, M. S. (2011). Serum levels of brain-derived neurotrophic factor and cortisol to sulfate of dehydroepiandrosterone molar ratio associated with clinical response to L-theanine as augmentation of antipsychotic therapy in schizophrenia and schizoaffective disorder patients. *Clinical Neuropharmacology, 34*, 155–160.

Mischoulon, D., & Fava, M. (2002). Role of S-adenosyl-L-methionine in the treatment of depression: A review of the evidence. *American Journal of Clinical Nutrition, 76*, 1158S–1161S.

Mischoulon, D., & Rosenbaum, J. F. (Eds.). (2002). *Natural medications for psychiatric disorders*. Philadelphia, PA: Lippincott Williams and Wilkins.

Mishra, L. C., Singh, B. B., & Dagenais, S. (2000). Scientific basis for the therapeutic use of *Withania somnifera* (ashwagandha): A review. *Alternative Medicine Review, 5*, 334–346.

Misner, B. (2006). Food alone may not provide sufficient micronutrients for preventing deficiency. *Journal of the International Society of Sports Nutrition, 3*, 51–55.

Mitchell, B. (2003). *Plant medicine in practice: Using the techniques of Dr. John Bastyr*. St. Louis, MO: Churchill Livingstone.

Mitte, K., Noack, P., Steil, R., & Hautzinger, M. (2005). A meta-analytic review of the efficacy of drug treatment in generalized anxiety disorder. *Journal of Clinical Psychopharmacology, 25*, 141–150.

Miyasaka, L. S., Atallah, A. N., & Soares, B. G. (2007). Passiflora for anxiety disorder. Retrieved from Cochrane Database of Systematic Reviews, CD004518.

Mlyniec, K., Oboszewska, U., & Nowak, G. (2011, May–June). Zinc deficiency induces treatment-resistant depression. Abstract presented at the 10th World Congress of Biological Psychiatry, Kyoto, Japan.

Mohajeri, D., Mousavi, G., Mesgari, M., Doustar, Y., & Nouri, M. H. K. (2007). Subacute toxicity of *Crocus sativus*, L. (saffron) stigma ethanolic extract in rats. *American Journal of Pharmacology & Toxicology, 2*, 189–193.

Möhler, H. (2012). The GABA system in anxiety and depression and its therapeutic potential. *Neuropharmacology, 62*, 42–53.

Montag, C., Buckholtz, J. W., Hartmann, P., Merz, M., Burk, C., Hennig, J., &

Reuter, M. (2008). COMT genetic variation affects fear processing: Psychophysiological evidence. *Behavioral Neuroscience, 122,* 901–909.

Monteleone, P., Beinat, L., Tanzillo, C., Maj, M., & Kemali, D. (1990). Effects of phosphatidylserine on the neuroendocrine response to physical stress in humans. *Neuroendocrinology, 52,* 243–248.

Monteleone, P., Maj, M., & Beinat, L. (1992). Blunting by chronic phosphatidylserine administration of the stress-induced activation of the hypothalamo-pituitary-adrenal axis in healthy men. *European Journal of Clinical Pharmacology, 42,* 385–388.

Morales, P., Simola, N., Bustamante, D., Lisboa, F., Fiedler, J., Gebicke-Haerter, P. J., Morelli, M., Tasker, R. A., Herrera-Marschitz, M. (2010, April). Nicotinamide prevents the long-term effects of perinatal asphyxia on apoptosis, non-spatial working memory and anxiety in rats. *Experimental Brain Research, 202,* 1–14.

Moran, J. M., Wig, G. S., Adams, R. B., Jr., Janata, P., & Kelley, W. M. (2004). Neural correlates of humor detection and appreciation. *Neuroimage, 21,* 1055–1060.

Morelli, V., & Zoorob, R. J. (2000). Alternative therapies: Part I. Depression, diabetes, obesity. *American Family Physician, 62,* 1051–1060.

Mori, M., Gähwiler, B. H., & Gerber, U. (2002). Beta-alanine and taurine as endogenous agonists at glycine receptors in rat hippocampus in vitro. *Journal of Physiology, 539,* 191–200

Morris, M. J., Na, E. S., & Johnson, A. K. (2008). Salt craving: The psychobiology of pathogenic sodium intake. *Physiology & Behavior, 94,* 709–721.

Morris, N. (2002). The effects of lavender (*Lavendula angustifolium*) baths on psychological well-being: two exploratory randomised control trials. *Complementary Therapies in Medicine, 10,* 223–228.

Moss, A., Wintering, N., Roggenkamp, H., Khalsa, D. S., Waldman, M. R., Monti, D., Newberg, A. B. (2012). Effects of an eight week meditation program on mood and anxiety in patients with memory loss. *Journal of Alternative and Complementary Medicine, 18,* 48–53.

Movafegh, A., Alizadeh, R., Hajimohamadi, F., Esfehani, F., & Nejatfar, M. (2008). Preoperative oral *Passiflora incarnata* reduces anxiety in ambulatory surgery patients: A double-blind, placebo-controlled study. *Anesthesia & Analgesia, 106,* 1728–1732.

Moyer, C. A., Round,s J., & Hannum, J. W. (2004). A meta-analysis of massage therapy research. *Psychological Bulletin, 130,* 3–18.

Mugunthan, K., McGuire, T., & Glasziou, P. (2011). Minimal interventions to decrease long-term use of benzodiazepines in primary care: a systematic review and meta-analysis. *British Journal of General Practice, 61*, e573–578.

Müller, W. E., Rolli, M., Schafer, C., & Hafner, U. (1997). Effects of *Hypericum* extract (LI 160) in biochemical models of antidepressant activity. *Pharmacopsychiatry, 30*, 102–107.

Murck, H. (2013). *Journal of Psychiatric Research, 47*, 955–965.

Nagamura, A., Furuchi, T., Miura, N., Hwang, G., & Kuge, S. (2002). Investigation of intracellular factors involved in methylmercury toxicity. *Thoku Journal Experimental Medicine, 196*, 65–70.

Nagashayana, N., Sankarankutty, P., Nampoothiri, M. R., Mohan, P. K., & Mohanakumar, K. P. (2000). Association of L-DOPA with recovery following Ayurveda medication in Parkinson's disease. *Journal of Neurological Sciences, 176*, 124–127.

Nardini, M., De Stefano, R., Iannuccelli, M., Borghesi, R., & Battistini, N. (1983). Treatment of depression with l-5-hydroxytryptophan combined with chlorimipramine, a double-blind study. *International Journal of Clinical Pharmacology Research, 3*, 239–250.

Narita, K., Murata, T., Hamada, T., Kosaka, H., Sudo, S., Mizukami, K., . . . Wada, Y. (2008). Associations between trait anxiety, insulin resistance, and atherosclerosis in the elderly: A pilot cross-sectional study. *Psychoneuroendocrinology, 33*, 305–312.

Naruszewicz, M., Zapolska-Downar, D., Kośmider, A., Nowicka, G., Kozłowska-Wojciechowska, M., Vikström, A., Törnqvist, M. (2009). Chronic intake of potato chips in humans increases the production of reactive oxygen radicals by leukocytes and increases plasma C-reactive protein: A pilot study. *American Journal of Clinical Nutrition, 89*, 773–777.

Nasca, C., Xenos, D., Barone, Y., Caruso, A., Scaccianoce, S., Matrisciano, F., . . . Nicoletti, F. (2013). L-Acetylcarnitine causes rapid antidepressant effects through the epigenetic induction of mGlu2 receptors. *Proceedings of the National Academy of Sciences of the USA, 110*, 4804–4809.

National Center for Complementary and Alternative Medicine. (2013a, May). Complementary, alternative, or integrative health: What's in a name? Retrieved from http://nccam.nih.gov/health/whatiscam.

National Center for Complementary and Alternative Medicine. (2013b, June). Yoga for health. Retrieved from http://nccam.nih.gov/health/yoga/introduction.htm.

National Center for Complementary and Alternative Medicine. (2014). Meditation: An Introduction. Retrieved from http://nccam.nih.gov/health/meditation/overview.htm.

National Health Service of England. (2013). Introduction. Retrieved from http://www.nhs.uk/conditions/leaky-gut-syndrome/Pages/Introduction .aspx.

National Resources Defense Council. (2014). Mercury in fish. Retrieved from http://www.nrdc.org/health/effects/mercury/guide.asp.

Nelson, R. P. (1988). Nonoperative management of impotence. *Journal of Urology*, *139*, 2–3.

Nemets, B., Stahl, Z., & Belmaker, R. H. (2002). Addition of omega-3 fatty acid to maintenance medication treatment for recurrent unipolar depressive disorder. *American Journal of Psychiatry*, *159*, 477–479.

Neri, D. F., Wiegmann, D., Stanny, R. R., Shappell, S. A., McCardie, A., & McKay, D. L. (1995). The effects of tyrosine on cognitive performance during extended wakefulness. *Aviation, Space, & Environmental Medicine*, *66*, 313–319.

Nguyen, D. D., Almirante, C. L. D., Swamy, S., Willard, L. A., Castillo, D., & Khardori, R. (2013, June). Poster. Effect of ashwagandha on adrenal hormones. The Endocrine Society Conference, San Francisco.

Nguyen, M., & Gregan, A. (2002). S-Adenosylmethionine and depression. *Australian Family Physician*, *31*, 339–343.

Nicolodi, M., & Sicuteri, F. (1996). Fibromyalgia and migraine, two faces of the same mechanism. Serotonin as the common clue for pathogenesis and therapy. *Advances in Experimental Medicine & Biology*, *398*, 373–379.

Nielsen, F. H., Johnson, L. K., & Zeng, H. (2010). Magnesium supplementation improves indicators of low magnesium status and inflammatory stress in adults older than 51 years with poor quality sleep. *Magnesium Research*, *23*, 158–168.

Nierenberg, A. A., Lund, H. G., & Mischoulon, D. (2008). St. John's wort: A critical evaluation of the evidence for antidepressant effects. In D. Mischoulon & J. F. Rosenbaum (Eds.), *Natural medications for psychiatry: Considering the alternatives*, pp. 27–29. Philadelphia: Lippincott Williams & Wilkins.

Noorbala, A. A., Akhondzadeh, S., Tamacebi-Pour, N., & Jamshidi, A. H. (2005). Hydro-alcoholic extract of *Crocus sativus*, L. versus fluoxetine in the treatment of mild to moderate depression: a double-blind, randomized pilot trial. *Ethnopharmacology*, *97*, 281–284.

Norrholm, S. D., & Ressler, K. J. (2009). Differential genetic and epigenetic regulation of catechol-O-methyltransferase is associated with impaired fear inhibition in posttraumatic stress disorder. *Neuroscience*, *164*, 272–287.

Nowak, G., Siwek, M., Dudek, D., Zieba, A., & Pilc, A. (2003). Effect of zinc supplementation on antidepressant therapy in unipolar depression: A preliminary placebo-controlled study. *Polish Journal of Pharmacology, 55,* 1143–1147.

O'Connor, T. G., Ben-Shlomo, Y., Heron, J., Golding, J., Adams, D., & Glover, V. (2005). Prenatal anxiety predicts individual differences in cortisol in pre-adolescent children. *Biological Psychiatry, 58,* 211–217.

Ogden, C. L., Carroll, M. D., Kit, B. K., & Flegal, K. M. (2012). Prevalence of obesity and trends in body mass index among U.S. children and adolescents, 1999–2010. *Journal of the American Medical Association, 307,* 483–490.

Olivier, D. K., & van Wyk, B. E. (2013). Bitterness values for traditional tonic plants of southern Africa. *Journal of Ethnopharmacology, 147,* 676–679.

O'Loan, J., Eyles, D. W., Kesby, J., K. O. P., McGrath, J. J., & Burne, T. H. (2007). Vitamin D deficiency during various stages of pregnancy in the rat: Its impact on development and behaviour in adult offspring. *Psychoneuroendocrinology, 32,* 227–234.

Olthof, M. R., & Verhoef, P. (2005). Effects of betaine intake on plasma homocysteine concentrations and consequences for health. *Current Drug Metabolism, 6,* 15–22.

O'Mahony, L., McCarthy, J., Kelly, P., Hurley, G., Luo, F., Chen, K., O'Sullivan, G. C., Kiely, B., Collins, J. K., Shanahan, F., Quigley, E. M. (2005). *Lactobacillus* and *Bifidobacterium* in irritable bowel syndrome: Symptom responses and relationship to cytokine profiles. *Gastroenterology, 128,* 541–551.

O'Neill, B. V., Croft, R. J., Leung, S., Oliver, C., Phan, K. L., & Nathan, P. J. (2007). High-dose glycine inhibits the loudness dependence of the auditory evoked potential (LDAEP) in healthy humans. *Psychopharmacology (Berlin), 195,* 85–93.

Otmani, S., Demazières, A., Staner, C., Jacob, N., Nir, T., Zisapel, N., & Staner, L. (2008, Dec.). Effects of prolonged-release melatonin, zolpidem, and their combination on psychomotor functions, memory recall, and driving skills in healthy middle aged and elderly volunteers. Hum *Psychopharmacology, 23,* 693–705.

Otmani, S., Metzger, D., Guichard, N., Danjou, P., Nir, T., Zisapel, N., & Katz, A. (2012). Effects of prolonged-release melatonin and zolpidem on postural stability in older adults. *Human Psychopharmacology, 27,* 270–276.

Oxman, T. E., & Sengupta, A. (2002). Treatment of minor depression. *American Journal of Geriatric Psychiatry, 10,* 256–264.

Pakfetrat, M., Malekmakan, L., Roozbeh, J., & Haghpanah, S. (2008). Magnesium and its relationship to C-reactive protein among hemodialysis patients. *Magnesium Research, 21*, 167–170.

Palmer, C., Ellis, K. A., O'Neill, B. V., Croft, R. J., Leung, S., Oliver, C., Wesnes K. A., & Nathan, P. J. (2008). The cognitive effects of modulating the glycine site of the NMDA receptor with high-dose glycine in healthy controls. *Journal of Human Psychopharmacology, 23*, 151–159.

Pancheri, P., Scapicchio, P., & Chiaie, R. D. (2002). A double-blind, randomized parallel-group, efficacy and safety study of intramuscular S-adenosyl-L-methionine 1,4-butanedisulphonate (SAMe) versus imipramine in patients with major depressive disorder. *International Journal of Neuropsychopharmacology, 5*, 287–294.

Panossian, A., Wikman, G., & Sarris, J. (2010). Rosenroot (*Rhodiola rosea*): Traditional use, chemical composition, pharmacology and clinical efficacy. *Phytomedicine, 17*, 481–493.

Park, S. H., & Mattson, R. H. (2009). Ornamental indoor plants in hospital rooms enhanced health outcomes of patients recovering from surgery. *Journal of Alternative & Complementary Medicine, 15*, 975–980.

Parker, G., Gibson, N. A., Brotchie, H., Heruc, G., Rees, A. M., & Hadzi-Pavlovic, D. (2006). Omega-3 fatty acids and mood disorders. *American Journal of Psychiatry, 163*, 969–978.

Parkin, D. M. (2011). The fraction of cancer attributable to lifestyle and environmental factors in the UK in 2010. *British Journal of Cancer, 105* (Suppl 2), Si–S81.

Pauzé, D. K., & Brooks, D. E. (2007). Lithium toxicity from an Internet dietary supplement. *Journal of Medical Toxicology, 3*, 61–62.

Pearson, S., Schmidt, M., Patton, G., Dwyer, T., Blizzard, L., Otahal, P., & Venn, A. (2010). Diabetes depression and insulin resistance: Cross-sectional associations in young adults. *Care, 33*, 1128–1133.

Peebles, K. A., Baker, R. K., Kurz, E. U., Schneider, B. J., & Kroll, D. J. (2001). Catalytic inhibition of human DNA topoisomerase II by hypericin, a naphthodianthrone from St. John's wort (*Hypericum perforatum*). *Biochemical Pharmacology, 62*, 1059–1070.

Peet, M. B., & Horrobin, D. F. (2003). A dose-ranging study of the effects of ethyl-eicosapentaenoate in patients with ongoing depression despite apparently adequate treatment with standard drugs. *Archives of General Psychiatry, 59*, 913–919.

Peet, M., Horrobin, D. F., & E-E Multicentre Study Group. (2002). A dose-ranging exploratory study of the effects of ethyl-eicosapentaenoate in patients with persistent schizophrenic symptoms. *Journal of Psychiatric Research, 36,* 7–18.

Pennington, J. A. (2000). Current dietary intakes of trace elements and minerals. In: J. Bogden & L. M. Klevay (Eds.), *Clinical nutrition of the essential trace elements & minerals,* pp. 49–67. Totowa, ON: Humana Press.

Perera, F., Vishnevetsky, J., Herbstman, J. B., Calafat, A. M., Xiong, W., Rauh, V., & Wang, S. (2012). Prenatal bisphenol a exposure and child behavior in an inner-city cohort. *Environmental Health Perspectives, 120,* 1190–1194.

Perfumi, M., & Mattioli, L. (2007). Adaptogenic and central nervous system effects of single doses of 3% rosavin and 1% salidroside *Rhodiola rosea,* L. extract in mice. *Phytotherapy Research, 21,* 37–43.

Petersen, M., Pedersen, H., Major-Pedersen, A., Jensen, T., & Marckmann, P. (2002). Effect of fish oil versus corn oil supplementation on LDL and HDL subclasses in type 2 diabetic patients. *Diabetes Care, 25,* 1704–1708.

Petersen, P. (1968). Psychiatric disorders in primary hyperparathyroidism. *Journal of Endocrinology & Metabolism, 28,* 1491–1495.

Pettegrew, J. W., Levine, J., Gershon, S., Stanley, J. A., Servan-Schreiber, D., Panchalingam, K., & McClure, R. J. (2002). 31P-MRS study of acetyl-L-carnitine treatment in geriatric depression: Preliminary results. *Bipolar Disorders, 4,* 61–66.

Pfeffer, C. R., Altemus, M., Heo, M., & Jiang, H. (2007). Salivary cortisol and psychopathology in children bereaved by the September 11, 2001 terror attacks. *Biological Psychiatry, 61,* 957–965.

Pfefferbaum, B., Tucker, P., North, C. S., & Jeon-Slaughter, H. (2012). Autonomic reactivity and hypothalamic pituitary adrenal axis dysregulation in spouses of Oklahoma City bombing survivors 7 years after the attack. *Comprehensive Psychiatry, 53,* 901–906.

Pham, N. (2014). Green tea and coffee consumption is inversely associated with depressive symptoms in a Japanese working population. *Public Health & Nutrition, 17,* 625–633.

Phosphatidylserine. (2008). *Alternative Medicine Review, 13,* 245–247.

Pigeon, W. R., Carr, M., Gorman, C., & Perlis, M. L. (2010). Effects of a tart cherry juice beverage on the sleep of older adults with insomnia: A pilot study. *Journal of Medicinal Food, 13,* 579–583.

Pilkington, K., Kirkwood, G., Rampes, H., Cummings, M., & Richardson, J. (2007). Acupuncture for anxiety and anxiety disorders—a systematic literature review. *Acupuncture in Medicine, 25,* 1–10.

Pilkington, K., Kirkwood, G., Rampes, H., Fisher, P., & Richardson, J. (2005).

Homeopathy for depression: A systematic review of the research evidence. *Homeopathy, 94,* 153–163.

Pittler, M. H., & Ernst, E. (2003). Kava extract for treating anxiety. *The Cochrane Database of Systematic Reviews,* 1, Article. no. CD003383.

Pope, H. G., Jr., Cohane, G. H., Kanayama, G., Siegel, A. J., & Hudson, J. I. (2003). Testosterone gel supplementation for men with refractory depression: A randomized, placebo-controlled trial. *American Journal of Psychiatry, 160,* 105–111.

Poyares, D. R., Guilleminault, C., Ohayon, M. M., & Tufik, S. (2002). Can valerian improve the sleep of insomniacs after benzodiazepine withdrawal? *Progress in Neuropsychopharmacology & Biological Psychiatry, 26,* 539–545.

Prange, A. J., Jr., & Loosen, P. T. (1982). Hormone therapy in depressive diseases. *Advances in Biochemical Psychopharmacology, 32,* 289–296.

Prange, A., Jr., Wilson, I. C., Lynn, C. W., Alltop, L. B., & Stikeleather, R. A. (1974). L-Tryptophan in mania. Contribution to a permissive hypothesis of affective disorders. *Archives of General Psychiatry, 30,* 56–62.

Praschak-Rieder, N., Willeit, M., Wilson, A. A., Houle, S., & Meyer, J. H. (2008). Seasonal variation in human brain serotonin transporter binding. *Archives of General Psychiatry, 65,* 1072–1078.

Primack, B., Swanier, B., Georgiopoulos, A., Land, S., & Fine, M. (2009). Association between media use in adolescence and depression in young adulthood. *Arch Gen Psychiatry, 66,* 2 , 181–188.

Quadbeck, H., Lehmann, E., & Tegeler, J. (1984). Comparison of the antidepressant action of tryptophan, tryptophan/5-hydroxytryptophan combination and nomifensine *Neuropsychobiology, 11,* 111–115.

Quinlan, J. F. (1938). Hypoglycemia: In relation to the anxiety states and the degenerative diseases. *California & Western Medicine, 49,* 446–450.

Rabin, R. C. (2009, October 8). Lower depression risk linked to Mediterranean diet. *New York Times.*

Ramanathan, K., Anusuyadevi, M., Shila, S., & Panneerselvam, C. (2005). Ascorbic acid and tocopherol as potent modulators of apoptosis on arsenic induced toxicity in rats. *Toxicology Letters, 156,* 297–306.

Rao, A. V., Bested, A. C., Beaulne, T. M., Katzman, M. A., Iorio, C., Berardi, J. M., & Logan, A. C. (2009). A randomized, double-blind, placebo-controlled pilot study of a probiotic in emotional symptoms of chronic fatigue syndrome. *Gut Pathogens, 1,* 6.

Rapin, J. R., & Wiernsperger, N. (2010). Possible links between intestinal permeability and food processing: A potential therapeutic niche for glutamine. *Clinics (Sao Paulo), 65,* 635–643.

Ray, K. K., Seshasai, S. R., Erqou, S., Sever, P., Jukema, J. W., Ford, I., & Sattar, N. (2010). Statins and all-cause mortality in high-risk primary prevention: A meta-analysis of 11 randomized controlled trials involving 65,229 participants. *Archives of Internal Medicine, 170,* 1024–1031.

Re, L., Corneli, C., Sturani, E., Paolucci, G., Rossini, F., Sonia León, O., . . . Tomassetti, Q. (2003). Effects of *Hypericum* extract on the acetylcholine release: A loose patch clamp approach. *Pharmacological Research, 48,* 55–60.

Reyes, H., Zapata, R., Hernández, I., Gotteland, M., Sandoval, L., Jirón, M. I., . . . Silva, J. J. (2006). Is a leaky gut involved in the pathogenesis of intrahepatic cholestasis of pregnancy? *Hepatology, 43,* 715–722.

Ridaura, V. K., Faith, J. J., Rey, F. E., Cheng, J., Duncan, A. E., Kau, A. L., Griffin, N. W., Lombard, V., Henrissat, B., Bain, J. R., Muehlbauer, M. J., Ilkayeva, O., Semenkovich, C. F., Funai, K., Hayashi, D. K., Lyle, B. J., Martini, M. C., Ursell, L. K., Clemente, J. C., Van Treuren, W., Walters, W. A., Knight, R., Newgard, C. B., Heath, A. C., Gordon, J. I. (2013). Gut microbiota from twins discordant for obesity modulate metabolism in mice. *Science, 341,* 1241214.

Ringdahl, E. N., Pereira, S. L., & Delzell, J. E., Jr. (2004). Treatment of primary insomnia. *Journal of the American Board of Family Medicine, 17,* 212–219.

Risch, N., Herrell, R., Lehner, T., Liang, K. Y., Eaves, L., Hoh, J., . . . Merikangas, K. R. (2009). Interaction between the serotonin transporter gene, stressful life events and risk of depression: A meta-analysis. *Journal of the American Medical Association, 301,* 2462–2471.

Ritsner, M. S., Miodownik, C., Ratner, Y., Shleifer, T., Mar, M., Pintov, L., & Lerner, V. (2011). L-Theanine relieves positive, activation, and anxiety symptoms in patients with schizophrenia and schizoaffective disorder: An 8-week, randomized, double-blind, placebo-controlled, 2-center study. *Journal of Clinical Psychiatry, 72,* 34–42.

Roberts, H. J. (1988). Reactions attributed to aspartame-containing products, 551 cases. *Journal of Applied Nutrition, 40,* 85–94.

Robinson, & Donald, S. (2007). The role of dopamine and norepinephrine in depression. *Primary Psychiatry, 14,* 21–23.

Robinson, J. P., & Martin, S. (2008). IT and activity displacement: Evidence from the general social survey. *Social Indicators Research, 91,* 115–139.

Rogler, G., & Rosano, G. (2014). The heart and the gut. *European Heart Journal, 35,* 426–430.

Rohini, V., Pandey, R. S., Janakiramaiah, N., Gangadhar, B. N., & Vedamurthachar, A. (2000). A comparative study of full and partial Sudarshan

Kriya yoga (SKY) in major depressive disorder. *NIMHANS Journal, 18,* 53–57.

Rondanelli, M., Opizzi, A., Monteferrario, F., Antoniello, N., Manni, R., & Klersy, C. (2011). The effect of melatonin, magnesium, and zinc on primary insomnia in long-term care facility residents in Italy: A double-blind, placebo-controlled clinical trial. *Journal of the American Geriatric Society, 59,* 82–90.

Rosh, P. J. (1997). Integrative thinking: The essence of good medical education and practice. *Integrative Physiological & Behavioral Science, 33,* 141–150.

Rotman School of Management. (2012). Definition of Integrative Thinking. Retrieved from http://www-2.rotman.utoronto.ca/integrativethinking/definition.htm.

Rowe, K., & Rowe, K. (1994). Synthetic food coloring and behavior: A dose response effect in a double-blind, placebo-controlled, repeated measures study. *Journal of Pediatrics, 125,* 691–698.

Rubio-Tapia, A., Kyle, R. A., Kaplan, E. L., Johnson, D. R., Page, W., Erdtmann, F., . . . Murray, J. A. (2009). Increased prevalence and mortality in undiagnosed celiac disease. *Gastroenterology, 137,* 88–93.

Russo, A. J. (2011). Decreased zinc and increased copper in individuals with anxiety. *Journal of Nutrition & Metabolic Insights, 4,* 1–5.

Sabelli, H. C., Fawcett, J., Gusovsky, F., Javaid, J. I., Wynn, P., Edwards, J., . . . Kravitz, H. (1986). Clinical studies on the phenylethylamine hypothesis of affective disorder: Urine and blood phenylacetic acid and phenylalanine dietary supplements. *Journal of Clinical Psychiatry, 47,* 66–70.

Salas-Salvadó, J., Casas-Agustench, P., Murphy, M. M., López-Uriarte, P., & Bulló, M. (2008). The effect of nuts on inflammation. *Asia Pacific Journal of Clinical Nutrition, 17* (Suppl. 1), 333–336.

Samokhvalov, A. V., Paton-Gay, C. L., Balchand, K., & Rehm, J. (2013). Phenibut dependence. *BMJ Case Reports, 2013,* bcr2012008381.

Samuels, N., Cornelius, G., & Shepherd, R. S. (2008). Acupuncture for psychiatric illness: A literature review. *Behavior & Medicine, 34,* 55–62.

Sanacora, G., Berman, R. M., Cappiello, A., Oren, D. A., Kugaya, A., . . . Charney, D. S. (2004). Addition of the a2-antagonist yohimbine to fluoxetine: effects on rate of antidepressant response. *Neuropsychopharmacology, 29,* 1166–1171.

Sánchez-Villegas, A., Delgado-Rodríguez, M., Alonso, A., Schlatter, J., Lahortiga, F., Serra Majem, L., & Martínez-González, M. A. (2009a). Association of the Mediterranean dietary pattern with the incidence of depression: The

Seguimiento Universidad de Navarra/University of Navarra follow-up (SUN) cohort. *Archives of General Psychiatry, 66,* 1090–1098.

Sánchez-Villegas, A., Doreste, J., Schlatter, J., Pla, J., Bes-Rastrollo, M., & Martínez-González, M. A. (2009b). Association between folate, vitamin B(6) and vitamin B(12) intake and depression in the SUN cohort study. *Journal of Human Nutrition & Diet, 22,* 122–133.

Sánchez-Villegas, A., Galbete, C., Martinez-González, M. A., Martinez, J. A., Razquin, C., Salas-Salvadó, J., . . . Martí, A. (2011). The effect of the Mediterranean diet on plasma brain-derived neurotrophic factor (BDNF) levels: The PREDIMED-NAVARRA randomized trial. *Nutritional Neuroscience, 14,* 195–201.

Sánchez-Villegas, A., Henríquez, P., Bes-Rastrollo, M., & Doreste, J. (2006). Mediterranean diet and depression. *Public Health & Nutrition, 9,* 1104–1109.

Sanmukhani, J., Anovadiya, A., & Tripathi, C. B. (2011). Evaluation of antidepressant like activity of curcumin and its combination with fluoxetine and imipramine: an acute and chronic study. *Acta Poloniae Pharmaceutica, 68,* 769–775.

Sanmukhani, J., Satodia, V., Trivedi, J., Patel, T., Tiwari, D., Panchal, B., . . . Tripathi, C. B. (2014). Efficacy and safety of curcumin in major depressive disorder: A randomized controlled trial. *Phytotherapy Research. 28,* 579–585.

Santarelli, L., Saxe, M., Gross, C., Surget, A., Battaglia, F., Dulawa, S., . . . Hen, R. (2003). Requirement of hippocampal neurogenesis for the behavioral effects of antidepressants. *Science, 301,* 805–809.

Saper, R. B., Kales, S. N., Paquin, J., Burns, M. J., Eisenberg, D. M., Davis, R. B., & Phillips, R. S. (2004). Heavy metal content of Ayurvedic herbal medicine products. *Journal of the American Medical Association, 292,* 2868–2873.

Sapolsky, R. M. (2001). Depression, antidepressants, and the shrinking hippocampus. *Proceedings of the National Academy of Sciences of the USA, 98,* 12320–12322.

Sarris, J., Kavanagh, D. J., Deed, G., & Bone, K. M. (2009). St. John's wort and Kava in treating major depressive disorder with comorbid anxiety: A randomised double-blind placebo-controlled pilot trial. *Human Psychopharmacology, 24,* 41–48.

Sartori, H. E. (1986). Lithium orotate in the treatment of alcoholism and related conditions. *Alcohol, 3,* 97–100.

Sartori, S. B., Whittle, N., Hetzenauer, A., & Singewald, N. (2012). Magnesium deficiency induces anxiety and HPA axis dysregulation: Modulation by therapeutic drug treatment. *Neuropharmacology, 62,* 304–312.

Schab, D., & Trinh, N. (2004). Do artificial food colours promote hyperactivity in children with hyperactivity in children with hyperactive syndromes? A meta analysis of double-blind placebo-controlled trials. *Journal of Developmental & Behavioral Pediatrics, 25,* 423–434.

Schildkraut, J. J. (1965). The catecholamine hypothesis of affective disorders: a review of supporting evidence. *Am J Psychiatry.*122, 5, 509–522.

Schmidt, P. J., Daly, R. C., Bloch, M., Smith, M. J., Danaceau, M. A., St. Clair, L. S., . . . Rubinow, D. R. (2005). Dehydroepiandrosterone monotherapy in midlife-onset major and minor depression. *Archives of General Psychiatry, 62,* 154–162.

Schneider, L. S., Small, G.W., & Clary, C.M.. (2001). Estrogen replacement therapy and antidepressant response to sertraline in older depressed women. *American Journal of Geriatric Psychiatry, 9,* 393–399.

Schoenfield, T. J., Rada, P., Pieruzzini, P. R., Hsueh, B., & Gould, E. (2013). Physical exercise prevents stress-induced activation of granule neurons and enhances local inhibitory mechanisms in the dentate gyrus. *Journal of Neuroscience, 33,* 7770–7777.

Schöttker, B., Haug, U., Schomburg, L., Köhrle, J., Perna, L., Müller, H., . . . Brenner, H. (2013). Strong associations of 25-hydroxyvitamin D concentrations with all-cause, cardiovascular, cancer, and respiratory disease mortality in a large cohort study. *American Journal of Clinical Nutrition, 97,* 782–793.

Schruers, K., van Diest, R., Overbeek, T., & Griez, E. (2002). Acute L-5-hydroxytryptophan administration inhibits carbon dioxide-induced panic in panic disorder patients. *Psychiatry Research, 113,* 237–243.

Seely, D. M., Wu,. P., & Mills, E. J. (2005). EDTA chelation therapy for cardiovascular disease: a systematic review. *BMC Cardiovascular Disorders, 5,* 32.

Sephton, S. E., Salmon, P., Weissbecker, I., Ulmer, C., Floyd, A., Hoover, K., & Studts, J. L. (2007). Mindfulness meditation alleviates depressive symptoms in women with fibromyalgia: Results of a randomized clinical trial. *Arthritis & Rheumatism, 57,* 77–85.

Severus, W. E., Littman, A. B., & Stoll, A. L. (2001). Omega-3 fatty acids, homocysteine, and the increased risk of cardiovascular mortality in major depression. *Harvard Review of Psychiatry, 9,* 280–293.

Shah, Z. A., Sharma, P., & Vohora, S. B. (2003). *Ginkgo biloba* normalises stress-elevated alterations in brain catecholamines, serotonin and plasma corticosterone levels. *European Neuropsychopharmacology, 13,* 321–325.

Shannahoff-Khalsa, D. S., Ray, L. E., Levine, S., Gallen, C. C., Schwartz, B. J., Sidorowich, J. J. (1999). Randomized controlled trial of yogic meditation techniques for patients with obsessive-compulsive disorder. *CNS Spectrums, 4,* 34–47.

Shastry, J. L. N. (2001). Ayurvedokta oushadha niruktamal., Chaukhambha Orientalia. Varanasi, India: .

Shaw, K., Turner, J., & Del Mar, C. (2002). Are tryptophan and 5-hydroxytryptophan effective treatments for depression? A meta-analysis. *Australian & New Zealand Journal of Psychiatry, 36,* 488–491.

Shealy, N. C., Cady, R. K., Veehoff, D., Houston, R., Burnette, M., Cox, R. H., et al. (1992). The neurochemistry of depression. *American Journal of Preventive Medicine, 2,* 13–16.

Shekhar, A., Truitt, W., Rainnie, D., & Sajdyk, T. (2005). Role of stress, corticotrophin releasing factor (CRF) and amygdala plasticity in chronic anxiety. *Stress, 8,* 209–219.

Shevchuk, N. A. (2008). Adapted cold shower as a potential treatment for depression. *Medial Hypotheses, 70,* 995–1001.

Shevchuk, N. A., & Radoja, S. (2007). Possible stimulation of anti-tumor immunity using repeated cold stress: A hypothesis. *Infectious Agents & Cancer, 2,* 20.

Shih, R. A., Glass, T. A., Bandeen-Roche, K., Carlson, M. C., Bolla, K. I., Todd, A. C., Schwartz, B. S. (2006). Environmental lead exposure and cognitive function in community-dwelling older adults. *Neurology, 67,* 1556–1562.

Shor-Posner, G. R., Lecusay, Miguez, M. J., Moreno-Black, G., Zhnag, G., Rodriguez, N., Burbano, X., Baum, M., Wilkie, F. (2003). Psychological burden in the era of HAART: Impact of selenium therapy. *International Journal of Psychiatry in Medicine, 33,* 55–69.

Shrivastava, S., Pucadyil, T. J., Paila, Y. D., Ganguly, S., & Chattopadhyay, A. (2010). Chronic cholesterol depletion using statin impairs the function and dynamics of human serotonin(1A) receptors. *Biochemistry, 49,* 5426–5435.

Siblerud, R. I. (1989). The relationship between mercury from dental amalgam and mental health. *American Journal of Psychotherapy, 43,* 575–587.

Skarupski, K. A., Tangney, C., Li., H., Ouyang, B., Evans, D. A., & Morris, M. C. (2010). Longitudinal association of vitamin B-6, folate, and vitamin B-12 with depressive symptoms among older adults over time. *American Journal of Clinical Nutrition, 92,* 330–335.

Slot, O. (2001). Changes in plasma homocysteine in arthritis patients starting treatment with low-dose methotrexate subsequently supplemented with folic acid. *Scandinavian Journal of Rheumatology, 30,* 305–307.

Smith, D. F., & Schou, M. (1979). Kidney function and lithium concentrations of rats given an injection of lithium orotate or lithium carbonate. *Journal of Pharmacy & Pharmacology, 31,* 161–163.

Smits, M. G., & Pandi-Perumal, S. R. (2005). Delayed sleep phase syndrome: a melatonin onset disorder. In S. R. Pandi-Perumal & D. P. Cardinali (Eds.), *Melatonin: Biological basis of its function in health & disease.* Retrieved from Landes Bioscience at http://www.landesbioscience.com/ curie/chapter/2420/.

Smoller, J. W., Allison, M., Cochrane, B. B., Curb, J. D., Perlis, R. H., Robinson, J. G., . . . Wassertheil-Smoller, S. (2009). Antidepressant use and risk of incident cardiovascular morbidity and mortality among postmenopausal women in the Women's Health Initiative study. *Archives of Internal Medicine, 169,* 2128–2139.

Smriga, M., & Torii, K. (2003). L-Lysine acts like a partial serotonin receptor 4 antagonist and inhibits serotonin-mediated intestinal pathologies and anxiety in rats. *Proceedings of the National Academy of Sciences of the USA, 100,* 15370–15375.

Smriga, M., Ando, T., Akutsu, M., Furukawa, Y., Miwa, K., & Morinaga, Y. (2007). Oral treatment with L-lysine and L-arginine reduces anxiety and basal cortisol levels in healthy humans. *BioMed Research International. 28,* 85–90.

Snydman, D. R. (2008). The safety of probiotics. *Clinical Infectious Diseases, 46* (Suppl 2), S104–S111, S144–S151.

Soczynska, J. K., Kennedy, S. H., Chow, C. S., Woldeyohannes, H. O., Konarski, J. Z., & McIntyre, R. S. (2008). Acetyl-L-carnitine and alpha-lipoic acid: possible neurotherapeutic agents for mood disorders. *Expert Opinion on Investigational Drugs, 17,* 827–843.

Solomon, B. L., Schaaf, M., & Smallridge, R. C. (1994). Psychologic symptoms before and after parathyroid surgery. *American Journal of Medicine, 96,* 101–106.

Sommerfield, A. J., Deary, I. J., & Frier, B. M. (2004). Acute hyperglycemia alters mood state and impairs cognitive performance in people with type 2 diabetes. *Diabetes Care, 27,* 2335–2340.

Song, C., Zhang, X. Y., & Manku, M. (2009). Increased phospholipase A2 activity and inflammatory response but decreased nerve growth factor expression in the olfactory bulbectomized rat model of depression: effects of chronic ethyl-eicosapentaenoate treatment. *Journal of Neuroscience, 29,* 14–22.

Spencer, S. J., & Tilbrook, A. (2009). Neonatal overfeeding alters adult anxiety and stress responsiveness. *Psychoneuroendocrinology, 34,* 1133–1143.

Stahl, S. M. (2008). L-Methylfolate: A vitamin for your monoamines. *Journal of Clinical Psychiatry, 69,* 1352–1353.

Staner, L. (2003). Sleep and anxiety disorders. *Dialogues in Clinical Neuroscience, 5,* 249–258.

Starr, L. R., & Davila, J. (2009). Clarifying co-rumination: Association with internalizing symptoms and romantic involvement among adolescent girls. Journal of Adolescence, 32, 19-37.

Steffens, D. C., McQuoid, D. R., & Krishnan, K. R. (2003). Cholesterol-lowering medication and relapse of depression. *Psychopharmacology Bulletin, 37,* 92–98.

Stokes, L., Letz, R., Gerr, F., Kolczak, M., McNeill, F. E., Chettle, D. R., & Kaye, W. E. (1998). Neurotoxicity in young adults 20 years after childhood exposure to lead: The Bunker Hill experience. *Occupational & Environmental Medicine, 55,* 507–516;

Stough, C., Scholey, A., Lloyd, J., Spong, J., Myers, S., & Downey, L. A. (2011). The effect of 90 day administration of a high dose vitamin B-complex on work stress. *Human Psychopharmacology, 26,* 470–476.

Straube, S., Moore, R. A., Derry, S., & McQuay, H. J. (2009). Vitamin D and chronic pain. *Pain, 141,* 10–13.

Streeter, C. (2010). Effects of yoga versus walking on mood, anxiety, and brain GABA levels: A randomized controlled MRS study. *Journal of Alternative & Complementary Medicine, 16,* 1145–1152.

Strous, R. D., Maayan, R., Lapidus, R., Stryjer, R., Lustig, M., Kotler, M., & Weizman, A. (2003). Dehydroepiandrosterone augmentation in the management of negative, depressive, and anxiety symptoms in schizophrenia. *Archives of General Psychiatry, 60,* 133–141.

Stumpf, W. E. (1995). Vitamin D sites and mechanisms of action: A histochemical perspective. Reflections on the utility of autoradiography and cytopharmacology for drug targeting. *Histochemistry & Cellular Biology, 104,* 417–427.

Sturniolo, G. C., Di Leo, V., Ferronato, A., D'Odorico, A., & D'Incà, R. (2001). Zinc supplementation tightens leaky gut in Crohn's disease. *Inflammatory Bowel Disease, 7,* 94–98.

Su, K. P., Huang, S. Y., Chiu, C. C., & Shen, W. W. (2003). Omega-3 fatty acids in major depressive disorder. A preliminary double-blind, placebo-controlled trial. *European Neuropsychopharmacology, 13,* 267–271.

Suarez, E. C. (1999). Relations of trait depression and anxiety to low lipid and lipoprotein concentrations in healthy young adult women. *Psychosomatic Medicine, 61,* 273–279.

Sublette, M. E., Milak, M. A., Hibbeln, J. R., Freed, P. J., Oauendo, M. A., Malone, K. M., . . . Mann, J. J. (2009). Plasma polyunsaturated fatty acids and regional cerebral glucose metabolism in major depression. *Prostaglandins Leukotrienes & Essential Fatty Acids, 80,* 57–64.

Suliman, S., Hemmings, S. M., & Seedat, S. (2013). Brain-derived neurotrophic factor (BDNF) protein levels in anxiety disorders: Systematic review and meta-regression analysis. *Frontiers in Integrative Neuroscience, 7,* 55.

Sun, Y., Chien, K. L., Hsu, H. C., Su, T. C., Chen, M. F., & Lee, Y. T. (2009). Use of serum homocysterine to predict stroke, coronary heart disease and death in ethnic Chinese. 12-year prospective cohort study. *Circulation Journal. 73,* 1423–1430.

Sutherland, E. R., Ellison, M. C., Kraft, M., & Martin, R. J. (2003). Elevated serum melatonin is associated with the nocturnal worsening of asthma. *Journal of Allergy & Clinical Immunology, 112,* 513–517.

Swaab, D. F., Bao, A. M., & Lucassen, P. J. (2005). The stress system in the human brain in depression and neurodegeneration. *Ageing Research Review, 4,* 141–194.

Taibi, D. M., Vitiello, M. V., Barsness, S., Elmer, G. W., Anderson, G. D., & Landis, C. A. (2009). Systematic review of Valerian as a sleep aid: Safe but not effective. *Sleep Medicine, 10,* 319–328.

Tajalizadekhoob, Y., Sharifi, F., Fakhrzadeh, H., Mirarefin, M., Ghaderpanahi, M., Badamchizade, Z., & Azimipour, S. (2011). The effect of low-dose omega 3 fatty acids on the treatment of mild to moderate depression in the elderly: A double-blind, randomized, placebo-controlled study. *European Archives of Psychiatry & Clinical Neuroscience, 261,* 539–549.

Takahashi, R., & Nakane, Y. (1978). Clinical trial of taurine in epilepsy. In A. Barbeau & R. J. Huxtable (Eds.), *Taurine and neurological disorders,* pp. 375–385. New York: Raven Press.

Takeda, A., Itoh, H., Imano, S., & Oku, N. (2006). Impairment of GABAergic neurotransmitter system in the amygdala of young rats after 4-week zinc deprivation. *Neurochemistry International, 49,* 746–750.

Tang, Y. Y., Ma, Y., Wang, J., Fan, Y., Feng, S., Lu, Q., Yu, Q., Sui, D., Rothbart, M. K., Fan, M., Posner, M.I. (2007). Short-term meditation training improves attention and self-regulation. *Proceedings of the National Academy of Sciences of the USA, 104,* 17152–17156.

Tannergren, C., Engman, H., Knutson, L., Hedeland, M., Bondesson, U., &

Lennernas, H. (2004). St John's wort decreases the bioavailability of R- and S-verapamil through induction of the first-pass metabolism. *Clinical Pharmacology & Therapeutics, 75,* 298–309.

Tanskanen, A., Tuomilehto, J., Viinamäki, H., Vartiainen, E., Lehtonen, J., & Puska, P. (2000). Heavy coffee drinking and the risk of suicide. *European Journal of Epidemiology, 16,* 789–791.

Taylor, M., Wilder, H., Bhagwagar, Z., & Geddes, J. (2004). Inositol for depressive disorders. Retrieved from the Cochrane Database of Systematic Reviews, 2: CD004049.

Terry, P., Lichtenstein, P., Feychting, M., Ahlbom, A., & Wolk, A. (2001). Fatty fish consumption and risk of prostate cancer. *Lancet, 357,* 1764–1766.

Teschke, R., Schwarzenboeck, A., & Akinci, A. (2008). Kava hepatotoxicity: A European view. *New Zealand Medical Journal, 121,* 90–98.

Thompson, E. A., & Reilly, D. (2002). The homeopathic approach to symptom control in the cancer patient: A prospective observational study. *Palliative Medicine, 16,* 227–233.

Thuret, S., Morisse, B., Ahmet, S., Aimone, L. J., Aimone, J. B., & Gage, F. H. (2007, November 7). Brain specific gene expression, adult neurogenesis and behaviour are altered by diet. Session 315.26/HHH26 presented at the Society for Neuroscience , San Diego.

Tochigi, M., Hibino, H., Otowa, T., Kato, C., Marui, T., Ohtani, T., . . . Sasaki, T. (2006). Association between dopamine D4 receptor (DRD4) exon III polymorphism and neuroticism in the Japanese population. *Neuroscience Letters, 398,* 333–336.

Toda, M., Morimoto, K., Nagasawa, S., & Kitamura, K. (2006). Change in salivary physiological stress markers by spa bathing. *Biomedical Research, 27,* 11–14.

Toffol, E., Kalleinen, N., Haukka, J., Vakkuri, O., Partonen, T., & Polo-Kantola, P. (2014). Melatonin in perimenopausal and postmenopausal women: Associations with mood, sleep, climacteric symptoms, and quality of life. *Menopause, 21,* 493–500.

Trivedi, M. H., Greer, T. L., Church, T. S., Carmody, T. J., Grannemann, B. D., Galper, D. I., . . . Blair, S. N. (2011). Exercise as an augmentation treatment for nonremitted major depressive disorder: A randomized, parallel dose comparison. *Journal of Clinical Psychiatry, 72,* 677–684.

Troisi, A., Moles, A., Panepuccia, L., Lo Russo, D., Palla, G., & Scucchi, S. (2002). Serum cholesterol levels and mood symptoms in the postpartum period. *Psychiatry Research, 3,* 213–219.

Tsai, J. F., Hsiao, S., & Wang, S. Y. (2007). Infrared irradiation has potential antidepressant effect. *Progress in Neuropsychopharmacology & Biological Psychiatry, 31*, 1397–1400.

Tsigos, C., & Chrousos, G. P. (2002). Hypothalamic-pituitary-adrenal axis, neuroendocrine factors and stress. *Journal of Psychosomatic Research, 53*, 865–871.

Tufik, S., Fujita, K., Seabra, M. L. V., & Lobo, L. L. (1994). Effects of a prolonged administration of valepotriates in rats on the mother and their offspring. *Journal of Ethnopharmacology, 41*, 39–44.

Turner, E. H., Loftis, J. M., & Blackwell, A. D. (2006). Serotonin a la carte: Supplementation with the serotonin precursor 5-hydroxytryptophan. *Pharmacology & Therapeutics, 109*, 325–338.

Ulrich, R. S. (1984). View through a window may influence recovery from surgery. *Science, 224*, 42–421.

Ulrich, R. S., Lundén, O., & Eltinge, J. L. (1993). Effects of exposure to nature and abstract pictures on patients recovering from heart surgery. *Psychophysiology, 30* (Suppl. 1), 7.

Uribarri, J., Cai, W., Sandu, O., Peppa, M., Goldberg, T., & Vlassara, H. (2005). Diet-derived advanced glycation end products are major contributors to the body's AGE pool and induce inflammation in healthy subjects. *Annals of the New York Academy of Sciences, 1043*, 461–466.

U.S. Department of Health and Human Services. (2002, Oct.). S-Adenosyl-L-Methionine for Treatment of Depression, Osteoarthritis, and Liver Disease. Agency for Healthcare Research and Quality. 64, 1–3. Retrieved from http://archive.ahrq.gov/clinic/tp/sametp.htm

U.S. Department of Health and Human Services. (2004, June). Celiac disease. Evidence Report/Technology Assessment 104. Retrieved from http://www.ahrq.gov/clinic/epcsums/celiacsum.htm.

U.S. Food & Drug Administration. (1996). CFR Part 880: Medical Devices; reclassification of acupuncture needles for the practice of acupuncture. Title 21. *Federal Register, 61*.1-2. Retrieved from http://www.gpo.gov/fdsys/pkg/FR-1996-12-06/pdf/96-31047.pdf

U.S. Food & Drug Administration. (2002). Consumer advisory: Kava-containing dietary supplements may be associated with severe liver injury. Retrieved http://www.fda.gov/Food/ResourcesForYou/Consumers/ucm085482.htm.

Vaarala, O., Atkinson, M. A., & Neu, J. (2008). The perfect storm for type 1 diabetes: The complex interplay between intestinal microbiota, gut permeability, and mucosal immunity. *Diabetes, 57*, 2555–2562.

van Ede, A. E., Laan, R. F., Rood, M. J., Huizinga, T. W., van de Laar, M. A., van Denderen, C. J., . . . van de Putte, L. B. (2001). Effect of folic or folinic acid

supplementation on the toxicity and efficacy of methotrexate in rheumatoid arthritis: A forty-eight week, multicenter, randomized, double-blind,
placebo-controlled study. *Arthritis & Rheumatism, 44*, 1515–1524.

van Honk, J., Peper, J. S., & Schutter, D. J. (2005). Testosterone reduces unconscious fear but not consciously experienced anxiety: Implications for the
disorders of fear and anxiety. *Biological Psychiatry, 58*, 218–225.

van Praag, H., Kempermann, G., & Gage, F. H. (1999). Running increases cell
proliferation and neurogenesis in the adult mouse dentate gyrus. *Nature
Neuroscience, 2*, 266–270.

Vaz Jdos, S., Kac, G., Emmett, P., Davis, J., Golding, J., & Hibbeln, J. (2013,
July). Dietary patterns, n-3 fatty acids intake from seafood and high levels
of anxiety symptoms during pregnancy: findings from the Avon Longitudinal Study of Parents and Children. *PLoS One, 12*, 8(7):e67671

Vaswani, K., Richard, C. W., III, & Tejwani, G. A. (1988). Cold swim stress-
induced changes in the levels of opioid peptides in the rat CNS and periph-
eral tissues. *Pharmacology, Biochemistry, & Behavior, 29*, 163–168.

Vaidya, A. B., Rajagopalan, T. G., Mankodi, N. A., Antarkar, D. S., Tathed, P.
S., Purohit, A. V., & Wadia, N. H. (1978) Treatment of Parkinson's disease
with the cowhage plant-Mucuna pruriens Bak. *Neurology India. 26*, 171–
176.

Vaz J. S., Kac, G., Emmett, P., Davis, J. M., Golding, J., & Hibbeln, J. Rl. (2013).
Dietary patterns, n-3 fatty acids intake from seafood and high levels of
anxiety symptoms during pregnancy: Findings from the Avon longitudinal
study of parents and children. *PLoS One, 8*, e67671.

Vegetarian Society. (2009). Omega 3 fats. Retrieved from http://www.vegsoc
.org/info/omega3.html.

Verdon, F., Burnand, B., Stubi, C. L., Bonard, C., Graff, M., Michaud, A., . . .
Favrat, B. (2003). Iron supplementation for unexplained fatigue in non-
anaemic women: Double blind randomised placebo controlled trial. *British
Medical Journal, 326*, 1124.

Vieth, R. (1999). Vitamin D supplementation, 25-hydroxy-vitamin D concentrations, and safety. *American Journal of Clinical Nutrition, 69*, 842–856.

Vieth, R., Kimball, S., Hu., A., & Walfish, P. G. (2004). Randomized comparison of the effects of the vitamin D3 adequate intake versus 100 mcg (4000
IU) per day on biochemical responses and the wellbeing of patients. *Nutrition Journal, 3*, 8.

Vigen, R., O'Donnell, Baron, A. E., Grunwald, G. K., Maddox, T. M., Bradley,
S. M., Barqawi, A., Woning, G., Wierman, M. E., Plomondon, M. E.,

Rumsfeld, J. S., Ho, P. M. (2013). Association of testosterone therapy with mortality, myocardial infarction, and stroke in men with low testosterone levels. *Journal of the American Medical Association, 310,* 1829–1835.

Vignes, M., Maurice, T., Lanté, F., Nedjar, M., Thethi, K., Guiramand, J., & Récasens, M. (2006). Anxiolytic properties of green tea polyphenol (-)-epigallocatechin gallate (EGCG). *Brain Research, 1110,* 102–115.

Villegas-Salas, E., Ponce de León, R., Juárez-Perez, M. A., & Grubb, G. S. (1997). Effect of vitamin B6 on the side effects of a low-dose combined oral contraceptive. *Contraception, 55,* 245–248.

Vogel, G. W., Vogel, F., McAbee, R. S., & Thurmond, A. J. (1980). Improvement of depression by REM sleep deprivation. New findings and a theory. *Archives of General Psychiatry, 37,* 247–253.

Vogelzangs, N., Beekman, A. T., de Jonge, P., & Penninx, B. W. (2013). Anxiety disorders and inflammation in a large adult cohort. *Translational Psychiatry, 3,* e249.

Vucenik, I., & Shamsuddin, A. M. (2003). Cancer inhibition by inositol hexaphosphate (IP6) and inositol: From laboratory to clinic. *Journal of Nutrition, 133,* 3778S–3784S.

Wagstaff, A. J., Ormrod, D., & Spencer, C. M. (2001). Tianeptine: A review of its use in depressive disorders. *CNS Drugs, 15,* 231–259.

Wang, H., Hong, Q., Wang, B.-S., Cui, Y.-Y., Zhu, L., Rong, Z.-X., & Chen, H.-Z. (2008). Is acupuncture beneficial in depression: A meta-analysis of 8 randomized controlled trials? *Journal of Affective Disorders, 111,* 125–134.

Wang, H. T., Chen, S. M., Lee, S. D., Hsu, M. C., Chen, K. N., Liou, Y. F., & Kuo, C. H. (2009). The role of DHEA-S in the mood adjustment against negative competition outcome in golfers. *Journal of Sports Science, 27,* 291–297.

Wang, X, Qin, X., Demirtas, H., Li, J., Mao, G., Huo, Y., Sun, N., Liu, L., Xu, X. (2007). Efficacy of folic acid supplementation in stroke prevention: A meta-analysis. *Lancet, 369,* 1876–1882.

Waring, W. S. (2006). Management of lithium toxicity. *Toxicology Review, 25,* 221–230.

Wassenaar, T. M., & Klein, G. (2008). Safety aspects and implications of regulation of probiotic bacteria in food and food supplements. *Journal of Food Protection, 71,* 1734–1741.

Watson, L. C., & Marx, C. E. (2002). New onset of neuropsychiatric symptoms in the elderly: Possible primary hyperparathyroidism. *Psychosomatics, 43,* 413–417.

Watson, W. P., Munter, T., & Golding, B. T. (2004). A new role for glutathione: Protection of vitamin B12 from depletion by xenobiotics. *Chemical Research in Toxicology, 17,* 1562–1567.

Waxman, E. A. (2005). N-Methyl-D-aspartate receptor subtypes: Multiple roles in excitotoxicity and neurological disease. *Neuroscientist, 11,* 37–49.

Weaver, I. C., Cervoni, N., Champagne, F. A., D'Alessio, A. C., Sharma, S., Seckl, J. R., . . . Meaney, M. J. (2004). Epigenetic programming by maternal behavior. *Nature Neuroscience, 7,* 847–854.

Weeks, B. S. (2009). Formulations of dietary supplements and herbal extracts for relaxation and anxiolytic action: Relarian. *Medical Science Monitor, 15,* RA256–RA262.

Weinstock, M. (2005). The potential influence of maternal stress hormones on development and mental health of the offspring. *Brain, Behavior, & Immunity, 19,* 296–308.

Weintraub, A. (2005). Yoga for depression. *LILIPOH,* Winter, 18–20.

Weizman, A., & Weizman, R. (2000). Serotonin transporter polymorphism and response to SSRIs in major depression and relevance to anxiety disorders and substance abuse. *Pharmacogenomics, 1,* 335–341.

Wells, S., Polglase, K., Andrews, H. B., Carrington, P., & Baker, A. H. (2003). Evaluation of a meridian-based intervention, Emotional Freedom Techniques (EFT), for reducing specific phobias of small animals. *Journal of Clinical Psychology, 59,* 943–966.

Wesensten, N. J., Balkin, T. J., Reichardt, R. M., Kautz, M. A., Saviolakis, G. A., & Belenky, G. (2005). Daytime sleep and performance following a zolpidem and melatonin cocktail. *Sleep, 28,* 93–103.

Westhoff, C., Truman, C., Kalmuss, D., Cushman, L., Davidson, A., Rulin, M., & Heartwell, S. (1998). Depressive symptoms and Depo-Provera. *Contraception, 57,* 237–240.

Wheatley, D. (2004). Triple-blind, placebo-controlled trial of *Ginkgo biloba* in sexual dysfunction due to antidepressant drugs. *Human Psychopharmacology, 19,* 545–548.

While, A., & Keen, L. (2012). The effects of statins on mood: A review of the literature. *European Journal of Cardiovascular Nursing, 11,* 85–96.

Wiebke, A. (2006). Androgen therapy in women. *European Journal of Endocrinology, 154,* 1–11.

Wion, D., MacGrogan, D., Neveu, I., Jehan, F., Houlgatte, R., & Brachet, P. (1991). 1,25-Dihydroxyvitamin D3 is a potent inducer of nerve growth factor synthesis. *Journal of Neuroscience Research, 28,* 110–114.

Winstock, A. R., Lea, T., & Copeland, J. (2009). Lithium carbonate in the management of cannabis withdrawal in humans: an open-label study. *Journal of Psycholpharmacology*. 23, 84-93.

*Withania somnifera.* (2004). *Alternative Medicine Review*, 9, 211–214.

Witt, C. M., Pach, D., Brinkhaus, B.,Wruck, K., Tag, B. Mank, S., Willich, S. N. (2009). Safety of acupuncture: Results of a prospective observational study with 229,230 patients and introduction of a medical information and consent form. *Forschende Komplementärmedizin*, 16, 91–97.

Witte, S., Loew, D., & Gaus, W. (2005). Meta-analysis of the efficacy of the acetonic kava-kava extract WS1490 in patients with non-psychotic anxiety disorders. *Phytotherapy Research*, 19, 183–188.

Woelk, H., & Schläfke, S. (2010). A multi-center, double-blind, randomised study of the Lavender oil preparation Silexan in comparison to lorazepam for generalized anxiety disorder. *Phytomedicine*, 17, 94–99.

Woolery, A., Myers, H., Sternlieb, B., & Zeltzer, L. (2004). A yoga intervention for young adults with elevated symptoms of depression. *Alternative Therapies in Health & Medicine*, 10, 60–63.

Wong, M.-L., Bongiorno, P. B., Rettori, V., McCann, S. M., & Licinio J. (1997). Interleukin (IL) 1b, IL-1 receptor antagonist, IL-b, and IL-13 gene expression in the central nervous system and anterior pituitary during systemic inflammation: Pathophysiological Implications. *Proceedings of the National Academy of Sciences of the USA*, 94, 227–232.

Wong, M. L., O'Kirwan, F., Hannestad J. P., Irizarry, K. J. L., Elashoff, D., & Licinio, J. (2004). St John's wort and imipramine-induced gene expression profiles identify cellular functions relevant to antidepressant action and novel pharmacogenetic candidates for the phenotype of antidepressant treatment response. *Molecular Psychiatry* 9, 237–251.

Wu, H., Jin, Y., Wei, J., Jin, H., Sha, D., & Wu, J. Y. (2005). Mode of action of taurine as a neuroprotector. *Brain Research*, 1038, 123–131.

Yaffe, K., Vittinghoff, E., Ensrud, K. E., Johnson, K. C., Diem, S., Hanes, V., & Grady, D. (2006). Effects of ultra-low-dose transdermal estradiol on cognition and health-related quality of life. *Archives of Neurology*, 63, 945–950.

Yam, D., Eliraz, A., & Berry, E. M. (1996). Diet and disease—the Israeli paradox: Possible dangers of high omega-6 polyunsaturated fatty acid diet. *Israel Journal of Medical Sciences*, 32, 1134–1143.

Yamamoto, K., Aso, Y., Nagata, S., Kasugai, K., & Maeda, S. (2008). Autonomic, neuro-immunological and psychological responses to wrapped warm footbaths—a pilot study. *Complementary Therapies in Clinical Practice*, 14, 195–203.

Yancheva, S., Ihl, R., Nikolova, G., Panayotov, P., Schlaefke, S., & Hoerr, R.

(2009). *Ginkgo biloba* extract EGb 761, donepezil or both combined in the treatment of Alzheimer's disease with neuropsychiatric features: A randomised, double-blind, exploratory trial. *Aging & Mental Health, 13*, 183–190.

Yarnell, E., & Russell, L. (2008). Common uses for crocus. *Naturopathic Doctor News & Review, 4*, 21.

Yehuda, R. (1997). Sensitization of the hypothalamic-pituitary-adrenal axis in posttraumatic stress disorder. *Annals of the New York Academy of Sciences, 821*, 57–75.

Yokogoshi, H., Roberts, C. H., Caballero, B., & Wurtman, R. J. (1984). Effects of aspartame and glucose administration on brain and plasma levels of large neutral amino acids and brain 5-hydroxyindoles. *American Journal of Clinical Nutrition, 40*, 1–7.

Yoshida, M., Takayanagi, Y., Inoue, K., Kimura, T., Young, L. J., Onaka, T., & Nishimori, K. J. (2009). Evidence that oxytocin exerts anxiolytic effects via oxytocin receptor expressed in serotonergic neurons in mice. *Neuroscience, 29*, 2259–2271.

Yoshimura, R., Ikenouchi-Sugita, A., Hori, H., Umene-Nakano, W., Hayashi, K., Katsuki, A., . . . Nakamura, J. (2010). Blood levels of brain-derived neurotrophic factor (BDNF) in major depressive disorder. *Seishin Shinkeigaku Zasshi, 112*, 982–985.

Yoto, A., Motoki, M., Murao, S., & Yokogoshi, H. (2012a). Effects of L-theanine or caffeine intake on changes in blood pressure under physical and psychological stresses. *Journal of Physiological Anthropology, 31*, 28.

Yoto, A., Murao, S., Motoki, M., Yokoyama, Y., Horie, N., Takeshima, K., . . . Yokogoshi, H. (2012b). Oral intake of γ-aminobutyric acid affects mood and activities of central nervous system during stressed condition induced by mental tasks. *Amino Acids, 43*, 1331–1337.

Your Dictionary. (2013). Retrieved from http://www.yourdictionary.com/supplement.

Zarate, C. (2013). Rapid antidepressant effects of yohimbine in major depression. Retrieved from http://clinicaltrials.gov/show/NCT00078715.

Zhang, G. J., Shi, Z. Y., Liu, S., Gong, S. H., Liu, J. Q., & Liu J. S. (2007). Clinical observation on treatment of depression electroacupuncture combined with Paroxetine. *Chinese Journal of Integrative Medicine, 113*, 228–230.

Zhang, J., Stewart, R., Phillips, M., Shi, Q., & Prince, M. (2009). Pesticide exposure and suicidal ideation in rural communities in Zhejiang Province, China. *Bulletin of the World Health Organization, 87*, 745–753.

Zhang, L., Kleiman-Weiner, M., Luo, R., Shi, Y., Martorell, R., Medina, A., & Rozelle, S. (2013). Multiple micronutrient supplementation reduces anemia and anxiety in rural China's elementary school children. *Journal of Nutrition, 143,* 640–647.

Zhao, X., Wang, C., Zhang, J. F., Liu, L., Liu, A. M., Ma, Q., . . . Xu, Y. (2014). Chronic curcumin treatment normalizes depression-like behaviors in mice with mononeuropathy: Involvement of supraspinal serotonergic system and GABAA receptor. *Psychopharmacology (Berlin), 231,* 2171–2187.

Zheng, J. S., Hu, X. J., Zhao, Y. M., Yang, J., & Li, D. (2013). Intake of fish and marine n-3 polyunsaturated fatty acids and risk of breast cancer: Meta-analysis of data from 21 independent prospective cohort studies. *British Medical Journal, 346,* f3706

Zhou, Y. J., Tan, F., & Deng, J. (2008) Update review of Passiflora. *Zhongguo Zhong Yao Za Zhi. 33,* 1789–1793.

Zhu, L., Bai, X., Teng, W. P., Shan, Z. Y., Wang, W. W., Fan, C. L., . . . Zhang, H. M. (2012). Effects of selenium supplementation on antibodies of autoimmune thyroiditis. *Zhonghua Yi Xue Za Zhi, 92,* 2256–2260.

Zielinski, M. R., Davis, J. M., Fadel, J. R., & Youngstedt, S. D. (2013). Influence of chronic moderate sleep restriction and exercise training on anxiety, spatial memory, and associated neurobiological measures in mice. *Behavioral Brain Research, 250,* 74–80.

Zucchi, F. C., Yao, Y., Ward, I. D., Ilnytskyy, Y., Olson, D. M., Benzies, K., . . . Metz, G. A. (2013). Maternal stress induces epigenetic signatures of psychiatric and neurological diseases in the offspring. *PLoS One, 8,* e56967.

# Index

Note: Italicized page locators refer to figures; tables are noted with *t*.